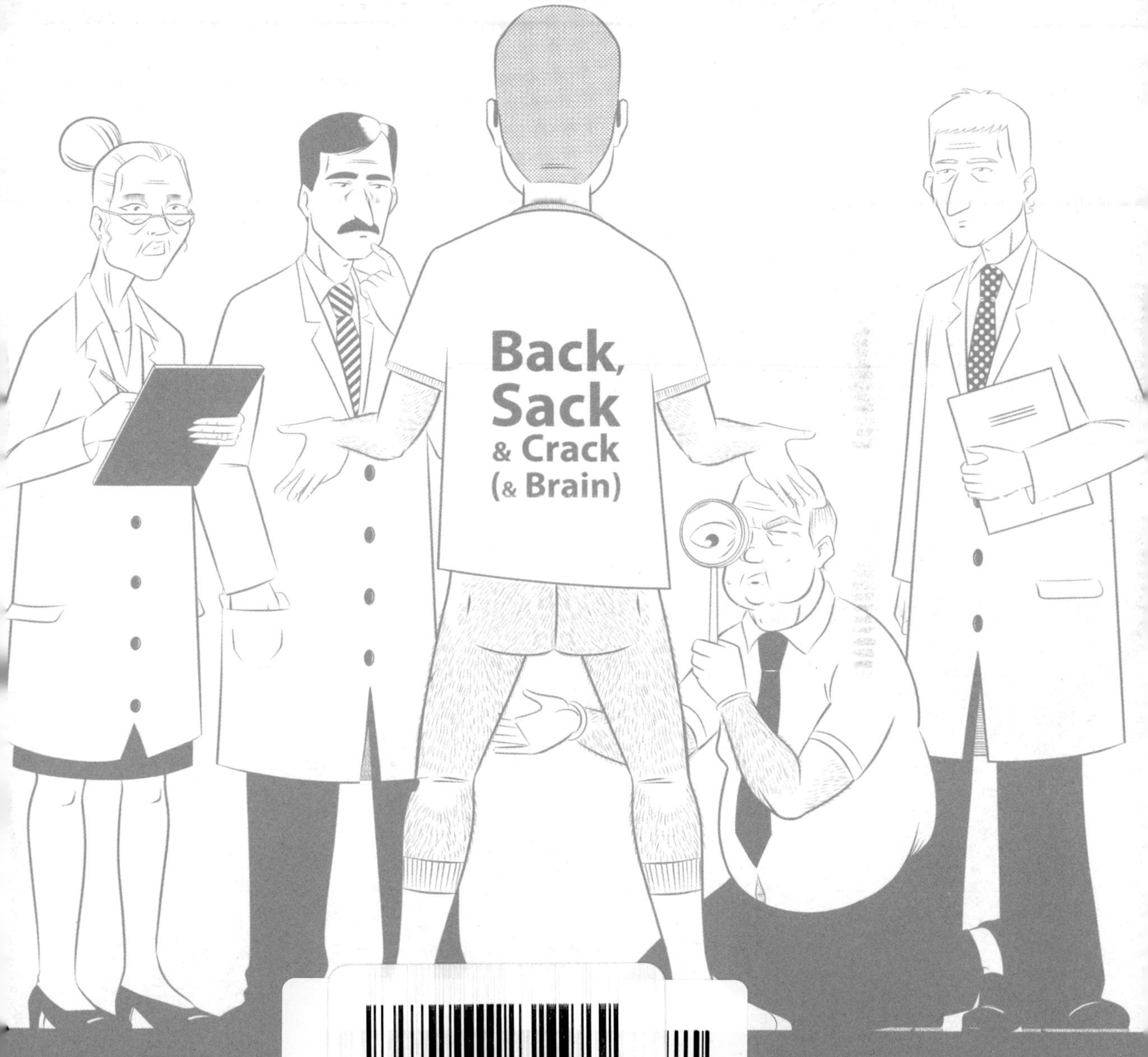
Back,
Sack
& Crack
(& Brain)

ROBINSON

First published in Great Britain in 2017 by Robinson

1 3 5 7 9 10 8 6 4 2

Copyright © Robert Wells, 2017

The moral right of the author has been asserted.

A CIP catalogue record for this book
is available from the British Library.

ISBN: 978-1-47213-675-6

Designed by Robert Wells
Lettered using Blambot font Digital Strip 2
Printed and bound in Great Britain by Bell & Bain Ltd, Glasgow G46 7UQ

Papers used by Robinson are from well-managed forests and other responsible sources.

Robinson
An imprint of
Little, Brown Book Group
Carmelite House
50 Victoria Embankment
London EC4Y 0DZ

An Hachette UK Company

www.hachette.co.uk

www.littlebrown.co.uk.

INTRODUCTION:

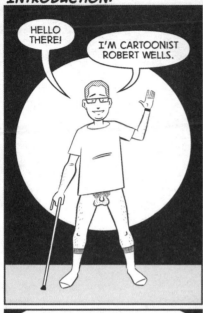

HELLO THERE!

I'M CARTOONIST ROBERT WELLS.

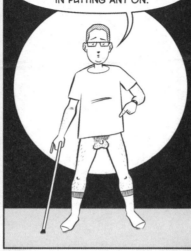

YOU MAY HAVE NOTICED THAT I'M NOT WEARING ANY TROUSERS OR UNDERPANTS TODAY. THERE JUST DIDN'T SEEM TO BE MUCH POINT IN PUTTING ANY ON.

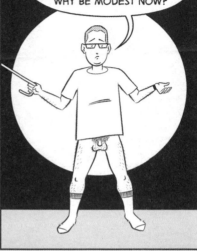

I MEAN, PRETTY SOON YOU ARE GOING TO BE SEEING PLENTY OF DRAWINGS OF MY BALLS ANYWAY, SO WHY BE MODEST NOW?

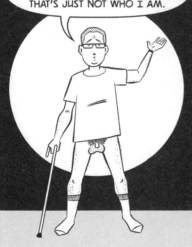

OH, I'M SURE I COULD TELL YOU ALL ABOUT MY EMBARRASSING HEALTH PROBLEMS WITHOUT DRAWING LOTS OF PICTURES OF MY BALLS, BUT THAT'S JUST NOT WHO I AM.

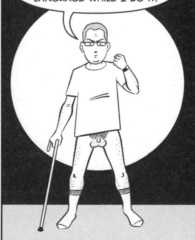

IF I'M GOING TO TELL YOU ABOUT MY BALLS, THEN BY GOD I'LL SHOW YOU MY BALLS – AND I'LL USE SOME FAIRLY SALTY LANGUAGE WHILE I DO IT!

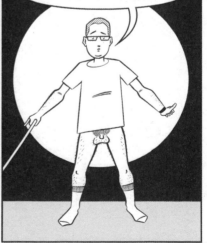

NOT THAT MY BALLS ARE THE ONLY THING – OR EVEN THE MOST EMBARRASSING THING – THAT I WANT TO TELL YOU ABOUT.

3

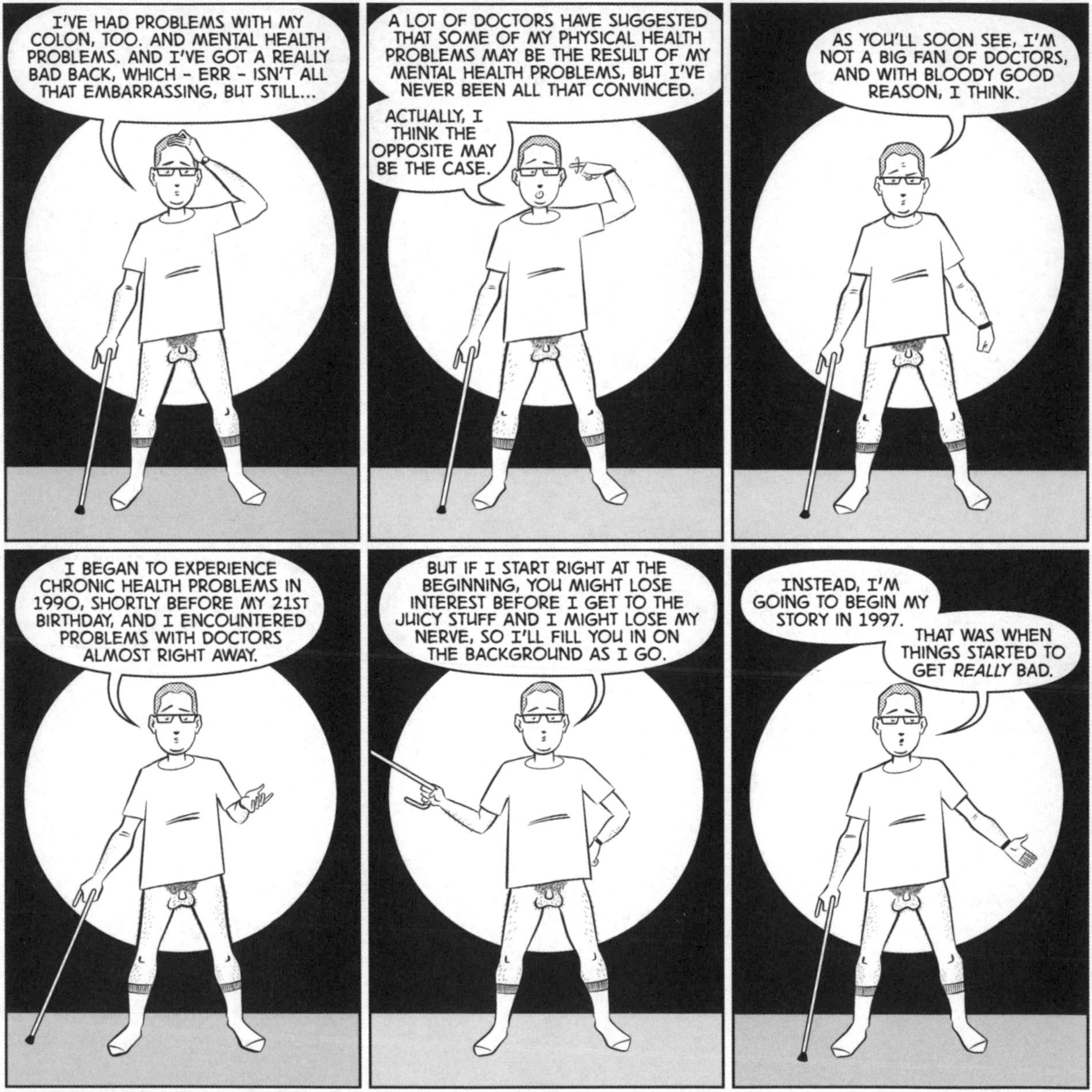
I'VE HAD PROBLEMS WITH MY COLON, TOO. AND MENTAL HEALTH PROBLEMS. AND I'VE GOT A REALLY BAD BACK, WHICH - ERR - ISN'T ALL THAT EMBARRASSING, BUT STILL...
A LOT OF DOCTORS HAVE SUGGESTED THAT SOME OF MY PHYSICAL HEALTH PROBLEMS MAY BE THE RESULT OF MY MENTAL HEALTH PROBLEMS, BUT I'VE NEVER BEEN ALL THAT CONVINCED.
ACTUALLY, I THINK THE OPPOSITE MAY BE THE CASE.
AS YOU'LL SOON SEE, I'M NOT A BIG FAN OF DOCTORS, AND WITH BLOODY GOOD REASON, I THINK.
I BEGAN TO EXPERIENCE CHRONIC HEALTH PROBLEMS IN 1990, SHORTLY BEFORE MY 21ST BIRTHDAY, AND I ENCOUNTERED PROBLEMS WITH DOCTORS ALMOST RIGHT AWAY.
BUT IF I START RIGHT AT THE BEGINNING, YOU MIGHT LOSE INTEREST BEFORE I GET TO THE JUICY STUFF AND I MIGHT LOSE MY NERVE, SO I'LL FILL YOU IN ON THE BACKGROUND AS I GO.
INSTEAD, I'M GOING TO BEGIN MY STORY IN 1997.
THAT WAS WHEN THINGS STARTED TO GET *REALLY* BAD.

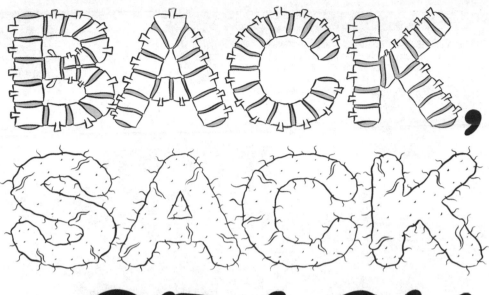

BACK, SACK & CRACK (& BRAIN)

A Rather Graphic Novel
by
Robert Wells

ROBINSON

1. WEAKNESS

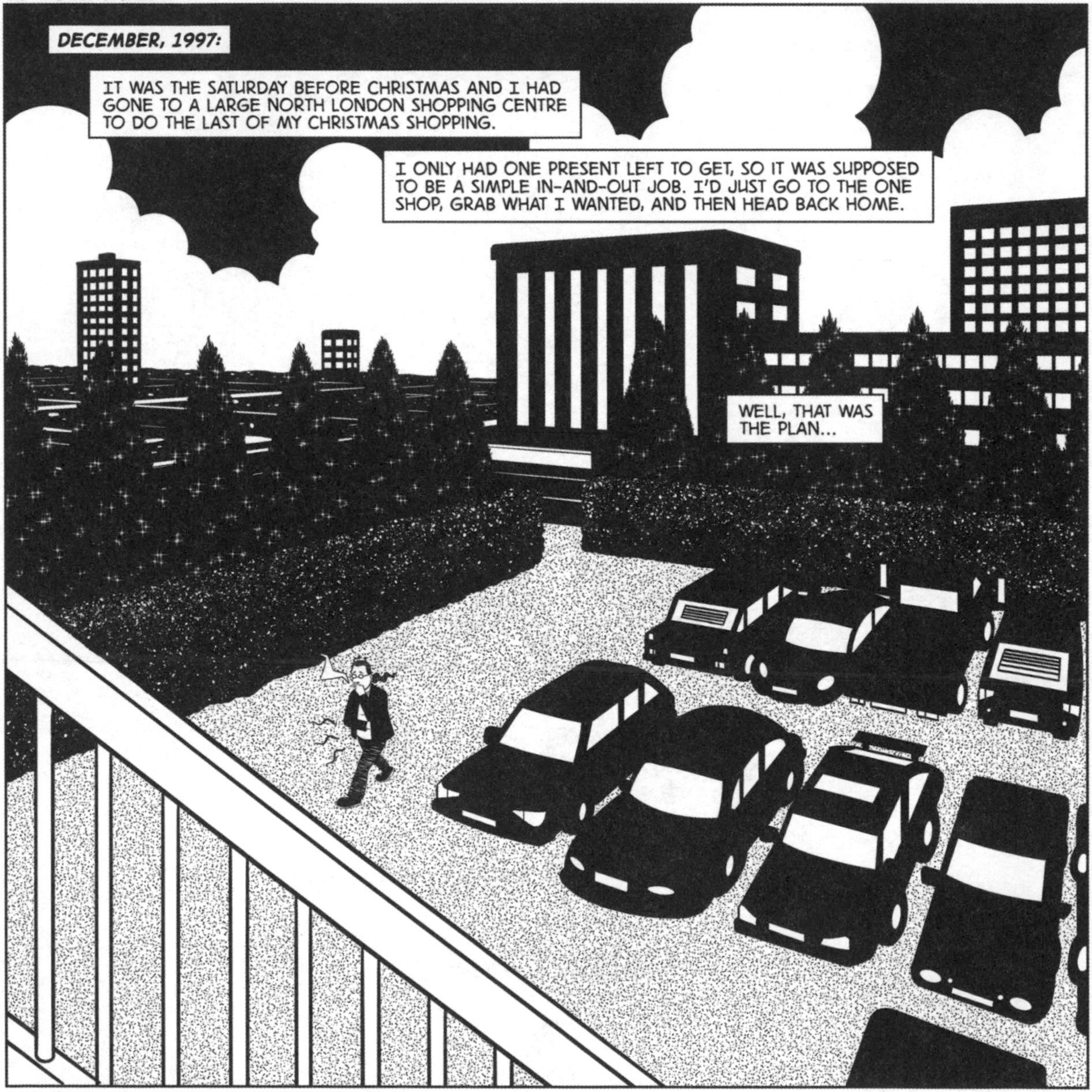
DECEMBER, 1997:
IT WAS THE SATURDAY BEFORE CHRISTMAS AND I HAD GONE TO A LARGE NORTH LONDON SHOPPING CENTRE TO DO THE LAST OF MY CHRISTMAS SHOPPING.
I ONLY HAD ONE PRESENT LEFT TO GET, SO IT WAS SUPPOSED TO BE A SIMPLE IN-AND-OUT JOB. I'D JUST GO TO THE ONE SHOP, GRAB WHAT I WANTED, AND THEN HEAD BACK HOME.
WELL, THAT WAS THE PLAN...

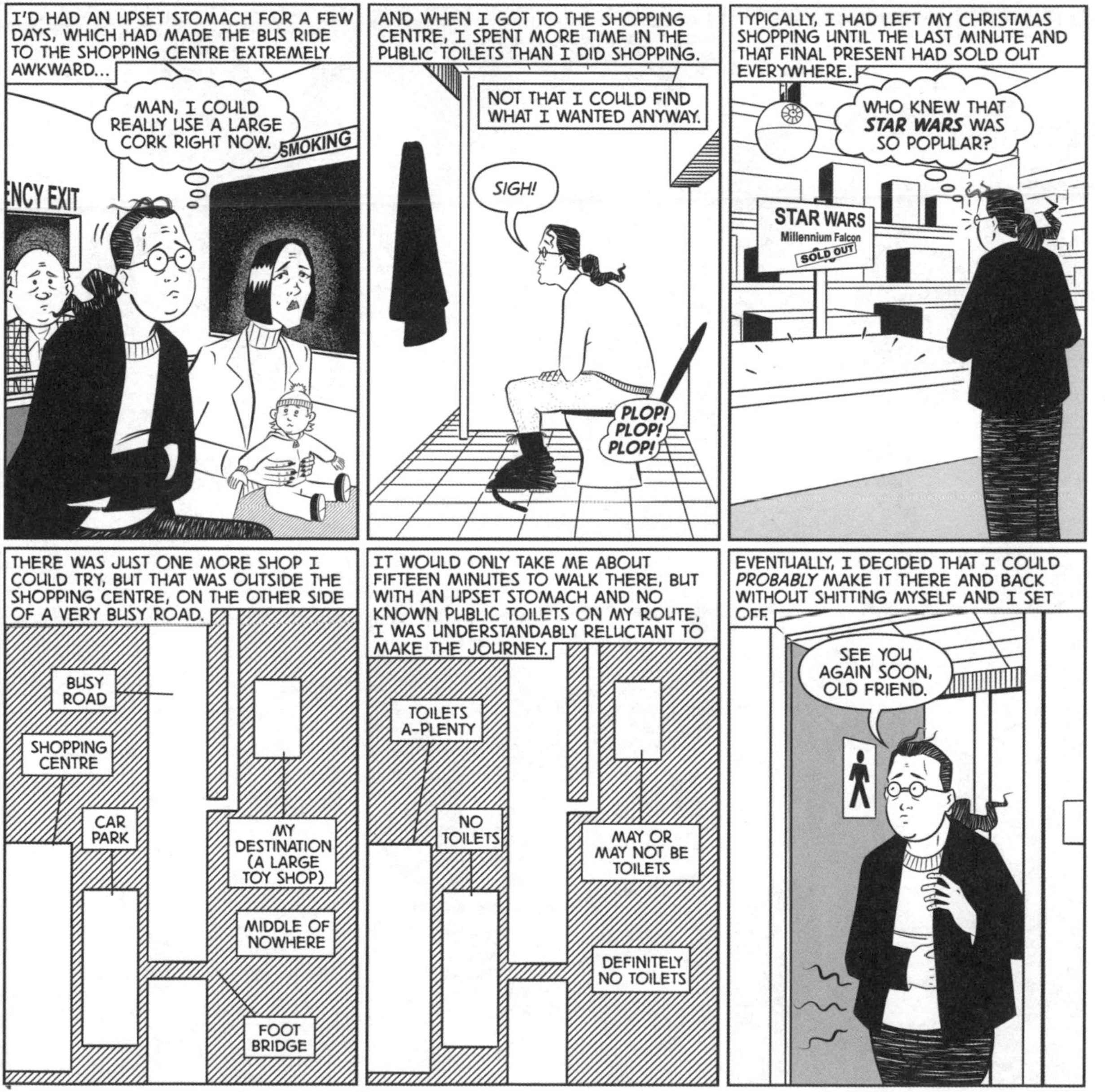

I'D HAD AN UPSET STOMACH FOR A FEW DAYS, WHICH HAD MADE THE BUS RIDE TO THE SHOPPING CENTRE EXTREMELY AWKWARD...
MAN, I COULD REALLY USE A LARGE CORK RIGHT NOW.
SMOKING
NCY EXIT
AND WHEN I GOT TO THE SHOPPING CENTRE, I SPENT MORE TIME IN THE PUBLIC TOILETS THAN I DID SHOPPING.
NOT THAT I COULD FIND WHAT I WANTED ANYWAY.
SIGH!
PLOP! PLOP! PLOP!
TYPICALLY, I HAD LEFT MY CHRISTMAS SHOPPING UNTIL THE LAST MINUTE AND THAT FINAL PRESENT HAD SOLD OUT EVERYWHERE.
WHO KNEW THAT STAR WARS WAS SO POPULAR?
STAR WARS
Millennium Falcon
SOLD OUT
THERE WAS JUST ONE MORE SHOP I COULD TRY, BUT THAT WAS OUTSIDE THE SHOPPING CENTRE, ON THE OTHER SIDE OF A VERY BUSY ROAD.
BUSY ROAD
SHOPPING CENTRE
CAR PARK
MY DESTINATION (A LARGE TOY SHOP)
MIDDLE OF NOWHERE
FOOT BRIDGE
IT WOULD ONLY TAKE ME ABOUT FIFTEEN MINUTES TO WALK THERE, BUT WITH AN UPSET STOMACH AND NO KNOWN PUBLIC TOILETS ON MY ROUTE, I WAS UNDERSTANDABLY RELUCTANT TO MAKE THE JOURNEY.
TOILETS A-PLENTY
NO TOILETS
MAY OR MAY NOT BE TOILETS
DEFINITELY NO TOILETS
EVENTUALLY, I DECIDED THAT I COULD PROBABLY MAKE IT THERE AND BACK WITHOUT SHITTING MYSELF AND I SET OFF.
SEE YOU AGAIN SOON, OLD FRIEND.

I LEFT THE SHOPPING CENTRE...

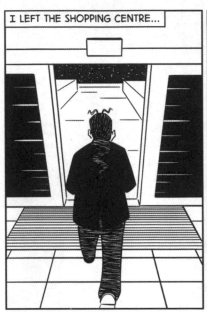

I CROSSED THE CAR PARK...

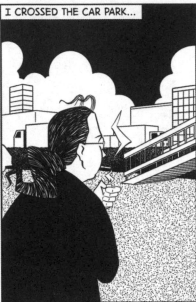

AND I STARTED TO WALK UP THE STEPS TO A FOOT BRIDGE THAT CROSSED THE BUSY ROAD.

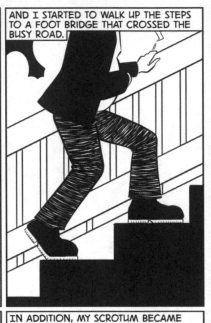

BUT BEFORE I GOT HALFWAY UP THE STEPS, SOMETHING STRANGE HAPPENED.

FUCK! M-MY BALLS!!!

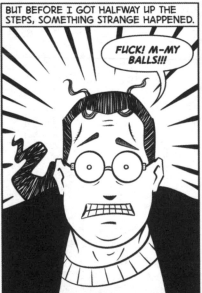

FROM OUT OF NOWHERE, I BEGAN TO EXPERIENCE PAINFUL SPASMS ON THE RIGHT SIDE OF MY GROIN.

WHAT THE FUCK IS WRONG WITH MY BALLS?

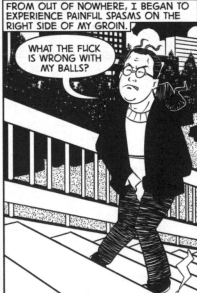

IN ADDITION, MY SCROTUM BECAME UNCOMFORTABLY TIGHT AND MY RIGHT TESTICLE FELT LIKE IT WAS MUCH TOO HIGH UP, WHICH WAS *EXTREMELY* UN-COMFORTABLE.

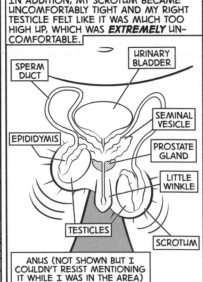

SPERM DUCT

URINARY BLADDER

EPIDIDYMIS

SEMINAL VESICLE

PROSTATE GLAND

LITTLE WINKLE

TESTICLES

SCROTUM

ANUS (NOT SHOWN BUT I COULDN'T RESIST MENTIONING IT WHILE I WAS IN THE AREA)

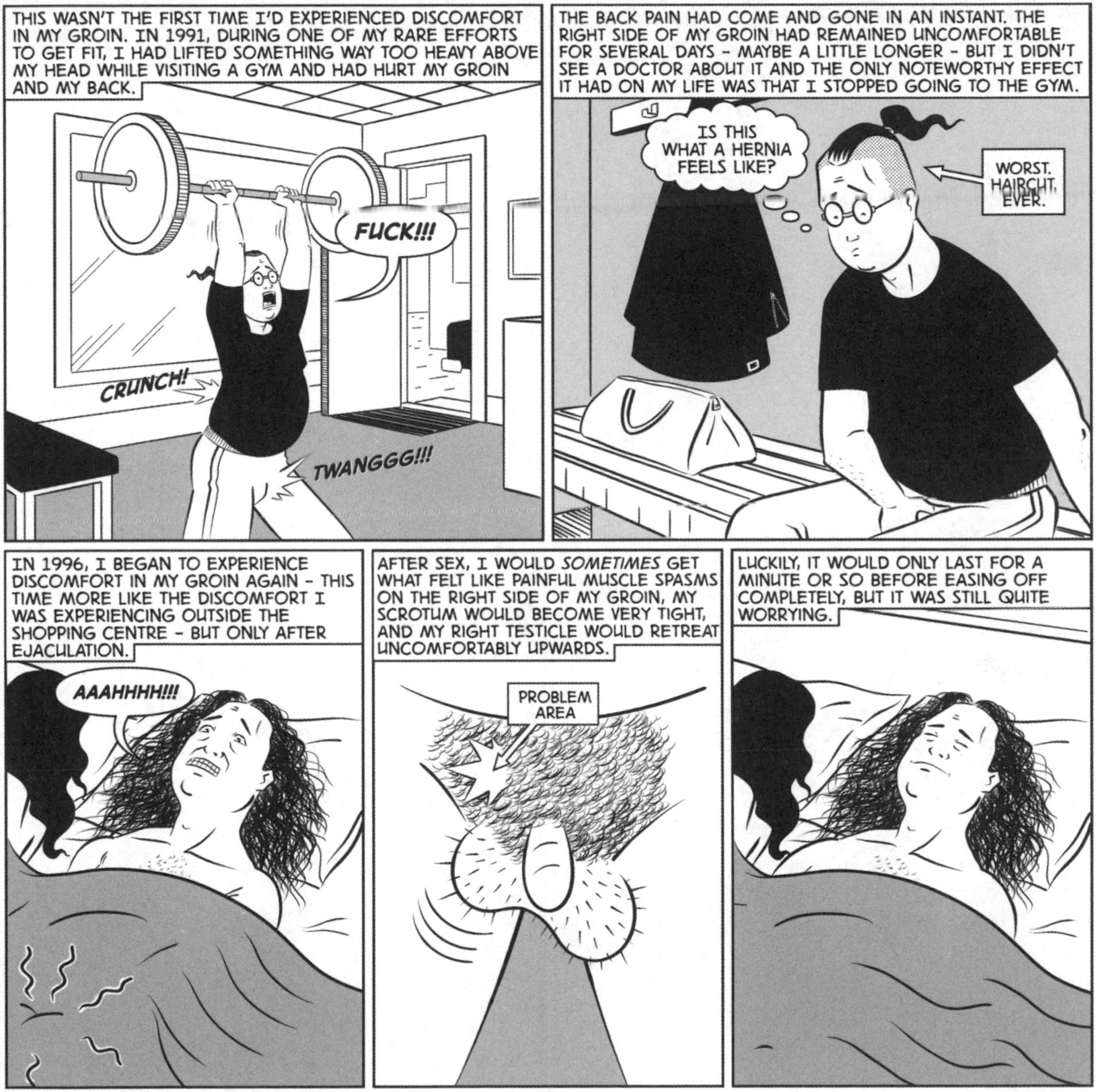
THIS WASN'T THE FIRST TIME I'D EXPERIENCED DISCOMFORT IN MY GROIN. IN 1991, DURING ONE OF MY RARE EFFORTS TO GET FIT, I HAD LIFTED SOMETHING WAY TOO HEAVY ABOVE MY HEAD WHILE VISITING A GYM AND HAD HURT MY GROIN AND MY BACK.
FUCK!!!
CRUNCH!
TWANGGG!!!
THE BACK PAIN HAD COME AND GONE IN AN INSTANT. THE RIGHT SIDE OF MY GROIN HAD REMAINED UNCOMFORTABLE FOR SEVERAL DAYS - MAYBE A LITTLE LONGER - BUT I DIDN'T SEE A DOCTOR ABOUT IT AND THE ONLY NOTEWORTHY EFFECT IT HAD ON MY LIFE WAS THAT I STOPPED GOING TO THE GYM.
IS THIS WHAT A HERNIA FEELS LIKE?
WORST. HAIRCUT. EVER.
IN 1996, I BEGAN TO EXPERIENCE DISCOMFORT IN MY GROIN AGAIN - THIS TIME MORE LIKE THE DISCOMFORT I WAS EXPERIENCING OUTSIDE THE SHOPPING CENTRE - BUT ONLY AFTER EJACULATION.
AAAHHHH!!!
AFTER SEX, I WOULD *SOMETIMES* GET WHAT FELT LIKE PAINFUL MUSCLE SPASMS ON THE RIGHT SIDE OF MY GROIN, MY SCROTUM WOULD BECOME VERY TIGHT, AND MY RIGHT TESTICLE WOULD RETREAT UNCOMFORTABLY UPWARDS.
PROBLEM AREA
LUCKILY, IT WOULD ONLY LAST FOR A MINUTE OR SO BEFORE EASING OFF COMPLETELY, BUT IT WAS STILL QUITE WORRYING.

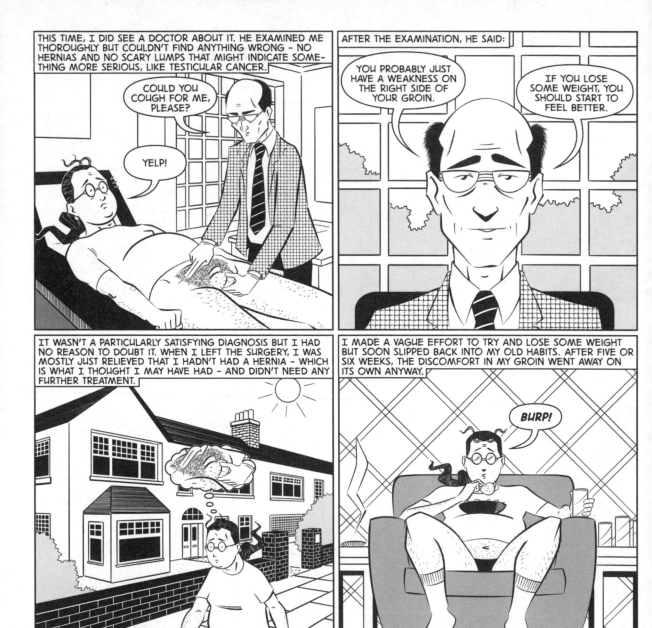

THIS TIME, I DID SEE A DOCTOR ABOUT IT. HE EXAMINED ME THOROUGHLY BUT COULDN'T FIND ANYTHING WRONG - NO HERNIAS AND NO SCARY LUMPS THAT MIGHT INDICATE SOMETHING MORE SERIOUS, LIKE TESTICULAR CANCER.

COULD YOU COUGH FOR ME, PLEASE?

YELP!

AFTER THE EXAMINATION, HE SAID:

YOU PROBABLY JUST HAVE A WEAKNESS ON THE RIGHT SIDE OF YOUR GROIN.

IF YOU LOSE SOME WEIGHT, YOU SHOULD START TO FEEL BETTER.

IT WASN'T A PARTICULARLY SATISFYING DIAGNOSIS BUT I HAD NO REASON TO DOUBT IT. WHEN I LEFT THE SURGERY, I WAS MOSTLY JUST RELIEVED THAT I HADN'T HAD A HERNIA - WHICH IS WHAT I THOUGHT I MAY HAVE HAD - AND DIDN'T NEED ANY FURTHER TREATMENT.

I MADE A VAGUE EFFORT TO TRY AND LOSE SOME WEIGHT BUT SOON SLIPPED BACK INTO MY OLD HABITS. AFTER FIVE OR SIX WEEKS, THE DISCOMFORT IN MY GROIN WENT AWAY ON ITS OWN ANYWAY.

BURP!

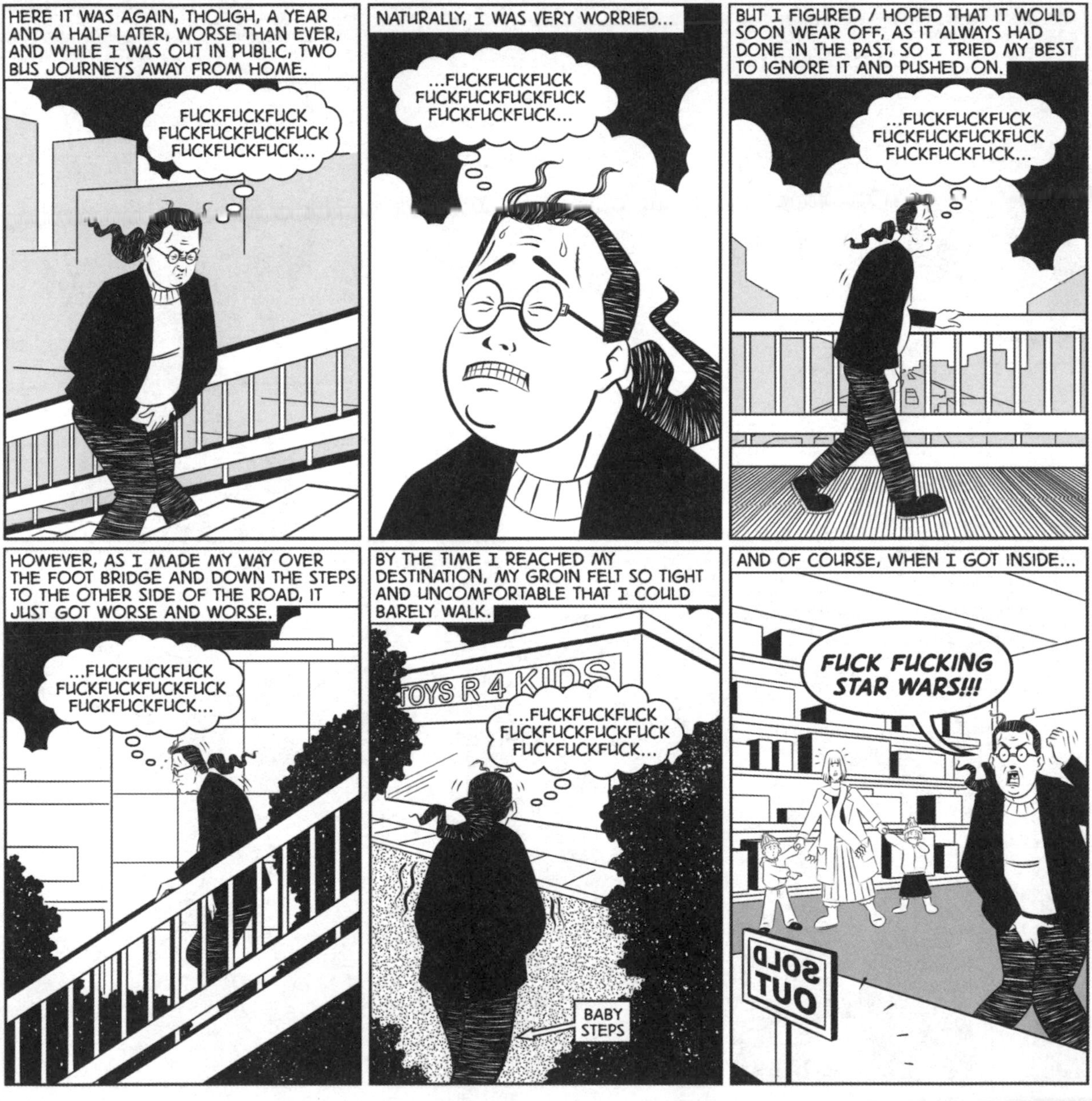
HERE IT WAS AGAIN, THOUGH, A YEAR AND A HALF LATER, WORSE THAN EVER, AND WHILE I WAS OUT IN PUBLIC, TWO BUS JOURNEYS AWAY FROM HOME.
FUCKFUCKFUCK FUCKFUCKFUCKFUCK FUCKFUCKFUCK...
NATURALLY, I WAS VERY WORRIED...
...FUCKFUCKFUCK FUCKFUCKFUCKFUCK FUCKFUCKFUCK...
BUT I FIGURED / HOPED THAT IT WOULD SOON WEAR OFF, AS IT ALWAYS HAD DONE IN THE PAST, SO I TRIED MY BEST TO IGNORE IT AND PUSHED ON.
...FUCKFUCKFUCK FUCKFUCKFUCKFUCK FUCKFUCKFUCK...
HOWEVER, AS I MADE MY WAY OVER THE FOOT BRIDGE AND DOWN THE STEPS TO THE OTHER SIDE OF THE ROAD, IT JUST GOT WORSE AND WORSE.
...FUCKFUCKFUCK FUCKFUCKFUCKFUCK FUCKFUCKFUCK...
BY THE TIME I REACHED MY DESTINATION, MY GROIN FELT SO TIGHT AND UNCOMFORTABLE THAT I COULD BARELY WALK.
TOYS R 4 KIDS
...FUCKFUCKFUCK FUCKFUCKFUCKFUCK FUCKFUCKFUCK...
BABY STEPS
AND OF COURSE, WHEN I GOT INSIDE...
FUCK FUCKING STAR WARS!!!
SOLD OUT

BEFORE I WENT BACK OUTSIDE, I BRIEFLY CONSIDERED ASKING SOMEONE IN THE SHOP IF THEY COULD CALL ME AN AMBULANCE*...

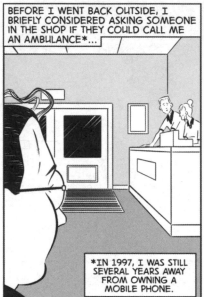

*IN 1997, I WAS STILL SEVERAL YEARS AWAY FROM OWNING A MOBILE PHONE.

BUT IN THE WARMTH OF THE SHOP, MY GROIN HAD RELAXED AND THE DISCOMFORT HAD EASED OFF A BIT.

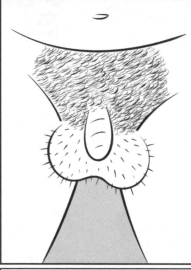

PLUS I WAS WORRIED THAT THE TEEN-AGERS WORKING ON THE CUSTOMER SERVICES DESK WOULD JUST LAUGH IF I TOLD THEM WHAT WAS WRONG WITH ME.

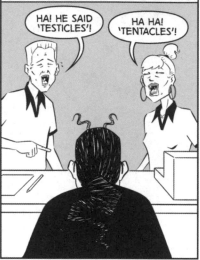

HA! HE SAID 'TESTICLES'!

HA HA! 'TENTACLES'!

CALLING AN AMBULANCE SEEMED A BIT EXTREME ANYWAY - I AGAIN THOUGHT I MIGHT HAVE HAD A HERNIA BUT DIDN'T THINK I WAS SERIOUSLY ILL - SO I MADE MY WAY BACK OUT INTO THE COLD AND HEADED BACK TOWARDS THE FOOT BRIDGE.

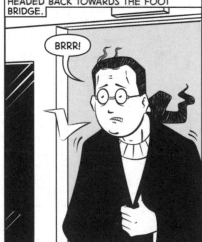

BRRR!

BUT AS I SHUFFLED ALONG, WITH ONE HAND ON MY GROIN TO MAKE SURE EVERYTHING WAS STILL WHERE IT SHOULD BE - A POSE I WOULD ADOPT FOR YEARS TO COME - MY GROIN JUST GOT TIGHTER...

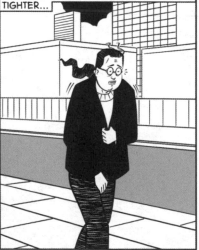

AND TIGHTER...

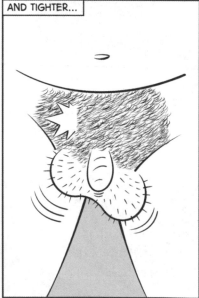

12

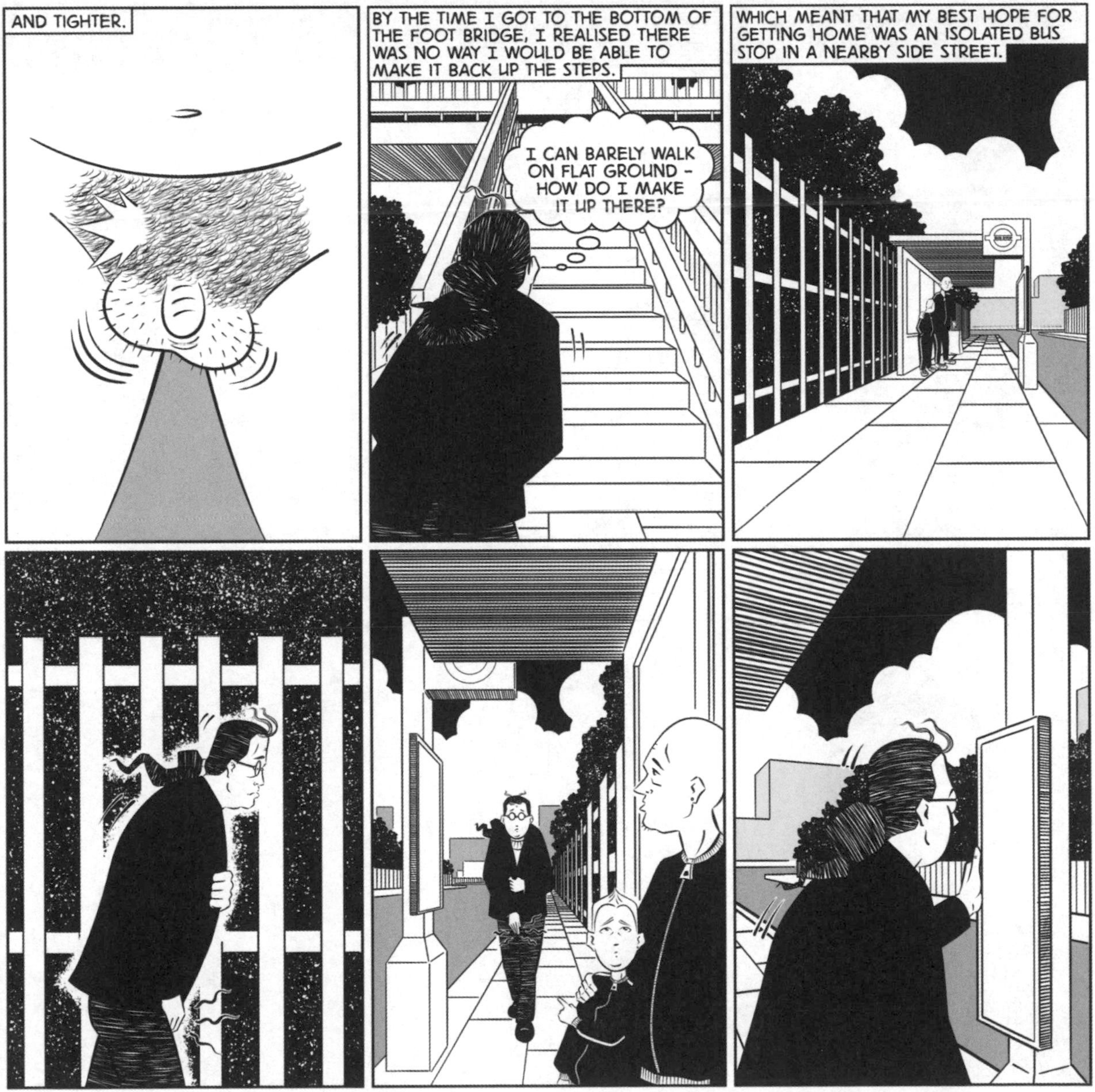
AND TIGHTER.
BY THE TIME I GOT TO THE BOTTOM OF THE FOOT BRIDGE, I REALISED THERE WAS NO WAY I WOULD BE ABLE TO MAKE IT BACK UP THE STEPS.
I CAN BARELY WALK ON FLAT GROUND - HOW DO I MAKE IT UP THERE?
WHICH MEANT THAT MY BEST HOPE FOR GETTING HOME WAS AN ISOLATED BUS STOP IN A NEARBY SIDE STREET.

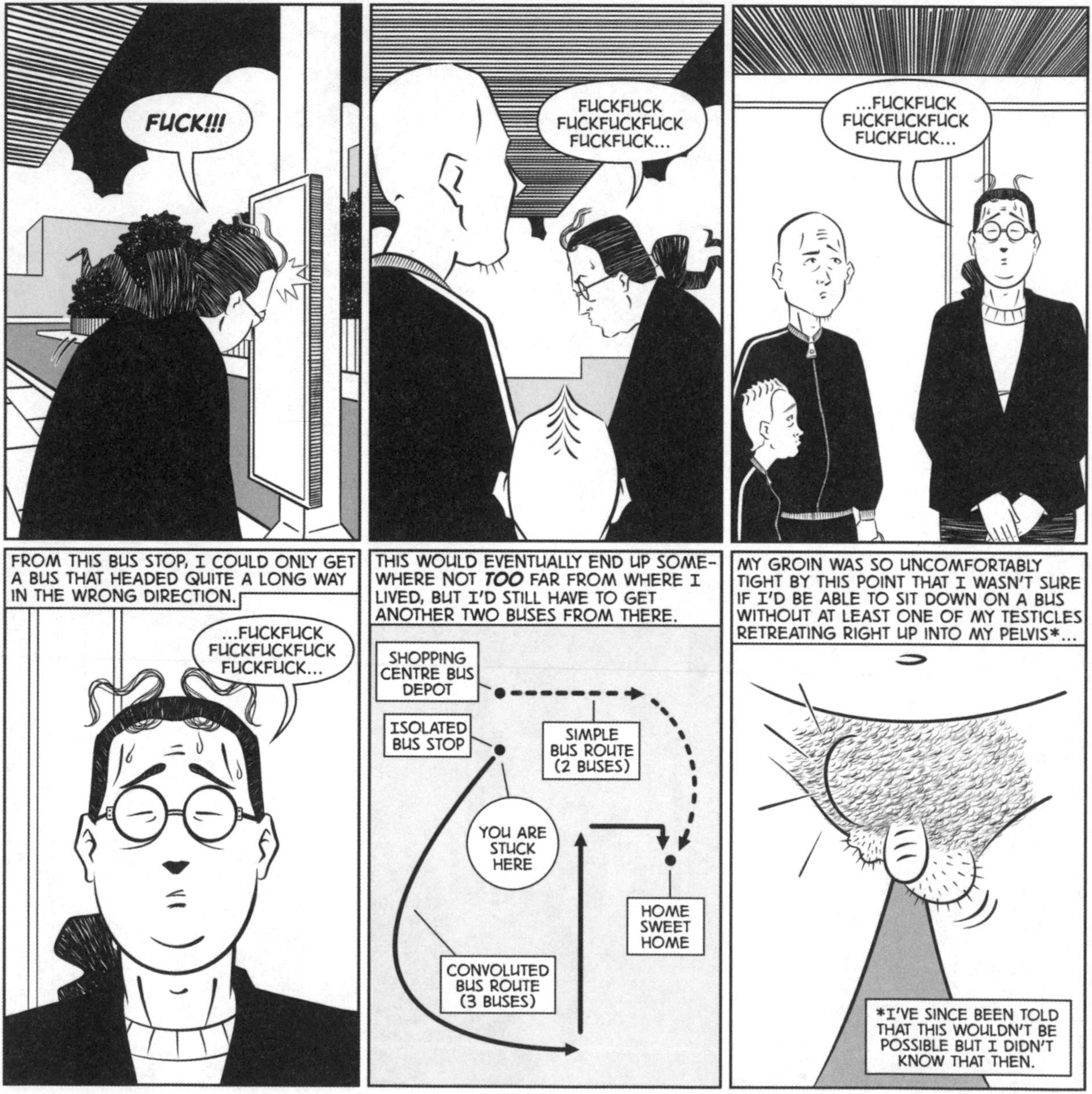
FUCK!!!
FUCKFUCK FUCKFUCKFUCK FUCKFUCK...
...FUCKFUCK FUCKFUCKFUCK FUCKFUCK...
FROM THIS BUS STOP, I COULD ONLY GET A BUS THAT HEADED QUITE A LONG WAY IN THE WRONG DIRECTION.
...FUCKFUCK FUCKFUCKFUCK FUCKFUCK...
THIS WOULD EVENTUALLY END UP SOMEWHERE NOT TOO FAR FROM WHERE I LIVED, BUT I'D STILL HAVE TO GET ANOTHER TWO BUSES FROM THERE.
SHOPPING CENTRE BUS DEPOT
ISOLATED BUS STOP
SIMPLE BUS ROUTE (2 BUSES)
YOU ARE STUCK HERE
HOME SWEET HOME
CONVOLUTED BUS ROUTE (3 BUSES)
MY GROIN WAS SO UNCOMFORTABLY TIGHT BY THIS POINT THAT I WASN'T SURE IF I'D BE ABLE TO SIT DOWN ON A BUS WITHOUT AT LEAST ONE OF MY TESTICLES RETREATING RIGHT UP INTO MY PELVIS*...
*I'VE SINCE BEEN TOLD THAT THIS WOULDN'T BE POSSIBLE BUT I DIDN'T KNOW THAT THEN.

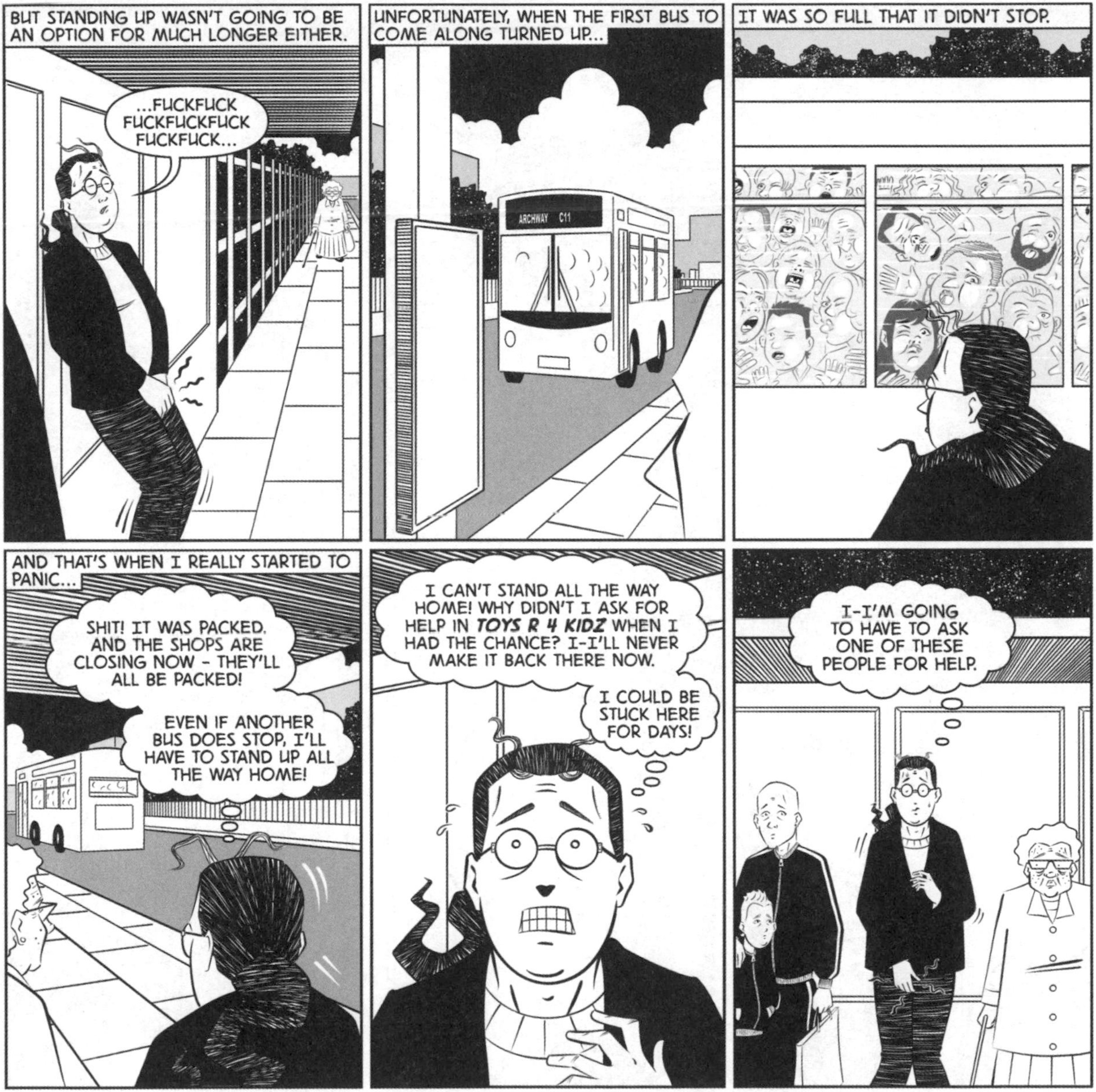
BUT STANDING UP WASN'T GOING TO BE AN OPTION FOR MUCH LONGER EITHER.
...FUCKFUCK FUCKFUCKFUCK FUCKFUCK...
UNFORTUNATELY, WHEN THE FIRST BUS TO COME ALONG TURNED UP...
ARCHWAY C11
IT WAS SO FULL THAT IT DIDN'T STOP.
AND THAT'S WHEN I REALLY STARTED TO PANIC...
SHIT! IT WAS PACKED. AND THE SHOPS ARE CLOSING NOW - THEY'LL ALL BE PACKED!
EVEN IF ANOTHER BUS DOES STOP, I'LL HAVE TO STAND UP ALL THE WAY HOME!
I CAN'T STAND ALL THE WAY HOME! WHY DIDN'T I ASK FOR HELP IN TOYS R 4 KIDZ WHEN I HAD THE CHANCE? I-I'LL NEVER MAKE IT BACK THERE NOW.
I COULD BE STUCK HERE FOR DAYS!
I-I'M GOING TO HAVE TO ASK ONE OF THESE PEOPLE FOR HELP.

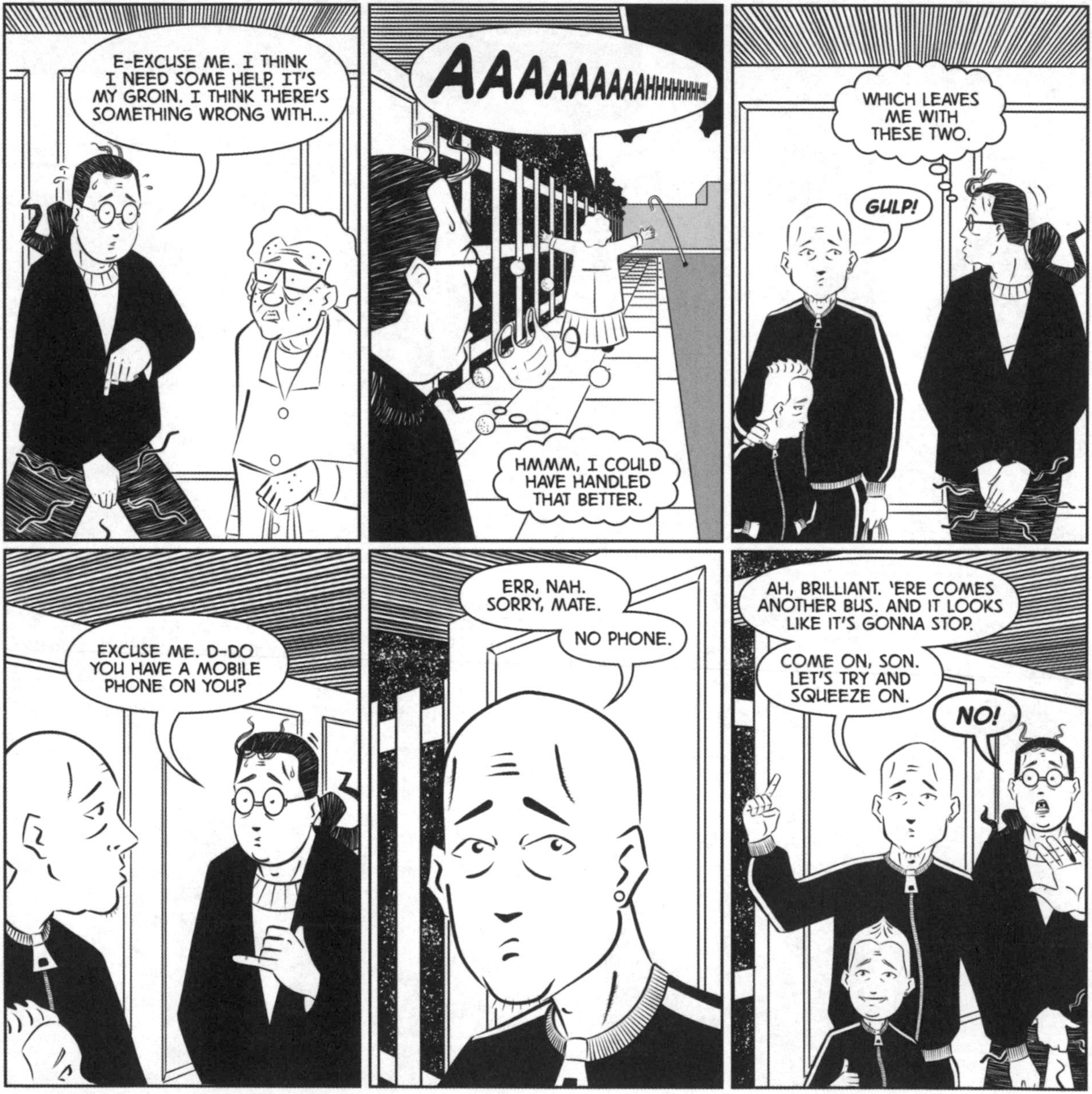
E-EXCUSE ME. I THINK I NEED SOME HELP. IT'S MY GROIN. I THINK THERE'S SOMETHING WRONG WITH...
AAAAAAAAAAHHHHHHH!!!
HMMM, I COULD HAVE HANDLED THAT BETTER.
WHICH LEAVES ME WITH THESE TWO.
GULP!
EXCUSE ME. D-DO YOU HAVE A MOBILE PHONE ON YOU?
ERR, NAH. SORRY, MATE.
NO PHONE.
AH, BRILLIANT. 'ERE COMES ANOTHER BUS. AND IT LOOKS LIKE IT'S GONNA STOP.
COME ON, SON. LET'S TRY AND SQUEEZE ON.
NO!

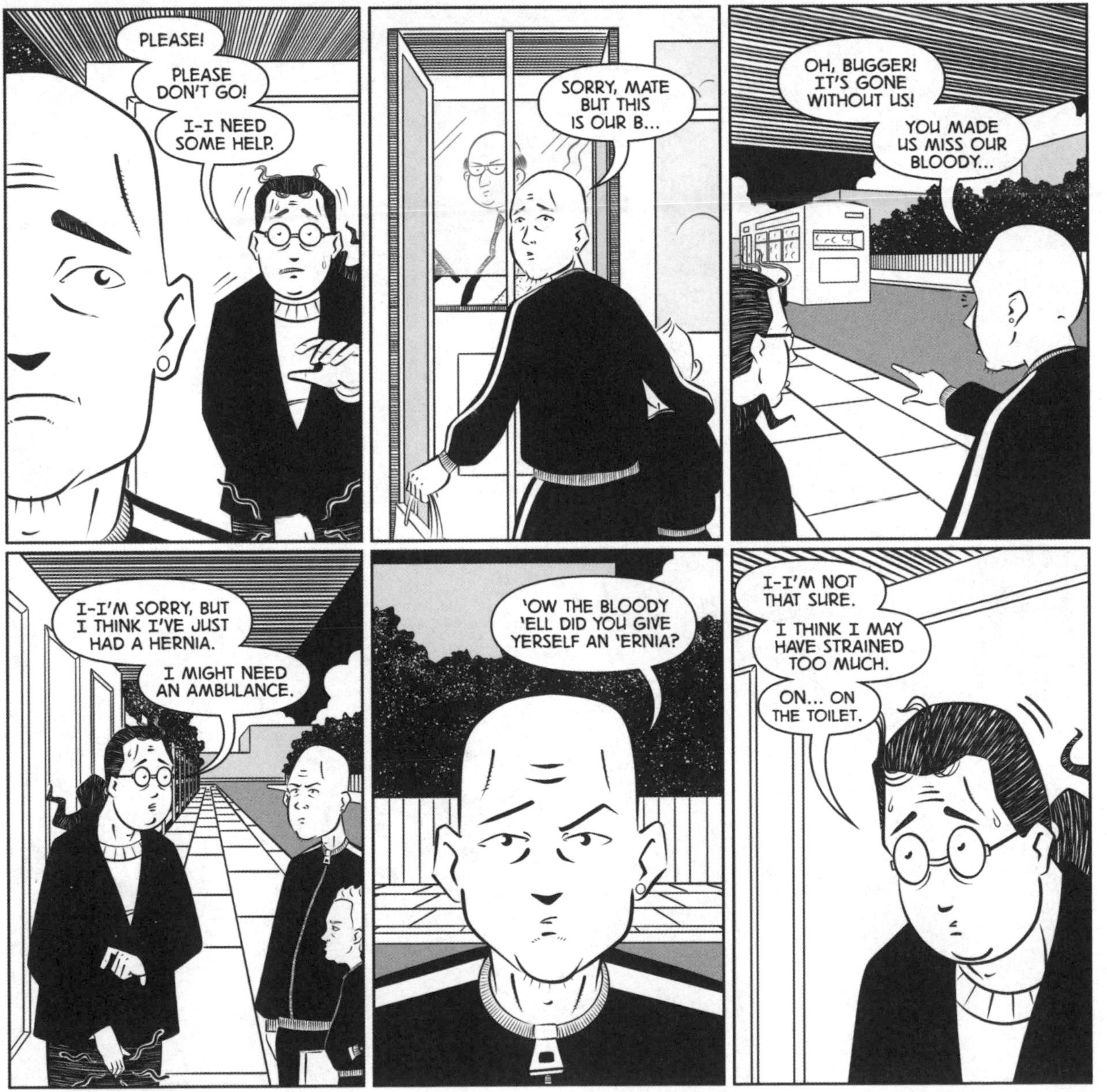
PLEASE!
PLEASE DON'T GO!
I-I NEED SOME HELP.
SORRY, MATE BUT THIS IS OUR B...
OH, BUGGER! IT'S GONE WITHOUT US!
YOU MADE US MISS OUR BLOODY...
I-I'M SORRY, BUT I THINK I'VE JUST HAD A HERNIA.
I MIGHT NEED AN AMBULANCE.
'OW THE BLOODY 'ELL DID YOU GIVE YERSELF AN 'ERNIA?
I-I'M NOT THAT SURE.
I THINK I MAY HAVE STRAINED TOO MUCH.
ON... ON THE TOILET.

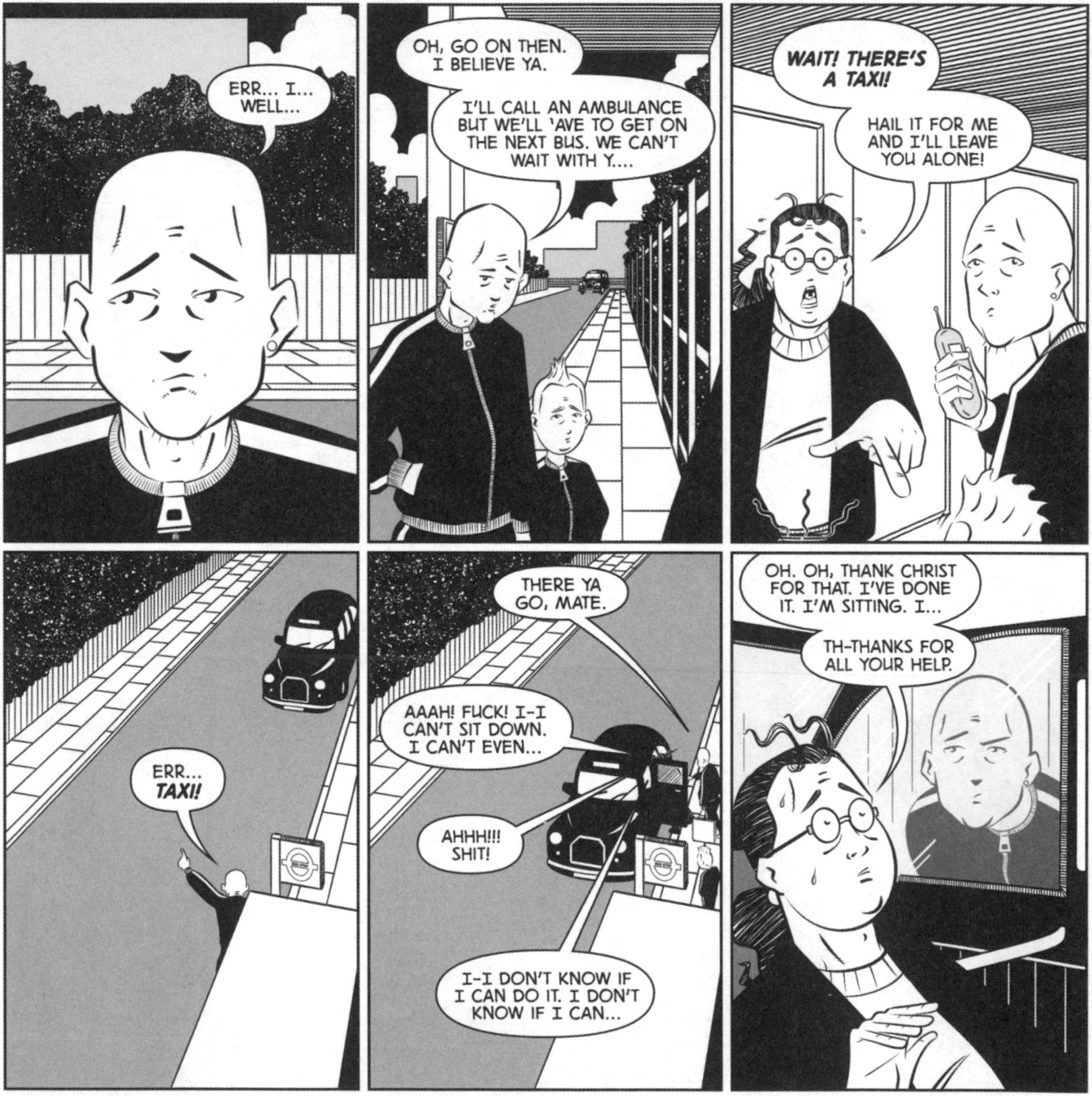
ERR... I... WELL...
OH, GO ON THEN. I BELIEVE YA.
I'LL CALL AN AMBULANCE BUT WE'LL 'AVE TO GET ON THE NEXT BUS. WE CAN'T WAIT WITH Y....
WAIT! THERE'S A TAXI!
HAIL IT FOR ME AND I'LL LEAVE YOU ALONE!
ERR... *TAXI!*
THERE YA GO, MATE.
AAAH! FUCK! I-I CAN'T SIT DOWN. I CAN'T EVEN...
AHHH!!! SHIT!
I-I DON'T KNOW IF I CAN DO IT. I DON'T KNOW IF I CAN...
OH. OH, THANK CHRIST FOR THAT. I'VE DONE IT. I'M SITTING. I...
TH-THANKS FOR ALL YOUR HELP.

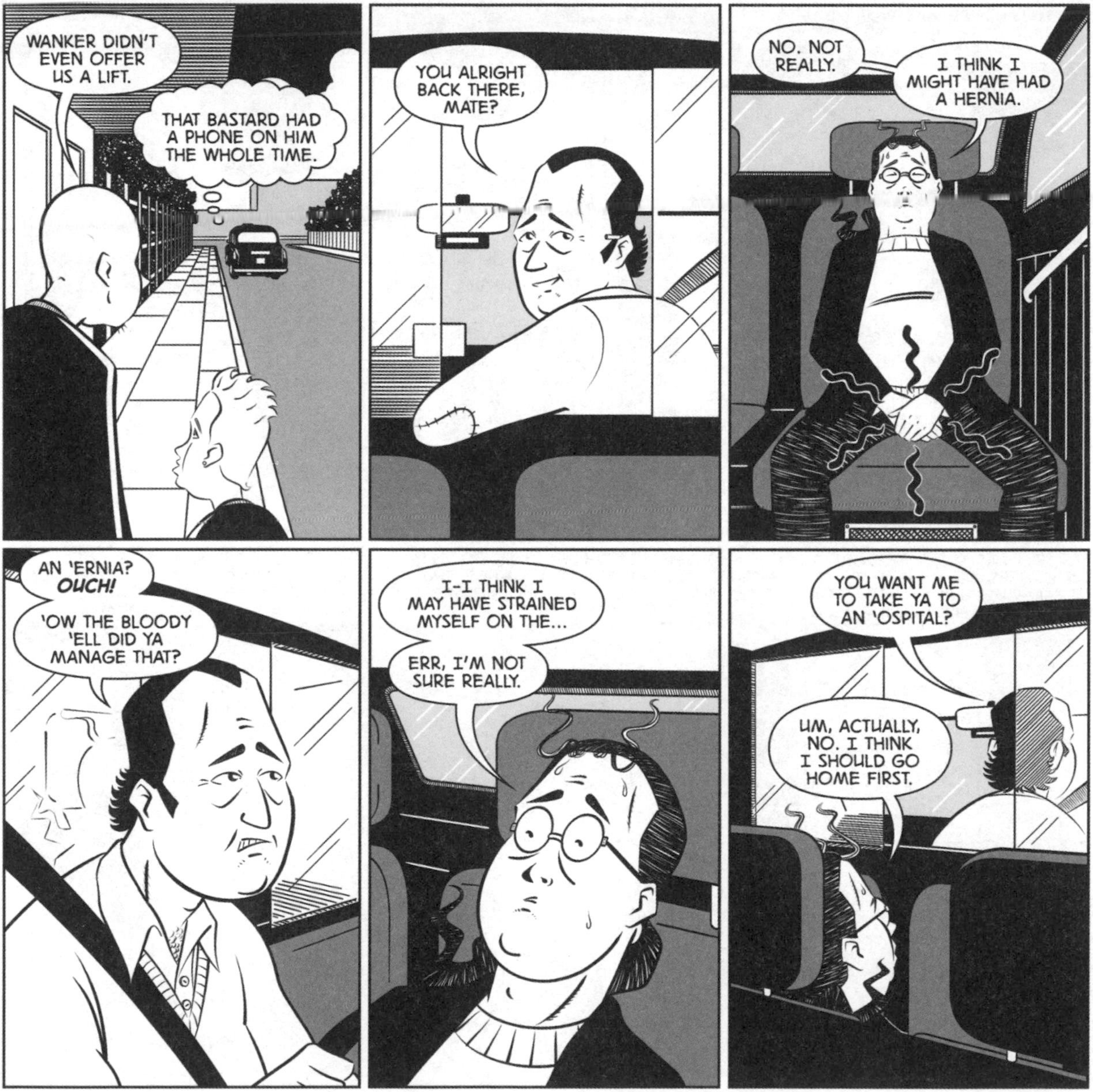
WANKER DIDN'T EVEN OFFER US A LIFT.
THAT BASTARD HAD A PHONE ON HIM THE WHOLE TIME.
YOU ALRIGHT BACK THERE, MATE?
NO. NOT REALLY.
I THINK I MIGHT HAVE HAD A HERNIA.
AN 'ERNIA? OUCH!
'OW THE BLOODY 'ELL DID YA MANAGE THAT?
I-I THINK I MAY HAVE STRAINED MYSELF ON THE...
ERR, I'M NOT SURE REALLY.
YOU WANT ME TO TAKE YA TO AN 'OSPITAL?
UM, ACTUALLY, NO. I THINK I SHOULD GO HOME FIRST.

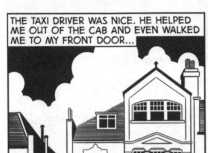

THE TAXI DRIVER WAS NICE. HE HELPED ME OUT OF THE CAB AND EVEN WALKED ME TO MY FRONT DOOR...

THERE YA GO, MATE.

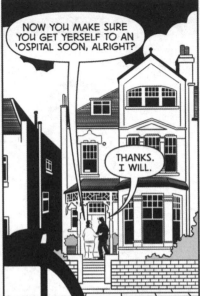

NOW YOU MAKE SURE YOU GET YERSELF TO AN 'OSPITAL SOON, ALRIGHT?

THANKS. I WILL.

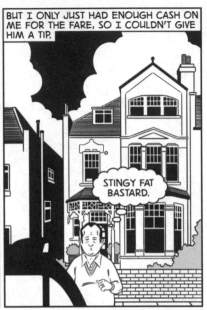

BUT I ONLY JUST HAD ENOUGH CASH ON ME FOR THE FARE, SO I COULDN'T GIVE HIM A TIP.

STINGY FAT BASTARD.

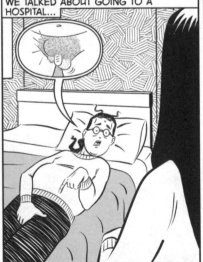

AS SOON AS I GOT INDOORS, I COLLAPSED ON THE BED, TOLD MY WIFE WHAT HAD HAPPENED, AND FOR A WHILE WE TALKED ABOUT GOING TO A HOSPITAL...

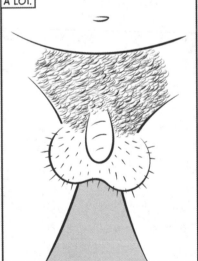

BUT AFTER I'D BEEN LYING DOWN IN OUR WARM FLAT FOR A WHILE, THE DISCOMFORT IN MY GROIN EASED OFF A LOT.

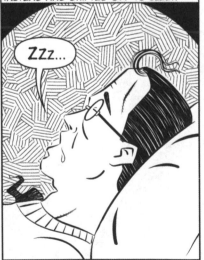

EVENTUALLY, IT EASED OFF SO MUCH THAT I DECIDED TO JUST GO AND SEE MY DOCTOR THE FOLLOWING WEEK INSTEAD AND DRIFTED OFF TO SLEEP.

ZZZ...

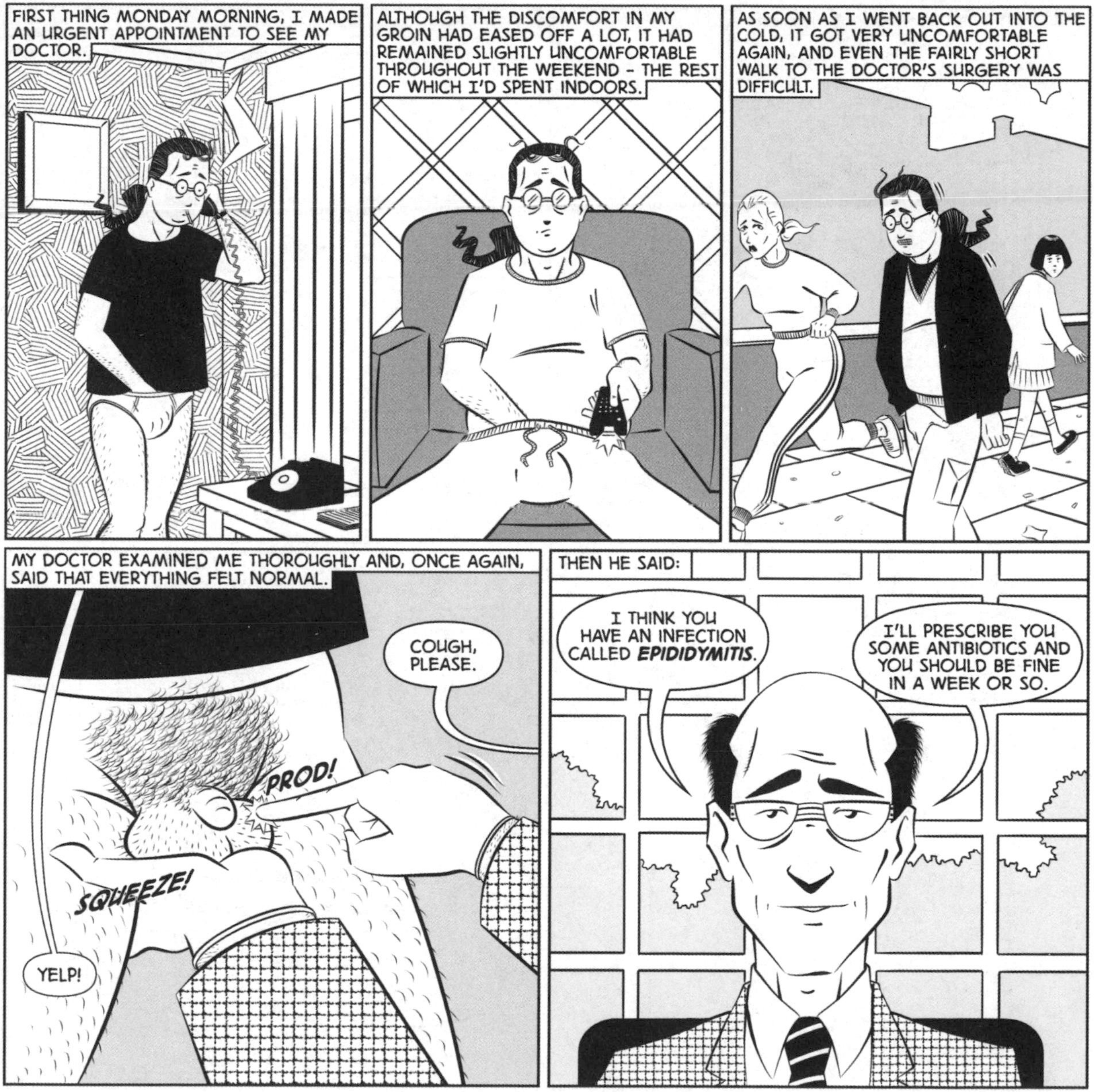
FIRST THING MONDAY MORNING, I MADE AN URGENT APPOINTMENT TO SEE MY DOCTOR.
ALTHOUGH THE DISCOMFORT IN MY GROIN HAD EASED OFF A LOT, IT HAD REMAINED SLIGHTLY UNCOMFORTABLE THROUGHOUT THE WEEKEND - THE REST OF WHICH I'D SPENT INDOORS.
AS SOON AS I WENT BACK OUT INTO THE COLD, IT GOT VERY UNCOMFORTABLE AGAIN, AND EVEN THE FAIRLY SHORT WALK TO THE DOCTOR'S SURGERY WAS DIFFICULT.
MY DOCTOR EXAMINED ME THOROUGHLY AND, ONCE AGAIN, SAID THAT EVERYTHING FELT NORMAL.
COUGH, PLEASE.
PROD!
SQUEEZE!
YELP!
THEN HE SAID:
I THINK YOU HAVE AN INFECTION CALLED ***EPIDIDYMITIS***.
I'LL PRESCRIBE YOU SOME ANTIBIOTICS AND YOU SHOULD BE FINE IN A WEEK OR SO.

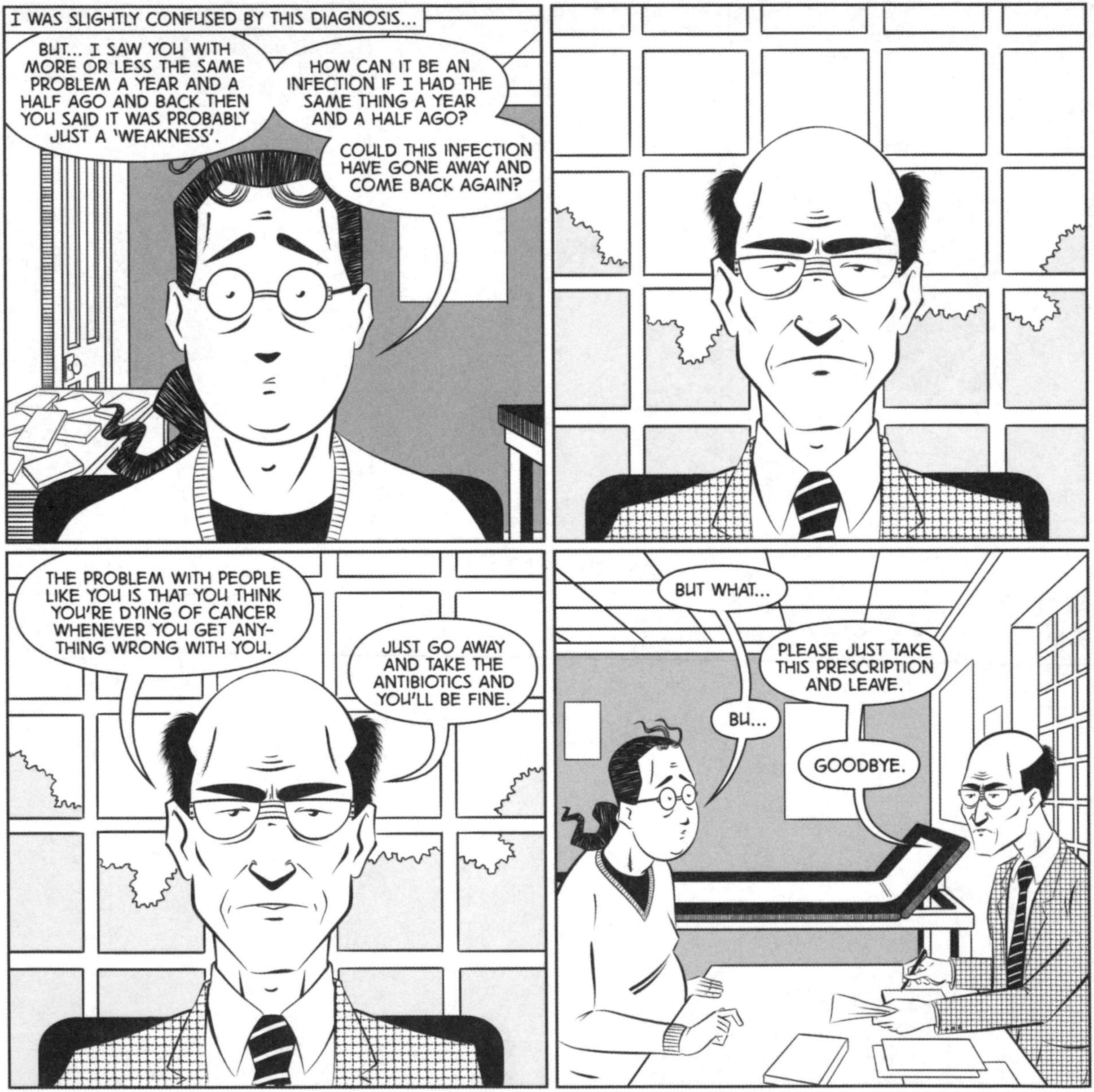
I WAS SLIGHTLY CONFUSED BY THIS DIAGNOSIS...
BUT... I SAW YOU WITH MORE OR LESS THE SAME PROBLEM A YEAR AND A HALF AGO AND BACK THEN YOU SAID IT WAS PROBABLY JUST A 'WEAKNESS'.
HOW CAN IT BE AN INFECTION IF I HAD THE SAME THING A YEAR AND A HALF AGO?
COULD THIS INFECTION HAVE GONE AWAY AND COME BACK AGAIN?
THE PROBLEM WITH PEOPLE LIKE YOU IS THAT YOU THINK YOU'RE DYING OF CANCER WHENEVER YOU GET ANY-THING WRONG WITH YOU.
JUST GO AWAY AND TAKE THE ANTIBIOTICS AND YOU'LL BE FINE.
BUT WHAT...
PLEASE JUST TAKE THIS PRESCRIPTION AND LEAVE.
BU...
GOODBYE.

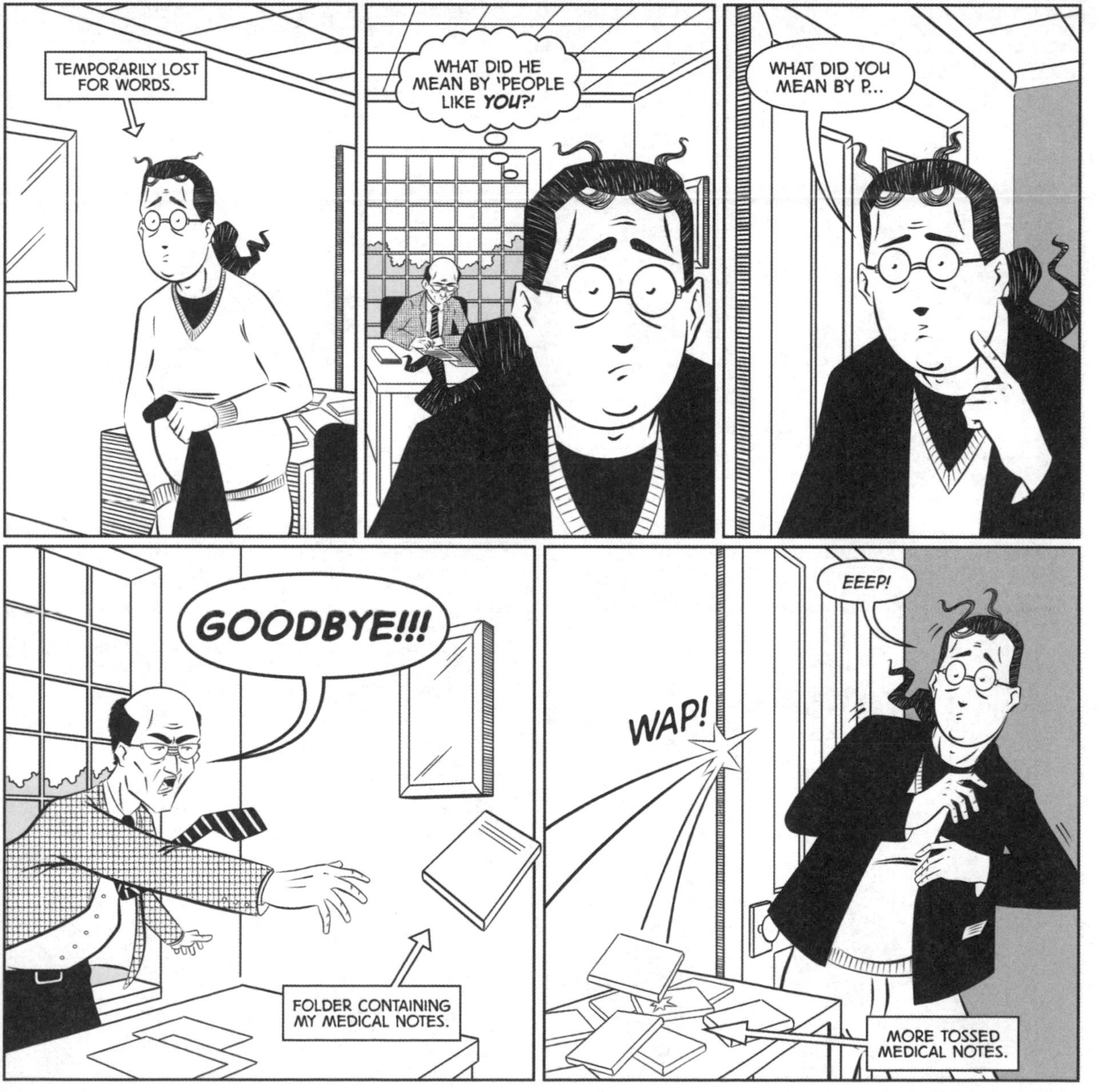
TEMPORARILY LOST FOR WORDS.
WHAT DID HE MEAN BY 'PEOPLE LIKE *YOU*?'
WHAT DID YOU MEAN BY P...
GOODBYE!!!
FOLDER CONTAINING MY MEDICAL NOTES.
WAP!
EEEP!
MORE TOSSED MEDICAL NOTES.

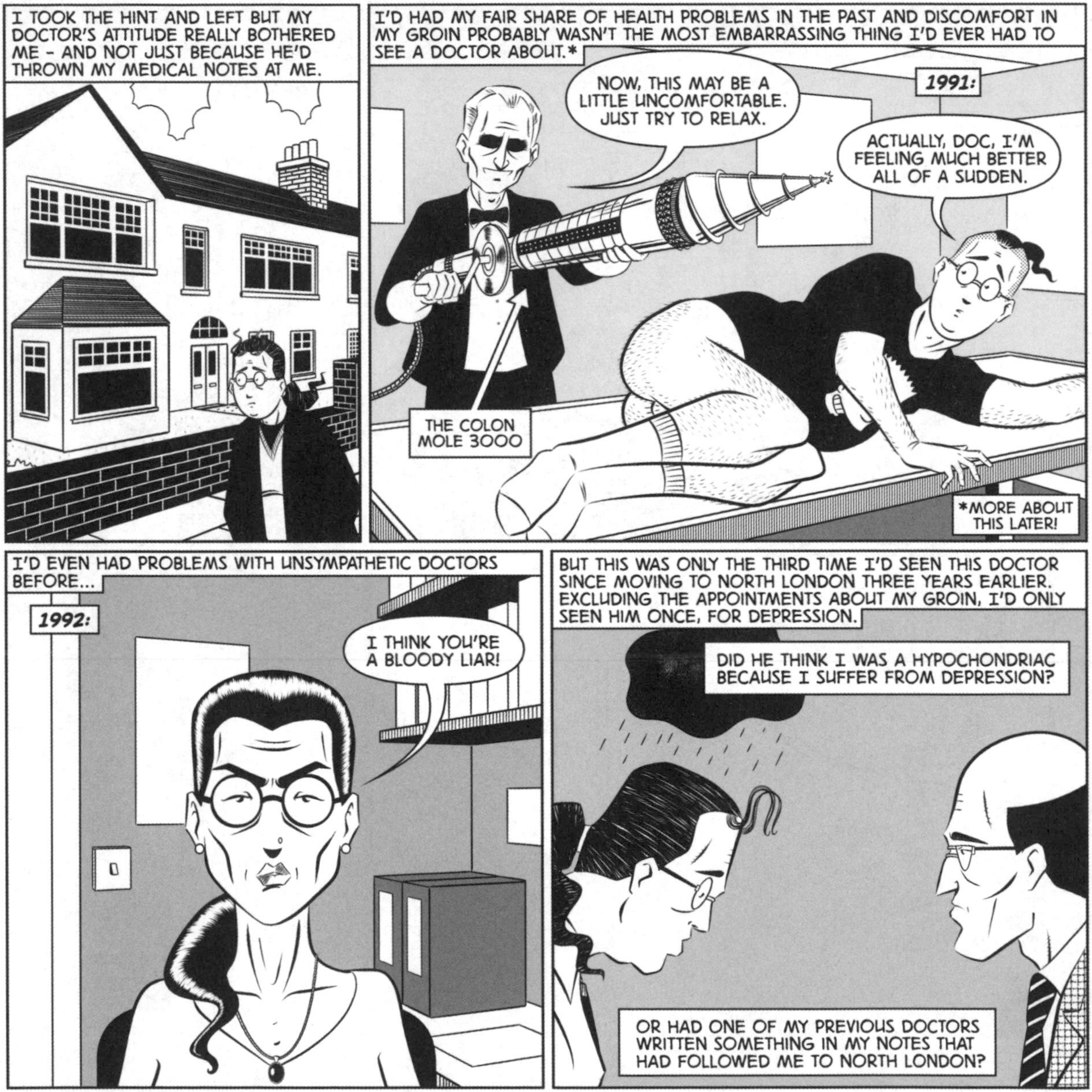
I TOOK THE HINT AND LEFT BUT MY DOCTOR'S ATTITUDE REALLY BOTHERED ME - AND NOT JUST BECAUSE HE'D THROWN MY MEDICAL NOTES AT ME.
I'D HAD MY FAIR SHARE OF HEALTH PROBLEMS IN THE PAST AND DISCOMFORT IN MY GROIN PROBABLY WASN'T THE MOST EMBARRASSING THING I'D EVER HAD TO SEE A DOCTOR ABOUT.*
1991:
NOW, THIS MAY BE A LITTLE UNCOMFORTABLE. JUST TRY TO RELAX.
ACTUALLY, DOC, I'M FEELING MUCH BETTER ALL OF A SUDDEN.
THE COLON MOLE 3000
*MORE ABOUT THIS LATER!
I'D EVEN HAD PROBLEMS WITH UNSYMPATHETIC DOCTORS BEFORE...
1992:
I THINK YOU'RE A BLOODY LIAR!
BUT THIS WAS ONLY THE THIRD TIME I'D SEEN THIS DOCTOR SINCE MOVING TO NORTH LONDON THREE YEARS EARLIER. EXCLUDING THE APPOINTMENTS ABOUT MY GROIN, I'D ONLY SEEN HIM ONCE, FOR DEPRESSION.
DID HE THINK I WAS A HYPOCHONDRIAC BECAUSE I SUFFER FROM DEPRESSION?
OR HAD ONE OF MY PREVIOUS DOCTORS WRITTEN SOMETHING IN MY NOTES THAT HAD FOLLOWED ME TO NORTH LONDON?

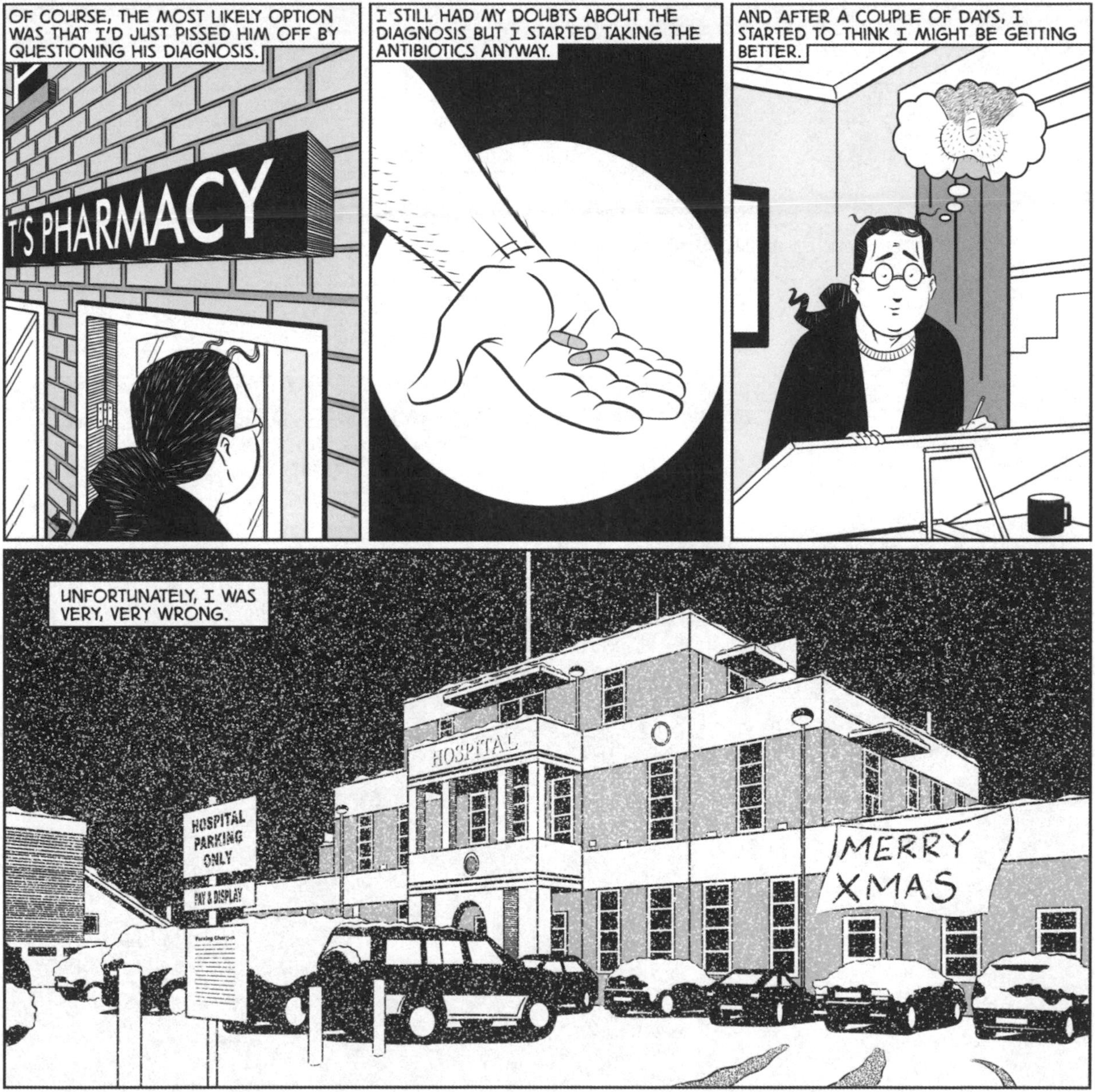
OF COURSE, THE MOST LIKELY OPTION WAS THAT I'D JUST PISSED HIM OFF BY QUESTIONING HIS DIAGNOSIS.
T'S PHARMACY
I STILL HAD MY DOUBTS ABOUT THE DIAGNOSIS BUT I STARTED TAKING THE ANTIBIOTICS ANYWAY.
AND AFTER A COUPLE OF DAYS, I STARTED TO THINK I MIGHT BE GETTING BETTER.
UNFORTUNATELY, I WAS VERY, VERY WRONG.
HOSPITAL
HOSPITAL PARKING ONLY
PAY & DISPLAY
Parking Charges
MERRY XMAS

2. THE BOXING DAY BALL

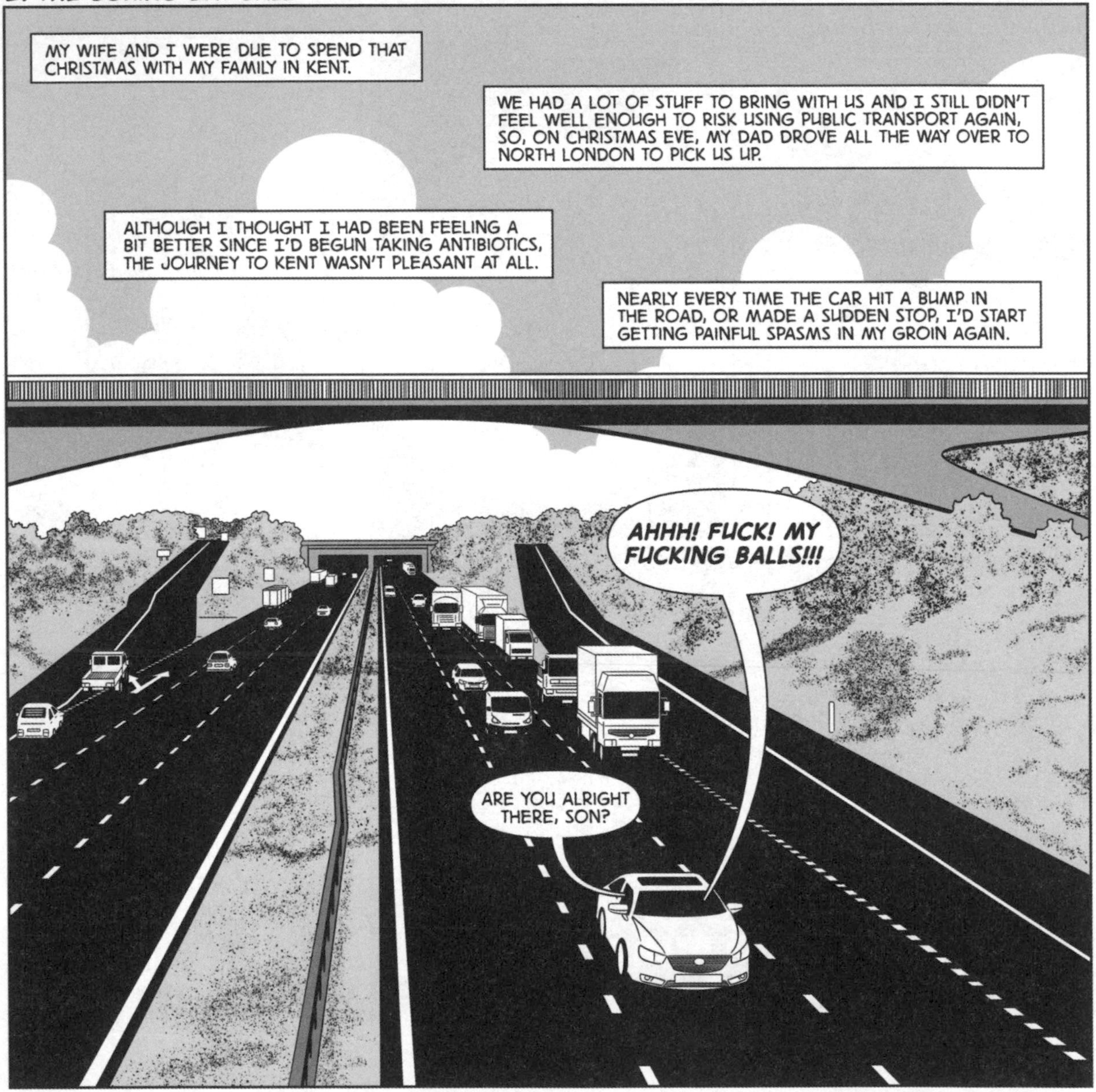

MY WIFE AND I WERE DUE TO SPEND THAT CHRISTMAS WITH MY FAMILY IN KENT.
WE HAD A LOT OF STUFF TO BRING WITH US AND I STILL DIDN'T FEEL WELL ENOUGH TO RISK USING PUBLIC TRANSPORT AGAIN, SO, ON CHRISTMAS EVE, MY DAD DROVE ALL THE WAY OVER TO NORTH LONDON TO PICK US UP.
ALTHOUGH I THOUGHT I HAD BEEN FEELING A BIT BETTER SINCE I'D BEGUN TAKING ANTIBIOTICS, THE JOURNEY TO KENT WASN'T PLEASANT AT ALL.
NEARLY EVERY TIME THE CAR HIT A BUMP IN THE ROAD, OR MADE A SUDDEN STOP, I'D START GETTING PAINFUL SPASMS IN MY GROIN AGAIN.
AHHH! FUCK! MY FUCKING BALLS!!!
ARE YOU ALRIGHT THERE, SON?

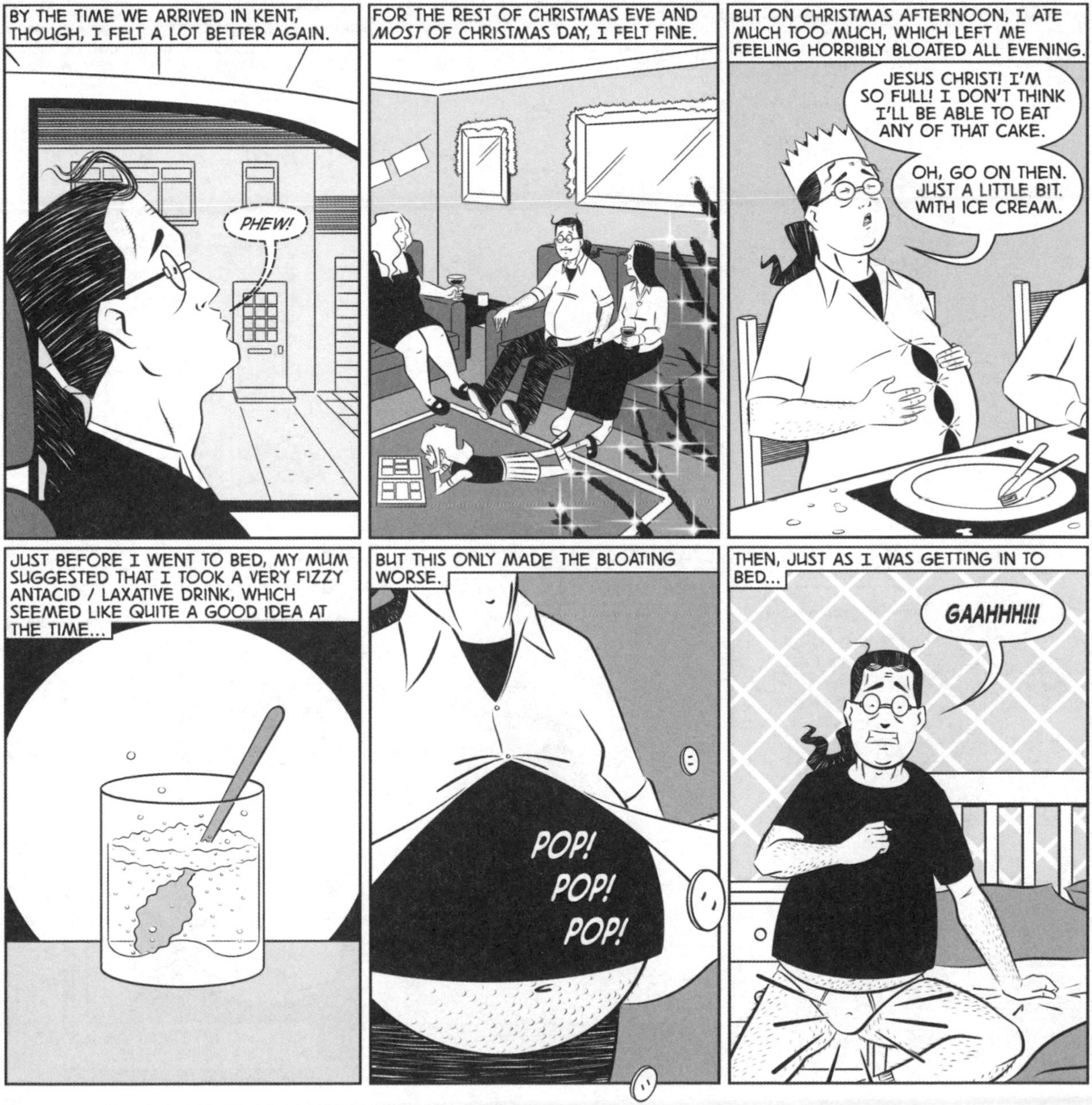

BY THE TIME WE ARRIVED IN KENT, THOUGH, I FELT A LOT BETTER AGAIN.
PHEW!
FOR THE REST OF CHRISTMAS EVE AND *MOST* OF CHRISTMAS DAY, I FELT FINE.
BUT ON CHRISTMAS AFTERNOON, I ATE MUCH TOO MUCH, WHICH LEFT ME FEELING HORRIBLY BLOATED ALL EVENING.
JESUS CHRIST! I'M SO FULL! I DON'T THINK I'LL BE ABLE TO EAT ANY OF THAT CAKE.
OH, GO ON THEN. JUST A LITTLE BIT. WITH ICE CREAM.
JUST BEFORE I WENT TO BED, MY MUM SUGGESTED THAT I TOOK A VERY FIZZY ANTACID / LAXATIVE DRINK, WHICH SEEMED LIKE QUITE A GOOD IDEA AT THE TIME...
BUT THIS ONLY MADE THE BLOATING WORSE.
POP! POP! POP!
THEN, JUST AS I WAS GETTING IN TO BED...
GAAHHH!!!

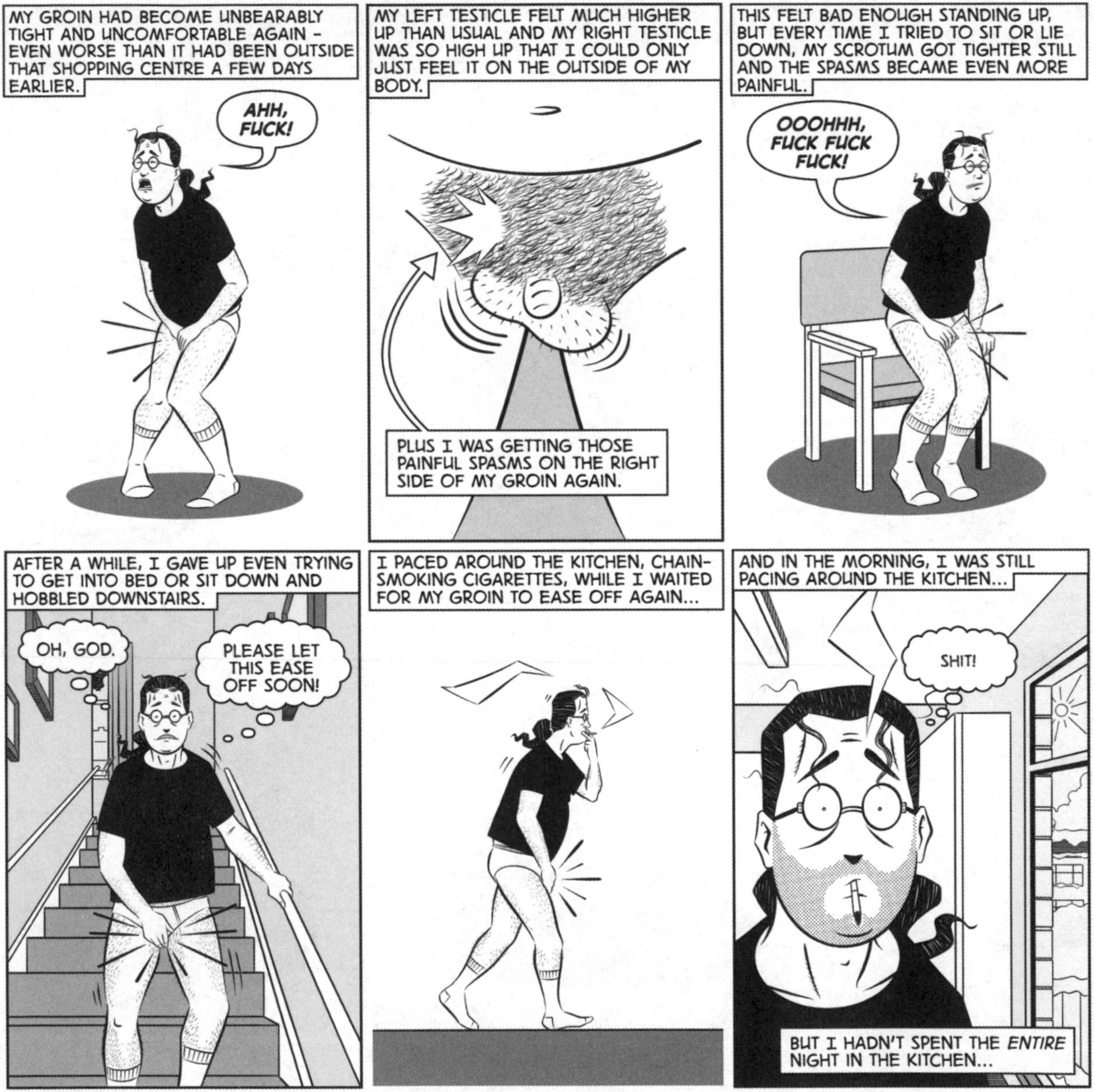
MY GROIN HAD BECOME UNBEARABLY TIGHT AND UNCOMFORTABLE AGAIN - EVEN WORSE THAN IT HAD BEEN OUTSIDE THAT SHOPPING CENTRE A FEW DAYS EARLIER.
AHH, FUCK!
MY LEFT TESTICLE FELT MUCH HIGHER UP THAN USUAL AND MY RIGHT TESTICLE WAS SO HIGH UP THAT I COULD ONLY JUST FEEL IT ON THE OUTSIDE OF MY BODY.
PLUS I WAS GETTING THOSE PAINFUL SPASMS ON THE RIGHT SIDE OF MY GROIN AGAIN.
THIS FELT BAD ENOUGH STANDING UP, BUT EVERY TIME I TRIED TO SIT OR LIE DOWN, MY SCROTUM GOT TIGHTER STILL AND THE SPASMS BECAME EVEN MORE PAINFUL.
OOOHHH, FUCK FUCK FUCK!
AFTER A WHILE, I GAVE UP EVEN TRYING TO GET INTO BED OR SIT DOWN AND HOBBLED DOWNSTAIRS.
OH, GOD.
PLEASE LET THIS EASE OFF SOON!
I PACED AROUND THE KITCHEN, CHAIN-SMOKING CIGARETTES, WHILE I WAITED FOR MY GROIN TO EASE OFF AGAIN...
AND IN THE MORNING, I WAS STILL PACING AROUND THE KITCHEN...
SHIT!
BUT I HADN'T SPENT THE *ENTIRE* NIGHT IN THE KITCHEN...

AT ABOUT 2:00AM, THE LAXATIVE DRINK I'D TAKEN BEFORE *TRYING* TO GET INTO BED KICKED IN AND I HAD TO HURRY BACK UPSTAIRS TO THE BATHROOM.

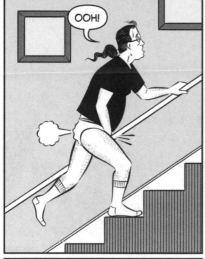

OOH!

THE TIGHTNESS IN MY GROIN MADE SITTING ON THE TOILET MORE OR LESS IMPOSSIBLE, SO I HAD TO TRY AND GO WHILE STANDING UP.

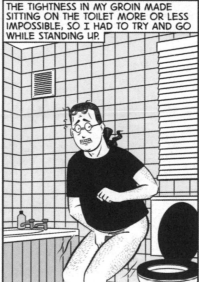

MY SHIT COMPLETELY MISSED THE TOILET AND LANDED ON THE BATHROOM CARPET...

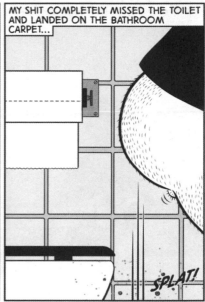

SPLAT!

AND THE PROCESS OF SQUEEZING OUT A SHIT – EVEN ONE THAT HAD BEEN LOOSENED BY A LAXATIVE – MADE MY GROIN TIGHTEN UP EVEN MORE.

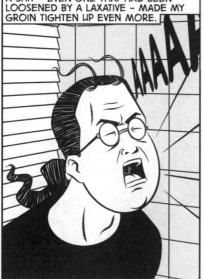

AAAA!

SQUATTING DOWN TO CLEAN UP MY OWN MESS WAS ALSO IMPOSSIBLE, SO I HAD TO CALL SOMEONE IN TO DO IT FOR ME.

AS MY DAD WAS THE ONLY OTHER PERSON IN THE HOUSE STILL AWAKE, HE GOT THE DIRTY JOB.

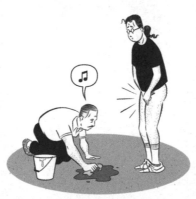

THEN HE HELPED ME PUT ON SOME JOGGING BOTTOMS AND I WENT BACK TO PACING AROUND THE KITCHEN.

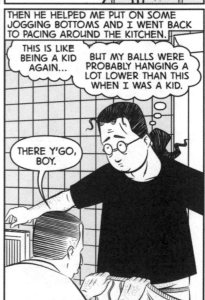

THIS IS LIKE BEING A KID AGAIN...

BUT MY BALLS WERE PROBABLY HANGING A LOT LOWER THAN THIS WHEN I WAS A KID.

THERE Y'GO, BOY.

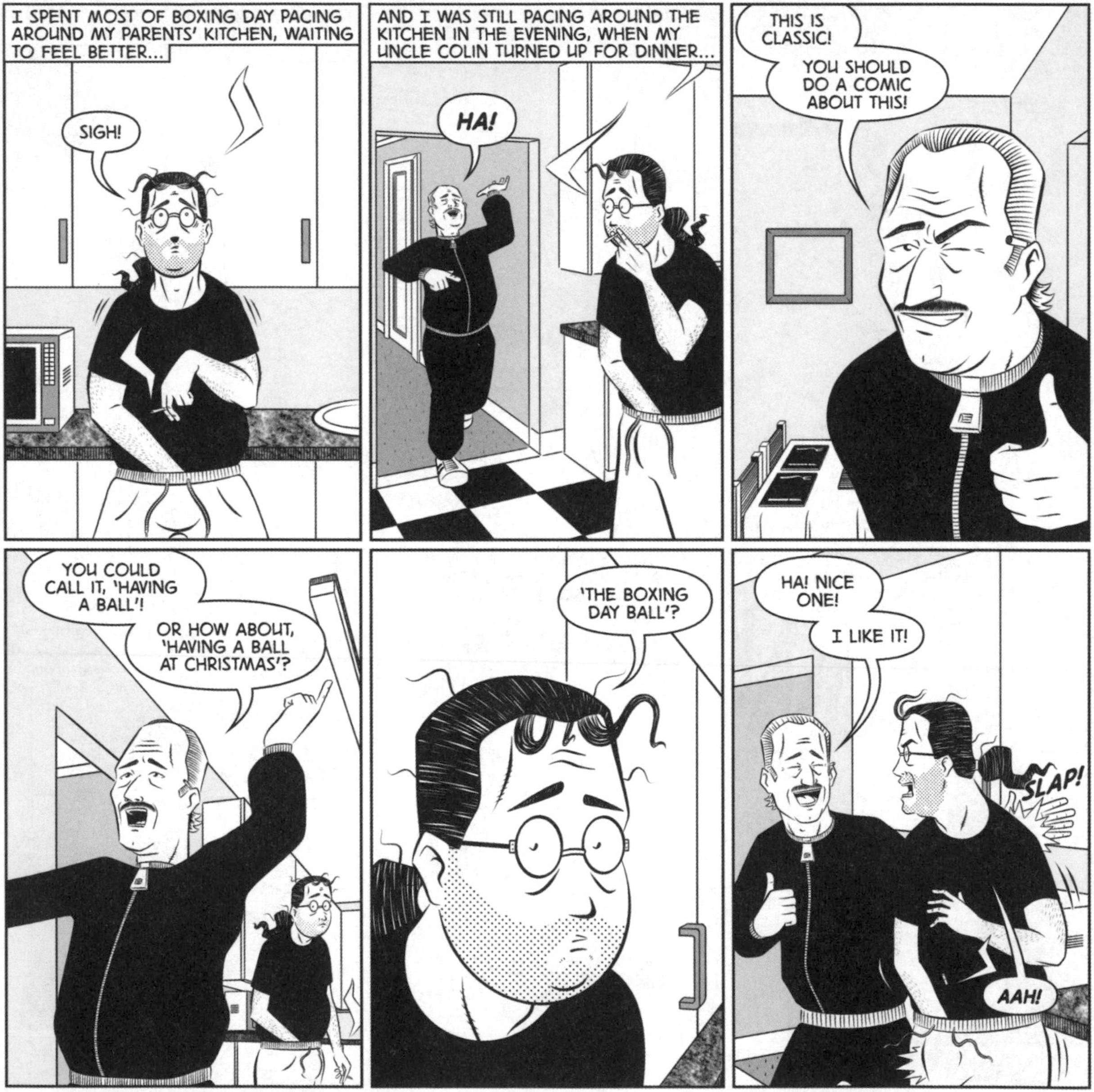
I SPENT MOST OF BOXING DAY PACING AROUND MY PARENTS' KITCHEN, WAITING TO FEEL BETTER...
SIGH!
AND I WAS STILL PACING AROUND THE KITCHEN IN THE EVENING, WHEN MY UNCLE COLIN TURNED UP FOR DINNER...
HA!
THIS IS CLASSIC!
YOU SHOULD DO A COMIC ABOUT THIS!
YOU COULD CALL IT, 'HAVING A BALL'!
OR HOW ABOUT, 'HAVING A BALL AT CHRISTMAS'?
'THE BOXING DAY BALL'?
HA! NICE ONE!
I LIKE IT!
SLAP!
AAH!

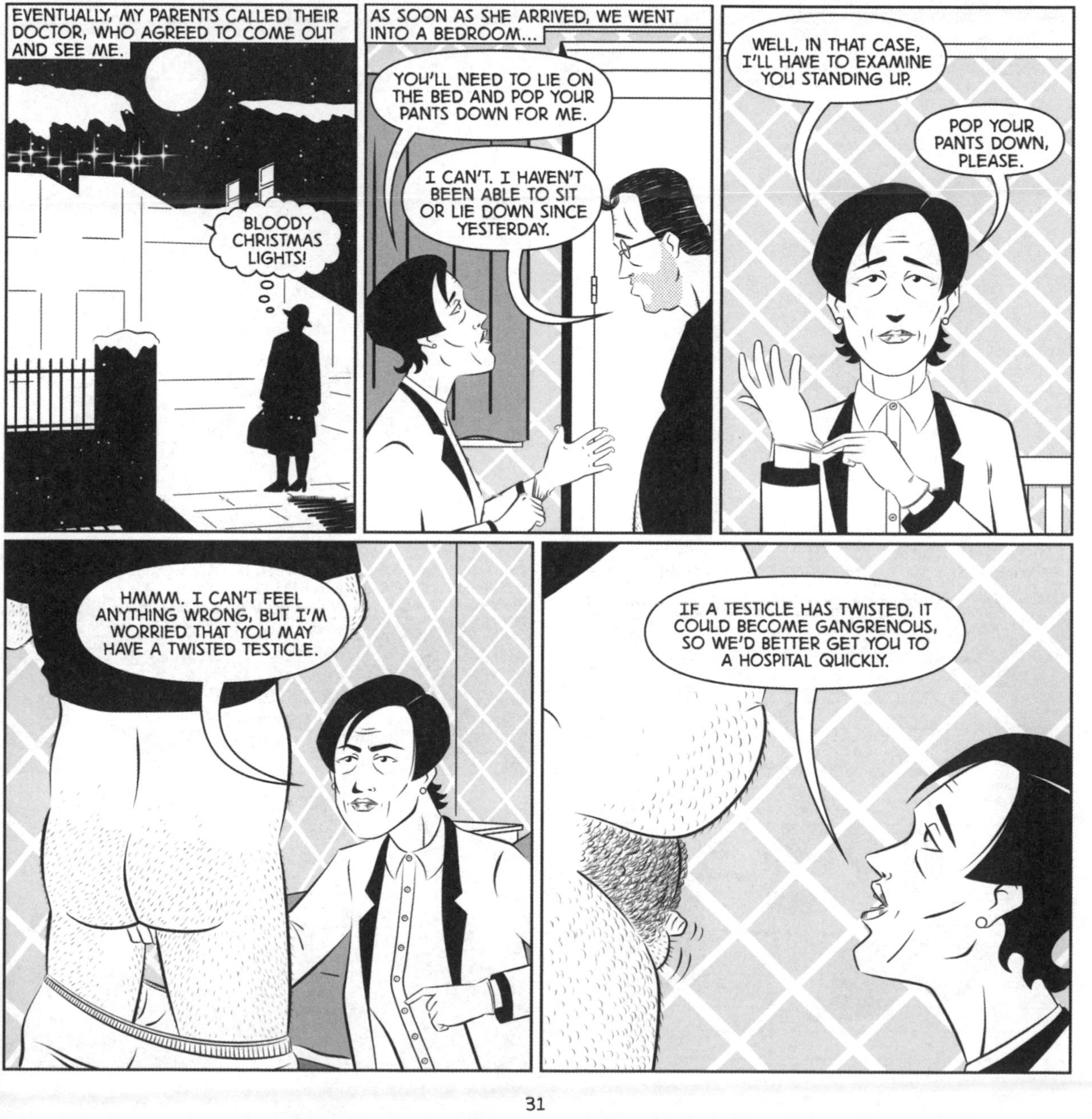
EVENTUALLY, MY PARENTS CALLED THEIR DOCTOR, WHO AGREED TO COME OUT AND SEE ME.
BLOODY CHRISTMAS LIGHTS!
AS SOON AS SHE ARRIVED, WE WENT INTO A BEDROOM...
YOU'LL NEED TO LIE ON THE BED AND POP YOUR PANTS DOWN FOR ME.
I CAN'T. I HAVEN'T BEEN ABLE TO SIT OR LIE DOWN SINCE YESTERDAY.
WELL, IN THAT CASE, I'LL HAVE TO EXAMINE YOU STANDING UP.
POP YOUR PANTS DOWN, PLEASE.
HMMM. I CAN'T FEEL ANYTHING WRONG, BUT I'M WORRIED THAT YOU MAY HAVE A TWISTED TESTICLE.
IF A TESTICLE HAS TWISTED, IT COULD BECOME GANGRENOUS, SO WE'D BETTER GET YOU TO A HOSPITAL QUICKLY.

THE TERM *TWISTED TESTICLE*, OR *TESTICULAR TORSION*, REFERS TO A TESTICLE THAT HAS TWISTED IN THE SCROTUM, RESULTING IN A TWIST IN THE SPERMATIC CORD.

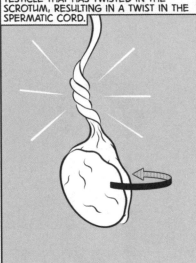

JUST AS A TWIST IN A HOSEPIPE WILL CUT OFF THE FLOW OF WATER, A TWIST IN THE SPERMATIC CORD CAN CUT OFF THE FLOW OF BLOOD TO A TESTICLE.

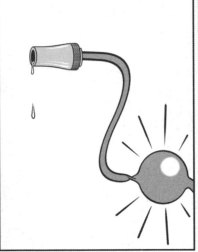

IF UNTREATED, THIS CAN LEAD TO THE DEATH (AND AMPUTATION) OF THE TESTICLE. THIS, THEN, WAS LOOKING LIKE AN EMERGENCY SITUATION.

RATHER THAN WAITING FOR AN AMBULANCE, MY DAD DROVE MY WIFE AND I TO THE HOSPITAL. COLIN TAGGED ALONG FOR A LAUGH.

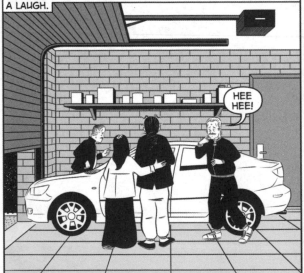

HEE HEE!

GETTING IN THE CAR AND FORCING MYSELF TO SIT DOWN FOR THE FIRST TIME IN NEARLY TWENTY-FOUR HOURS WAS EXTREMELY DIFFICULT. GETTING OUT OF THE CAR AT THE OTHER END WAS ALMOST AS BAD.

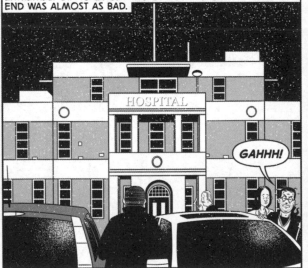

HOSPITAL

GAHHH!

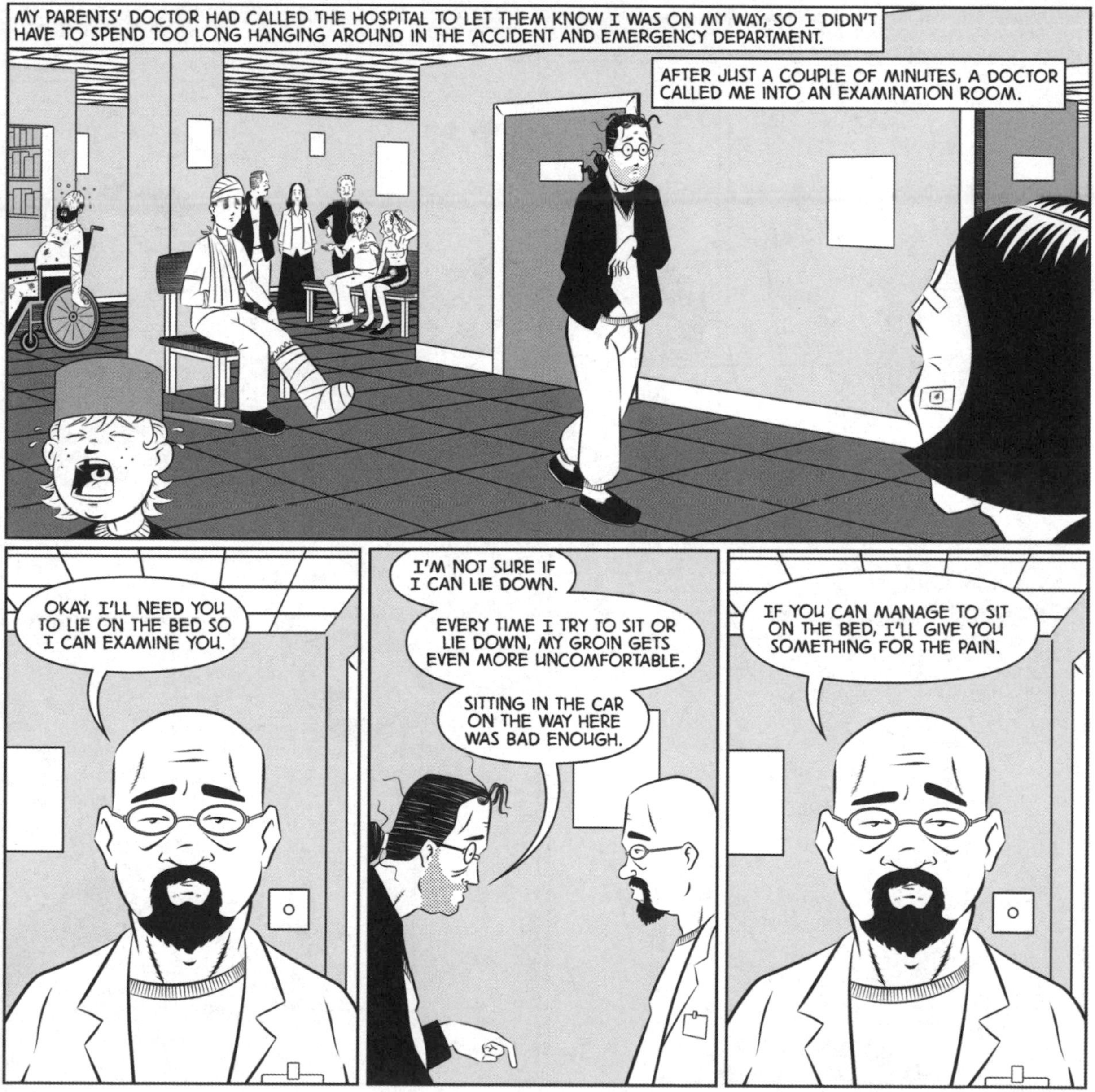

MY PARENTS' DOCTOR HAD CALLED THE HOSPITAL TO LET THEM KNOW I WAS ON MY WAY, SO I DIDN'T HAVE TO SPEND TOO LONG HANGING AROUND IN THE ACCIDENT AND EMERGENCY DEPARTMENT.
AFTER JUST A COUPLE OF MINUTES, A DOCTOR CALLED ME INTO AN EXAMINATION ROOM.
OKAY, I'LL NEED YOU TO LIE ON THE BED SO I CAN EXAMINE YOU.
I'M NOT SURE IF I CAN LIE DOWN.
EVERY TIME I TRY TO SIT OR LIE DOWN, MY GROIN GETS EVEN MORE UNCOMFORTABLE.
SITTING IN THE CAR ON THE WAY HERE WAS BAD ENOUGH.
IF YOU CAN MANAGE TO SIT ON THE BED, I'LL GIVE YOU SOMETHING FOR THE PAIN.

I MANAGED TO SIT ON THE EDGE OF THE BED AND THE DOCTOR INJECTED SOME MORPHINE INTO MY ARM.

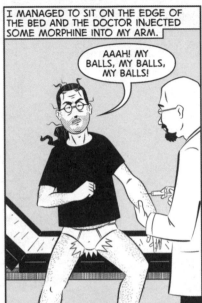

AAAH! MY BALLS, MY BALLS, MY BALLS!

ALMOST IMMEDIATELY, A WARM GLOW HIT ME IN THE CHEST AND SPREAD THROUGHOUT MY BODY.

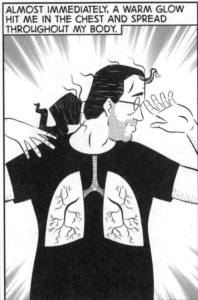

WITHIN A MINUTE, I WAS PAIN-FREE AND LYING DOWN. MY TESTICLES STILL FELT MUCH HIGHER UP THAN THEY SHOULD HAVE BEEN, BUT FOR A WHILE, I DIDN'T PARTICULARLY CARE.

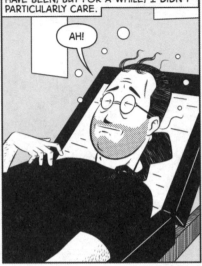

AH!

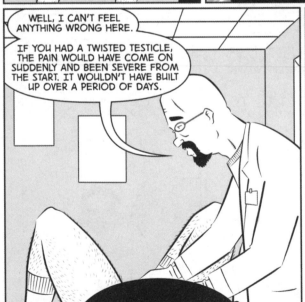

WELL, I CAN'T FEEL ANYTHING WRONG HERE.

IF YOU HAD A TWISTED TESTICLE, THE PAIN WOULD HAVE COME ON SUDDENLY AND BEEN SEVERE FROM THE START. IT WOULDN'T HAVE BUILT UP OVER A PERIOD OF DAYS.

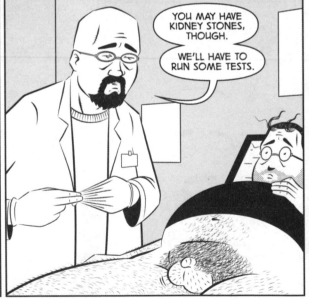

YOU MAY HAVE KIDNEY STONES, THOUGH.

WE'LL HAVE TO RUN SOME TESTS.

OVER THE NEXT COUPLE OF HOURS, I WAS WHEELED FROM ROOM TO ROOM WHILE VARIOUS TESTS WERE CONDUCTED. FIRST, I WAS INJECTED WITH A DYE THAT WOULD PASS THROUGH MY KIDNEYS INTO MY BLADDER AND SENT FOR AN X-RAY.

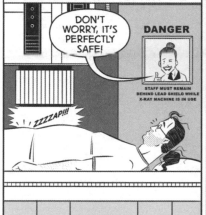

DON'T WORRY, IT'S PERFECTLY SAFE!

DANGER

STAFF MUST REMAIN BEHIND LEAD SHIELD WHILE X-RAY MACHINE IS IN USE

ZZZZAP!!!

NO SIGN OF KIDNEY STONES.

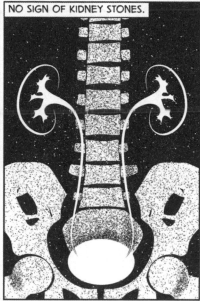

THEY DID THIS TWICE, JUST TO BE SURE.

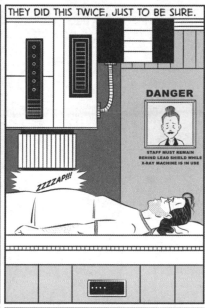

DANGER

STAFF MUST REMAIN BEHIND LEAD SHIELD WHILE X-RAY MACHINE IS IN USE

ZZZZAP!!!

STILL NO SIGN OF KIDNEY STONES.

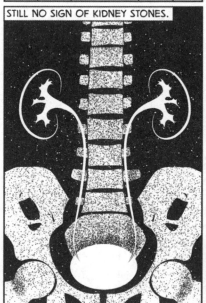

EVENTUALLY, I FOUND MYSELF LYING ON A TROLLEY IN A CORRIDOR WHILE A TEAM OF DOCTORS DISCUSSED MY CASE.

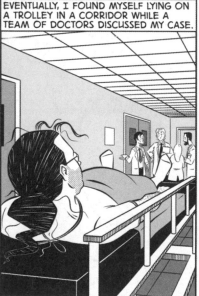

IN RETROSPECT, IT WAS OBVIOUS THAT THEY DIDN'T HAVE A CLUE WHAT WAS WRONG WITH ME.

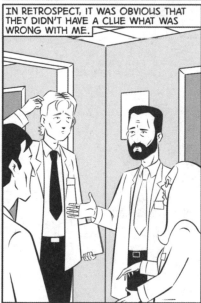

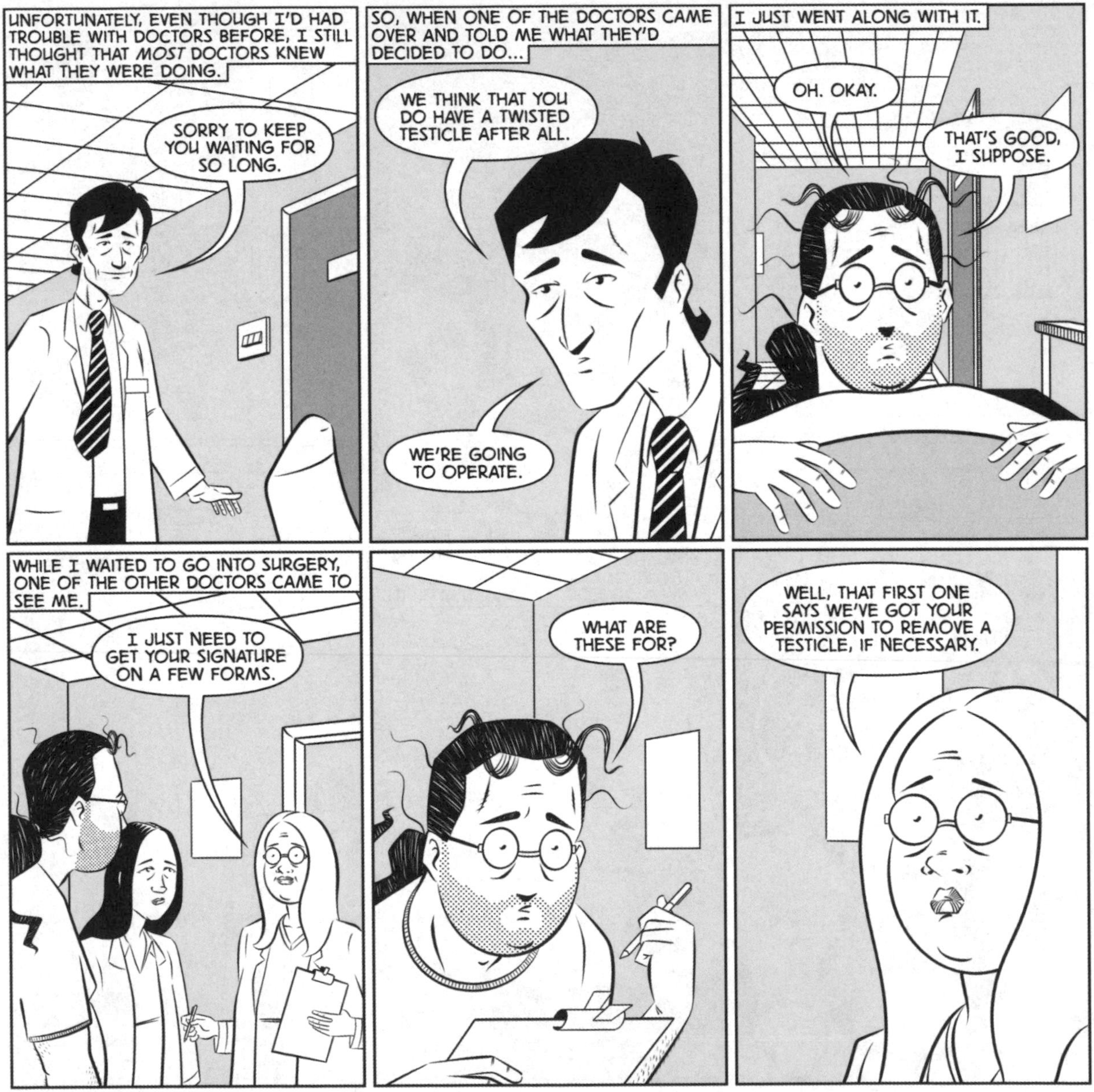
UNFORTUNATELY, EVEN THOUGH I'D HAD TROUBLE WITH DOCTORS BEFORE, I STILL THOUGHT THAT *MOST* DOCTORS KNEW WHAT THEY WERE DOING.
SORRY TO KEEP YOU WAITING FOR SO LONG.
SO, WHEN ONE OF THE DOCTORS CAME OVER AND TOLD ME WHAT THEY'D DECIDED TO DO...
WE THINK THAT YOU DO HAVE A TWISTED TESTICLE AFTER ALL.
WE'RE GOING TO OPERATE.
I JUST WENT ALONG WITH IT.
OH. OKAY.
THAT'S GOOD, I SUPPOSE.
WHILE I WAITED TO GO INTO SURGERY, ONE OF THE OTHER DOCTORS CAME TO SEE ME.
I JUST NEED TO GET YOUR SIGNATURE ON A FEW FORMS.
WHAT ARE THESE FOR?
WELL, THAT FIRST ONE SAYS WE'VE GOT YOUR PERMISSION TO REMOVE A TESTICLE, IF NECESSARY.

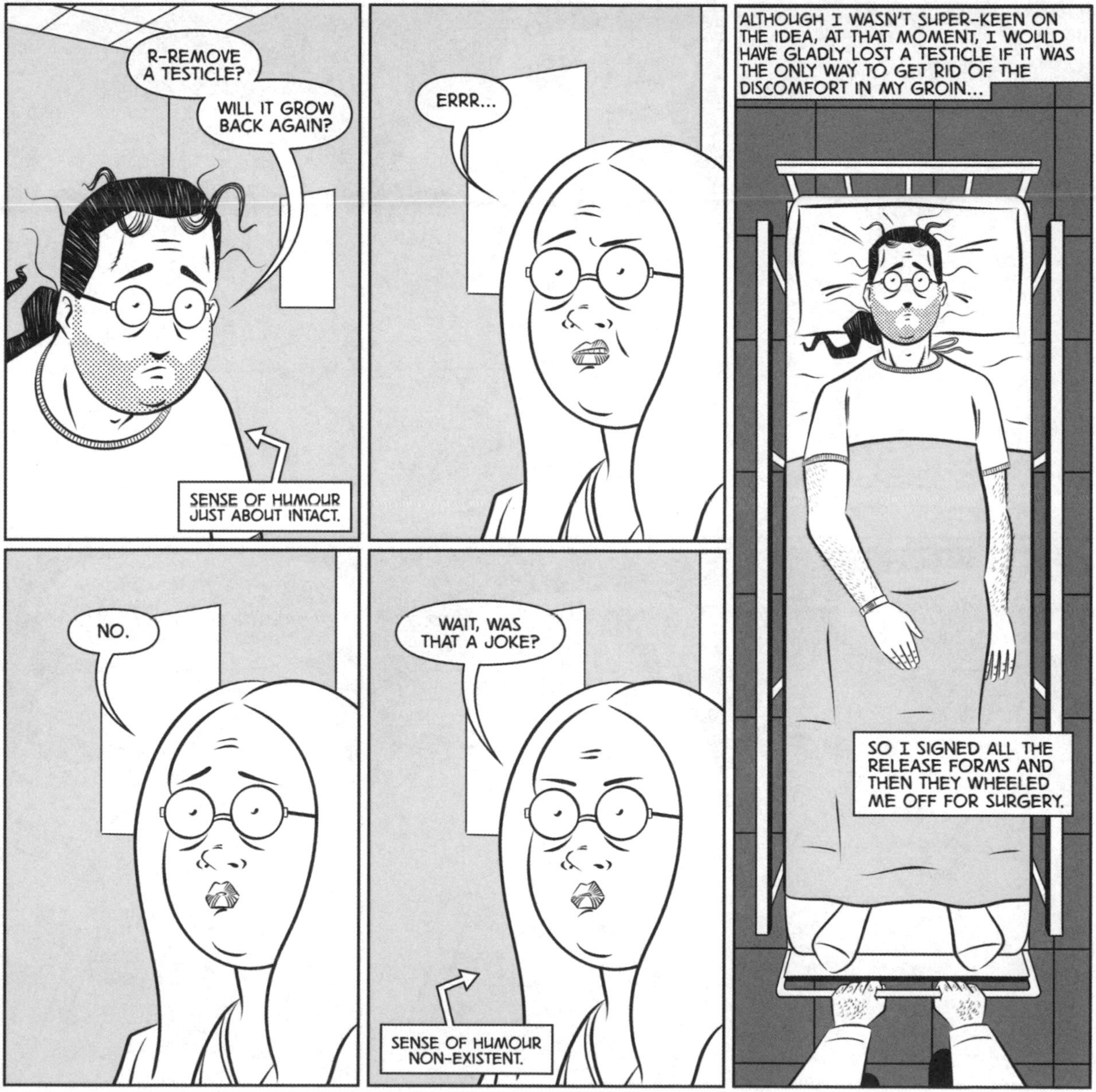
R-REMOVE A TESTICLE?
WILL IT GROW BACK AGAIN?
SENSE OF HUMOUR JUST ABOUT INTACT.
ERRR...
ALTHOUGH I WASN'T SUPER-KEEN ON THE IDEA, AT THAT MOMENT, I WOULD HAVE GLADLY LOST A TESTICLE IF IT WAS THE ONLY WAY TO GET RID OF THE DISCOMFORT IN MY GROIN...
NO.
WAIT, WAS THAT A JOKE?
SENSE OF HUMOUR NON-EXISTENT.
SO I SIGNED ALL THE RELEASE FORMS AND THEN THEY WHEELED ME OFF FOR SURGERY.

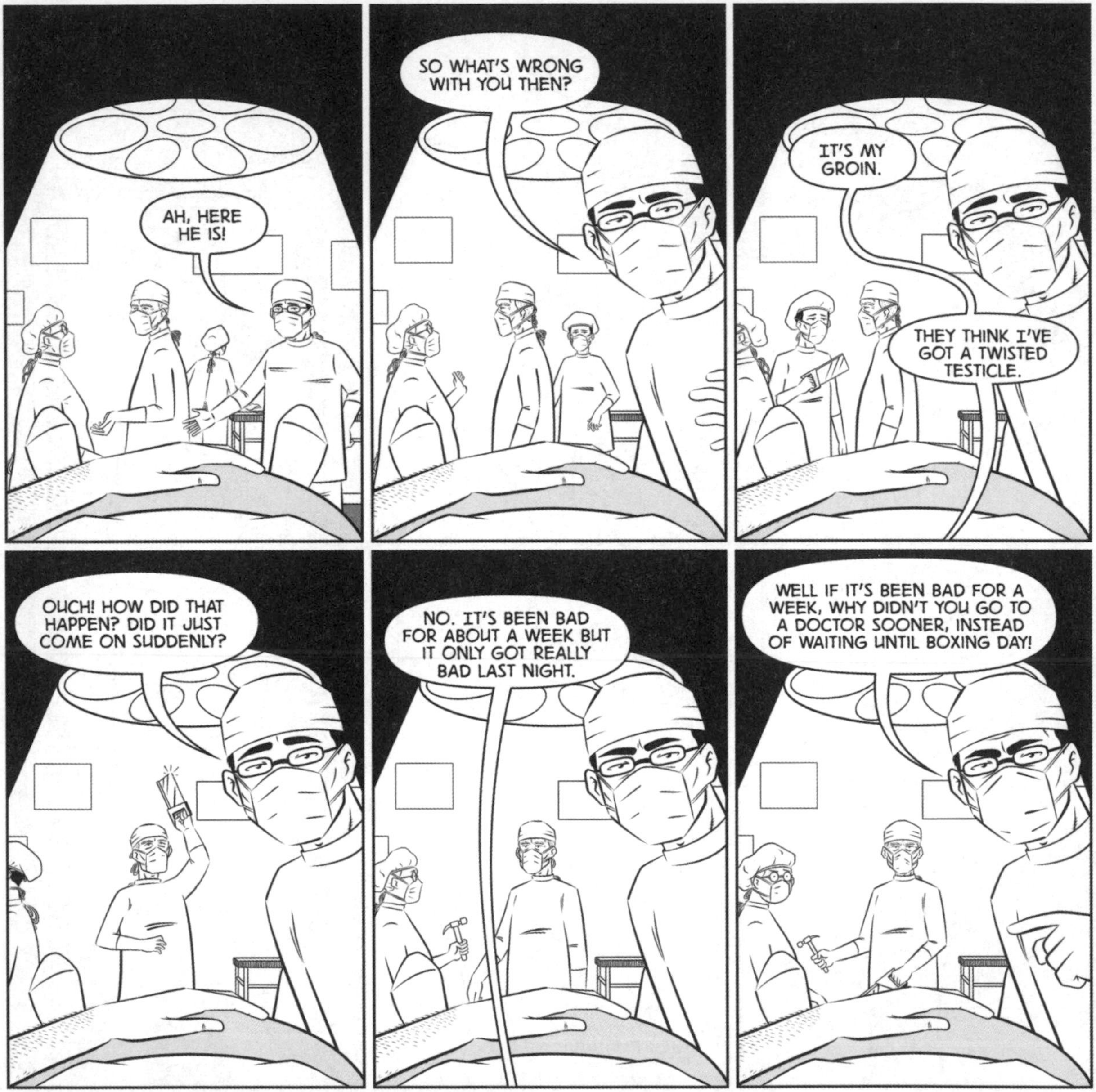
AH, HERE HE IS!
SO WHAT'S WRONG WITH YOU THEN?
IT'S MY GROIN.
THEY THINK I'VE GOT A TWISTED TESTICLE.
OUCH! HOW DID THAT HAPPEN? DID IT JUST COME ON SUDDENLY?
NO. IT'S BEEN BAD FOR ABOUT A WEEK BUT IT ONLY GOT REALLY BAD LAST NIGHT.
WELL IF IT'S BEEN BAD FOR A WEEK, WHY DIDN'T YOU GO TO A DOCTOR SOONER, INSTEAD OF WAITING UNTIL BOXING DAY!

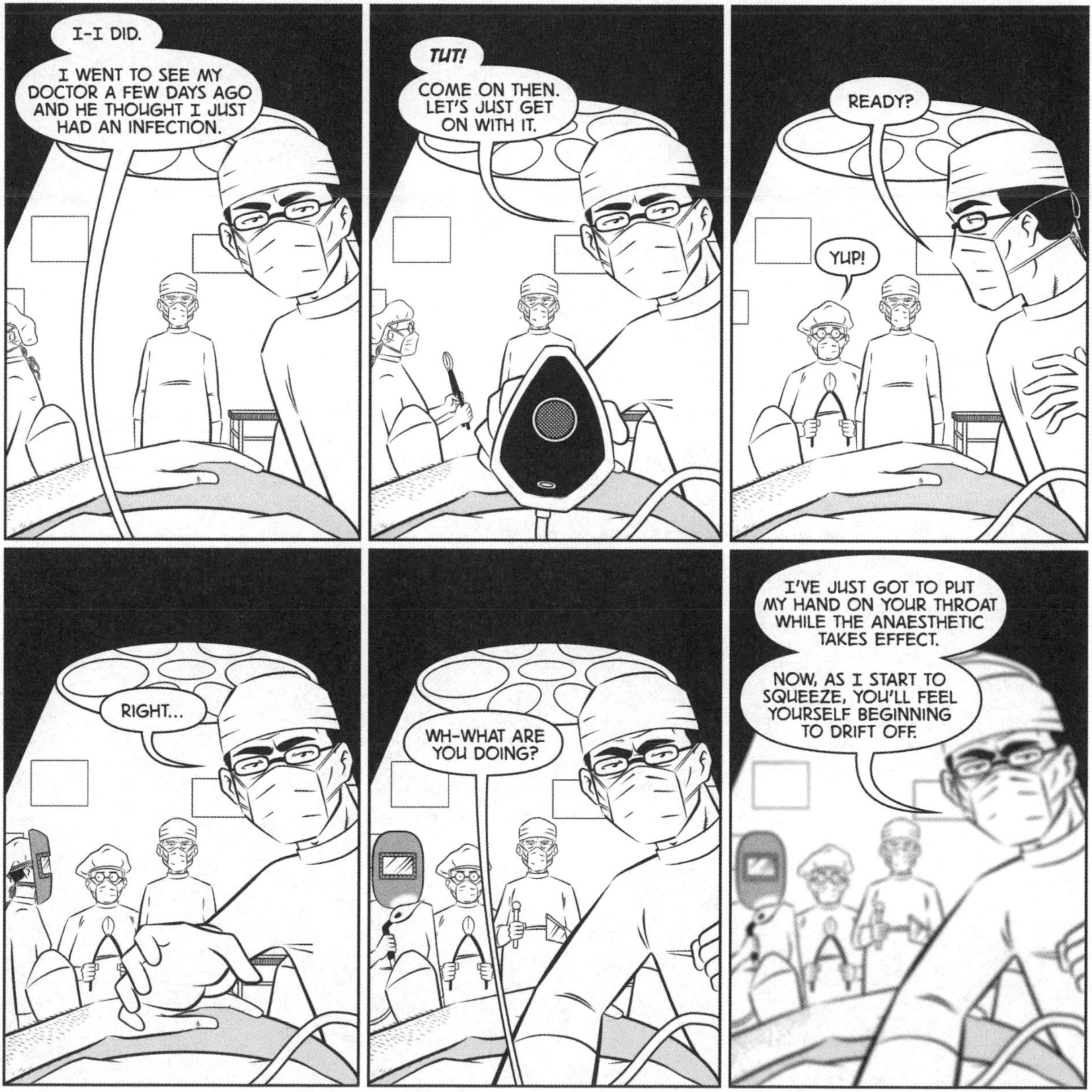
I-I DID.
I WENT TO SEE MY DOCTOR A FEW DAYS AGO AND HE THOUGHT I JUST HAD AN INFECTION.
TUT!
COME ON THEN. LET'S JUST GET ON WITH IT.
READY?
YUP!
RIGHT...
WH-WHAT ARE YOU DOING?
I'VE JUST GOT TO PUT MY HAND ON YOUR THROAT WHILE THE ANAESTHETIC TAKES EFFECT.
NOW, AS I START TO SQUEEZE, YOU'LL FEEL YOURSELF BEGINNING TO DRIFT OFF.

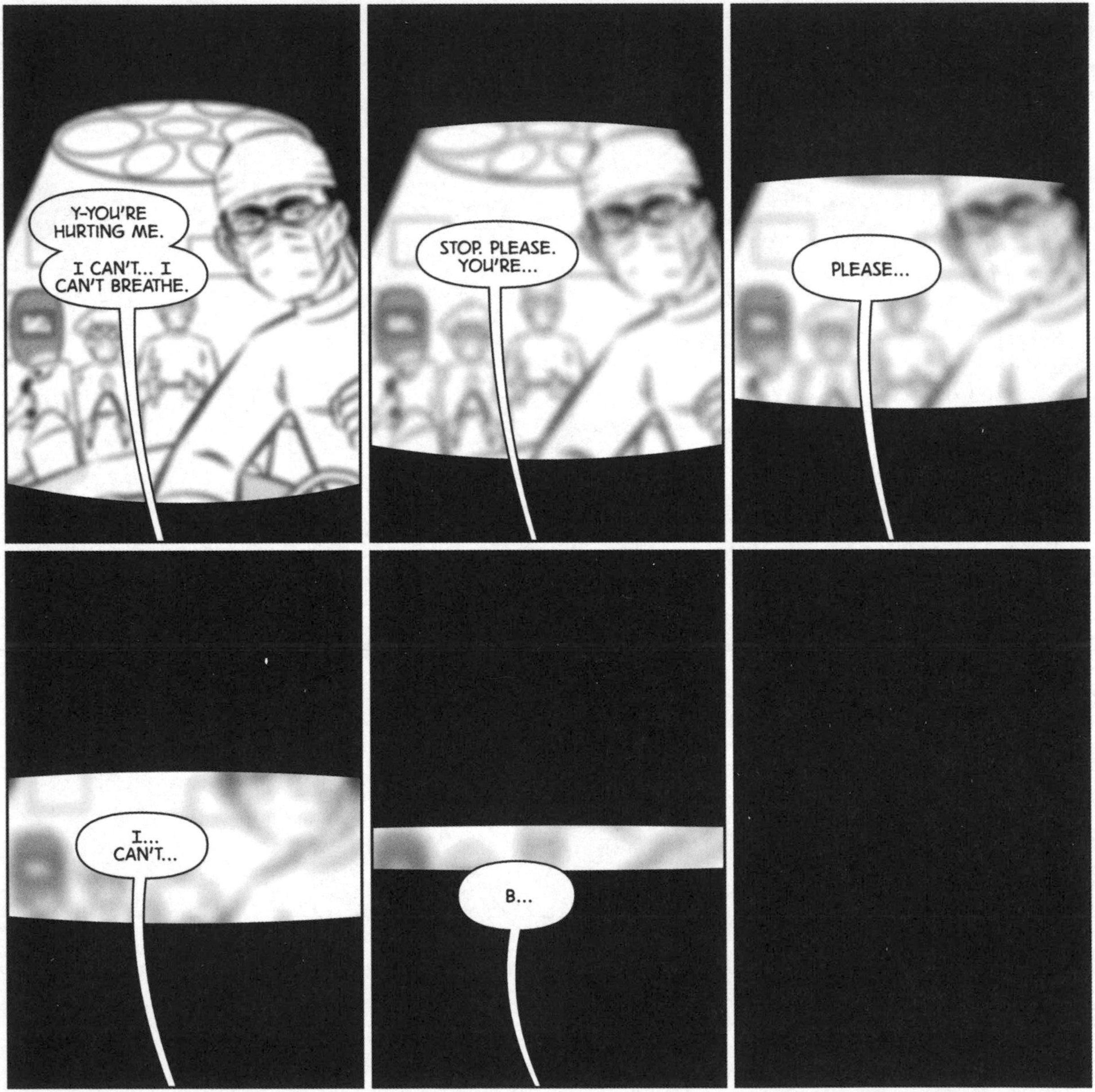
Y-YOU'RE HURTING ME.
I CAN'T... I CAN'T BREATHE.
STOP. PLEASE. YOU'RE...
PLEASE...
I... CAN'T...
B...

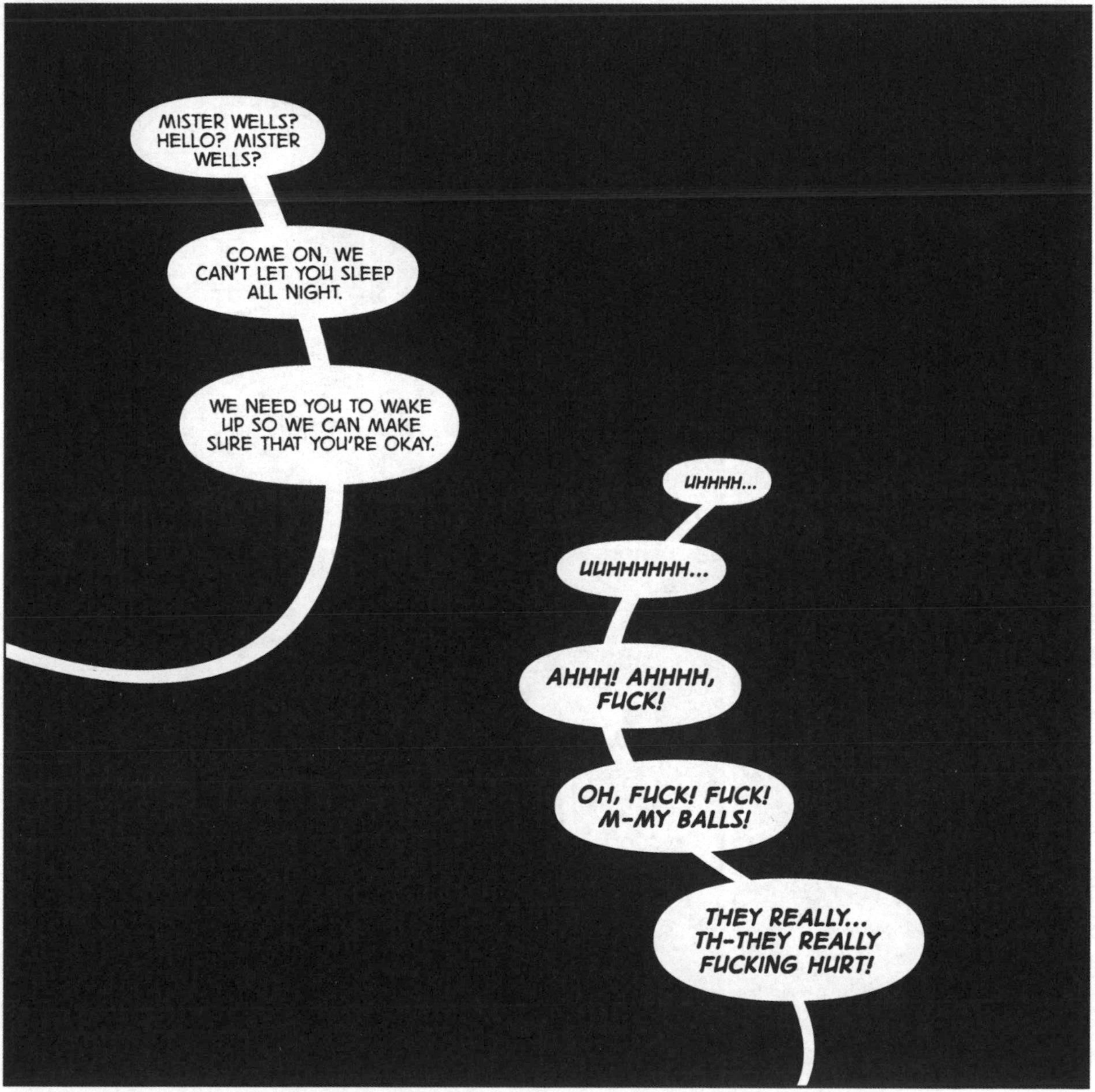
MISTER WELLS? HELLO? MISTER WELLS?
COME ON, WE CAN'T LET YOU SLEEP ALL NIGHT.
WE NEED YOU TO WAKE UP SO WE CAN MAKE SURE THAT YOU'RE OKAY.
UHHHH...
UUHHHHHH...
AHHH! AHHHH, FUCK!
OH, FUCK! FUCK! M-MY BALLS!
THEY REALLY... TH-THEY REALLY FUCKING HURT!

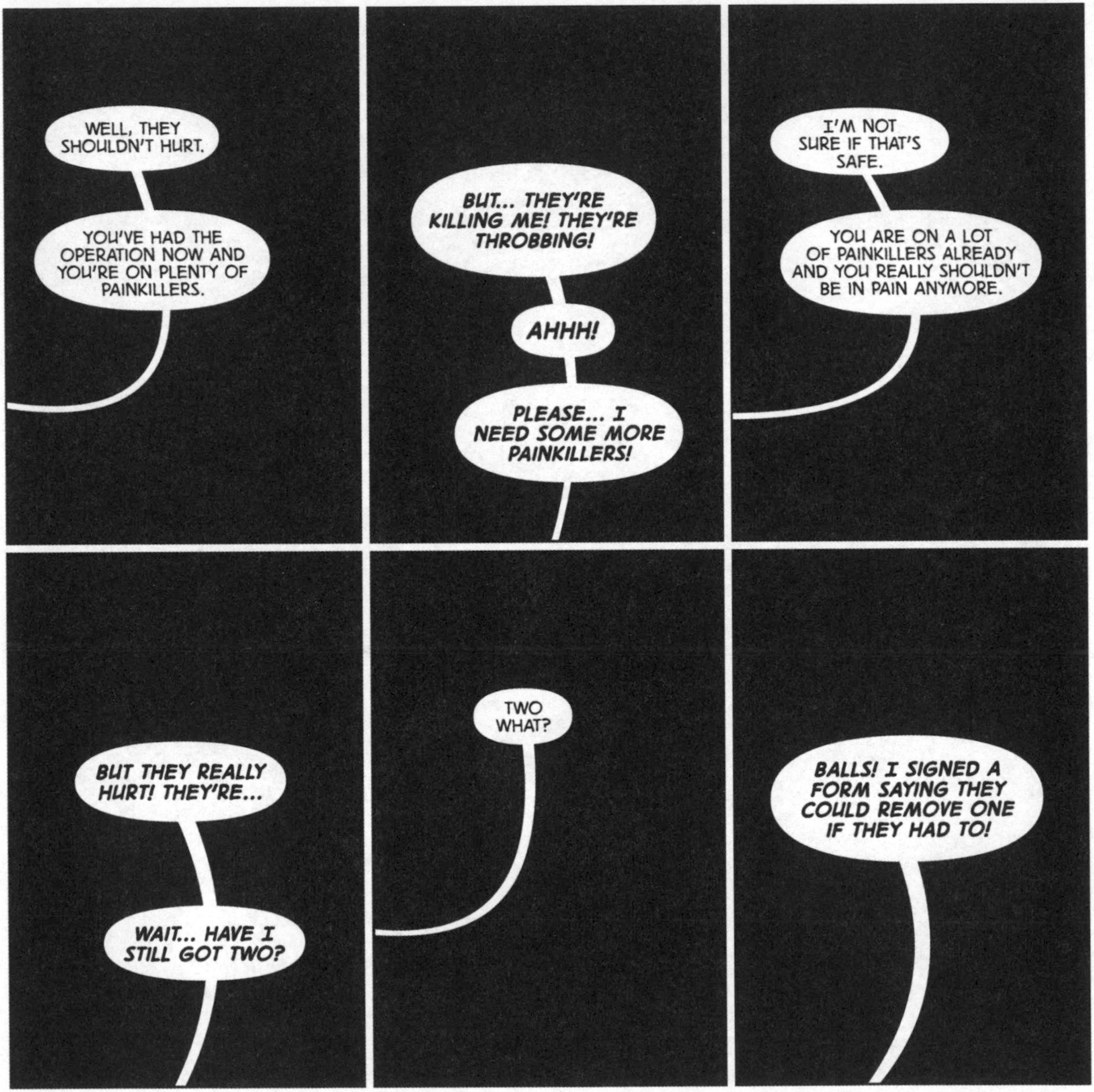
WELL, THEY SHOULDN'T HURT.
YOU'VE HAD THE OPERATION NOW AND YOU'RE ON PLENTY OF PAINKILLERS.
BUT... THEY'RE KILLING ME! THEY'RE THROBBING!
AHHH!
PLEASE... I NEED SOME MORE PAINKILLERS!
I'M NOT SURE IF THAT'S SAFE.
YOU ARE ON A LOT OF PAINKILLERS ALREADY AND YOU REALLY SHOULDN'T BE IN PAIN ANYMORE.
BUT THEY REALLY HURT! THEY'RE...
WAIT... HAVE I STILL GOT TWO?
TWO WHAT?
BALLS! I SIGNED A FORM SAYING THEY COULD REMOVE ONE IF THEY HAD TO!

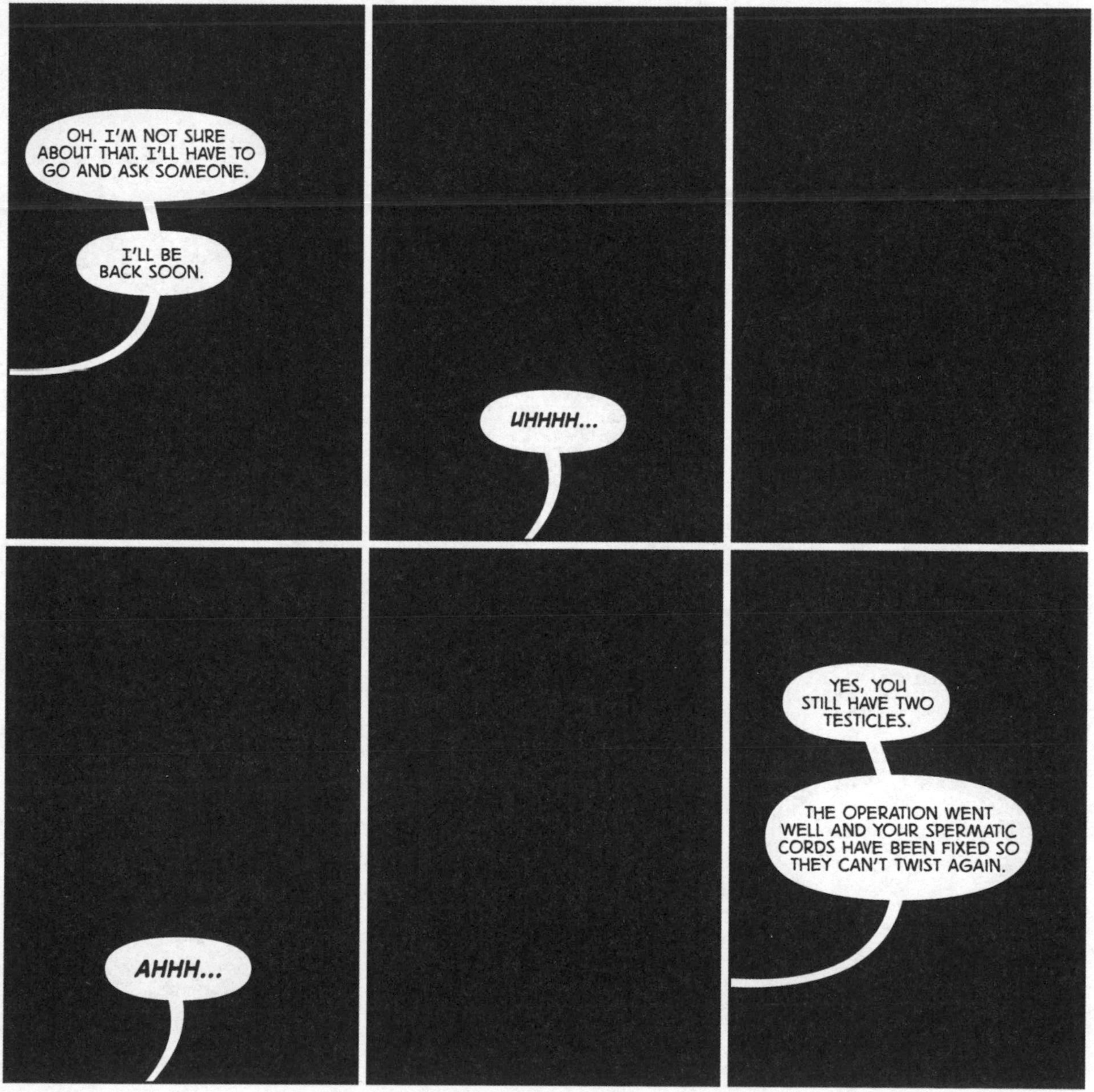

OH. I'M NOT SURE ABOUT THAT. I'LL HAVE TO GO AND ASK SOMEONE.
I'LL BE BACK SOON.
UHHHH...
AHHH...
YES, YOU STILL HAVE TWO TESTICLES.
THE OPERATION WENT WELL AND YOUR SPERMATIC CORDS HAVE BEEN FIXED SO THEY CAN'T TWIST AGAIN.

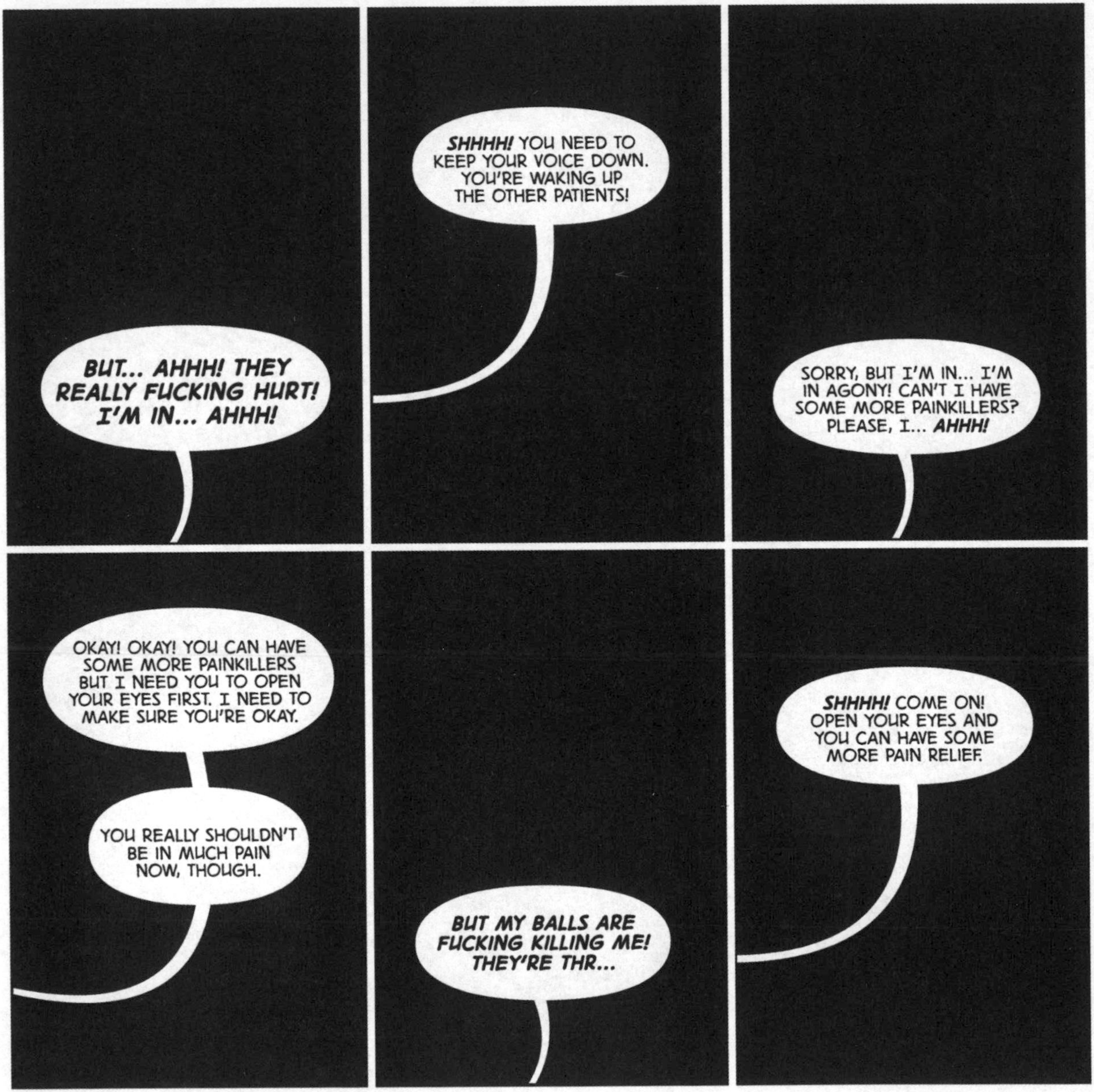
BUT... AHHH! THEY REALLY FUCKING HURT! I'M IN... AHHH!
SHHHH! YOU NEED TO KEEP YOUR VOICE DOWN. YOU'RE WAKING UP THE OTHER PATIENTS!
SORRY, BUT I'M IN... I'M IN AGONY! CAN'T I HAVE SOME MORE PAINKILLERS? PLEASE, I... AHHH!
OKAY! OKAY! YOU CAN HAVE SOME MORE PAINKILLERS BUT I NEED YOU TO OPEN YOUR EYES FIRST. I NEED TO MAKE SURE YOU'RE OKAY.
YOU REALLY SHOULDN'T BE IN MUCH PAIN NOW, THOUGH.
BUT MY BALLS ARE FUCKING KILLING ME! THEY'RE THR...
SHHHH! COME ON! OPEN YOUR EYES AND YOU CAN HAVE SOME MORE PAIN RELIEF.

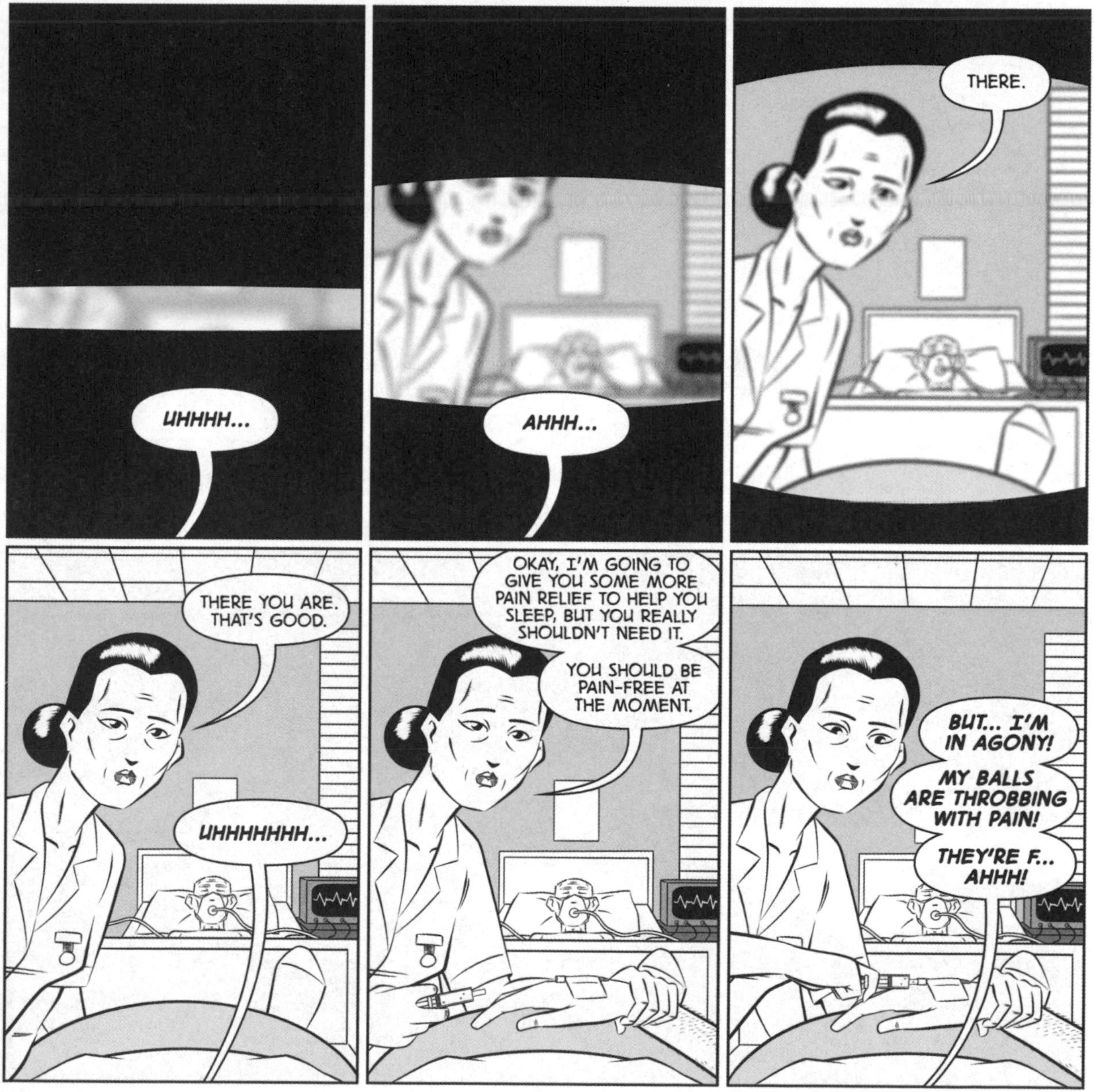
UHHHH...
AHHH...
THERE.
THERE YOU ARE. THAT'S GOOD.
UHHHHHHH...
OKAY, I'M GOING TO GIVE YOU SOME MORE PAIN RELIEF TO HELP YOU SLEEP, BUT YOU REALLY SHOULDN'T NEED IT.
YOU SHOULD BE PAIN-FREE AT THE MOMENT.
BUT... I'M IN AGONY!
MY BALLS ARE THROBBING WITH PAIN!
THEY'RE F... AHHH!

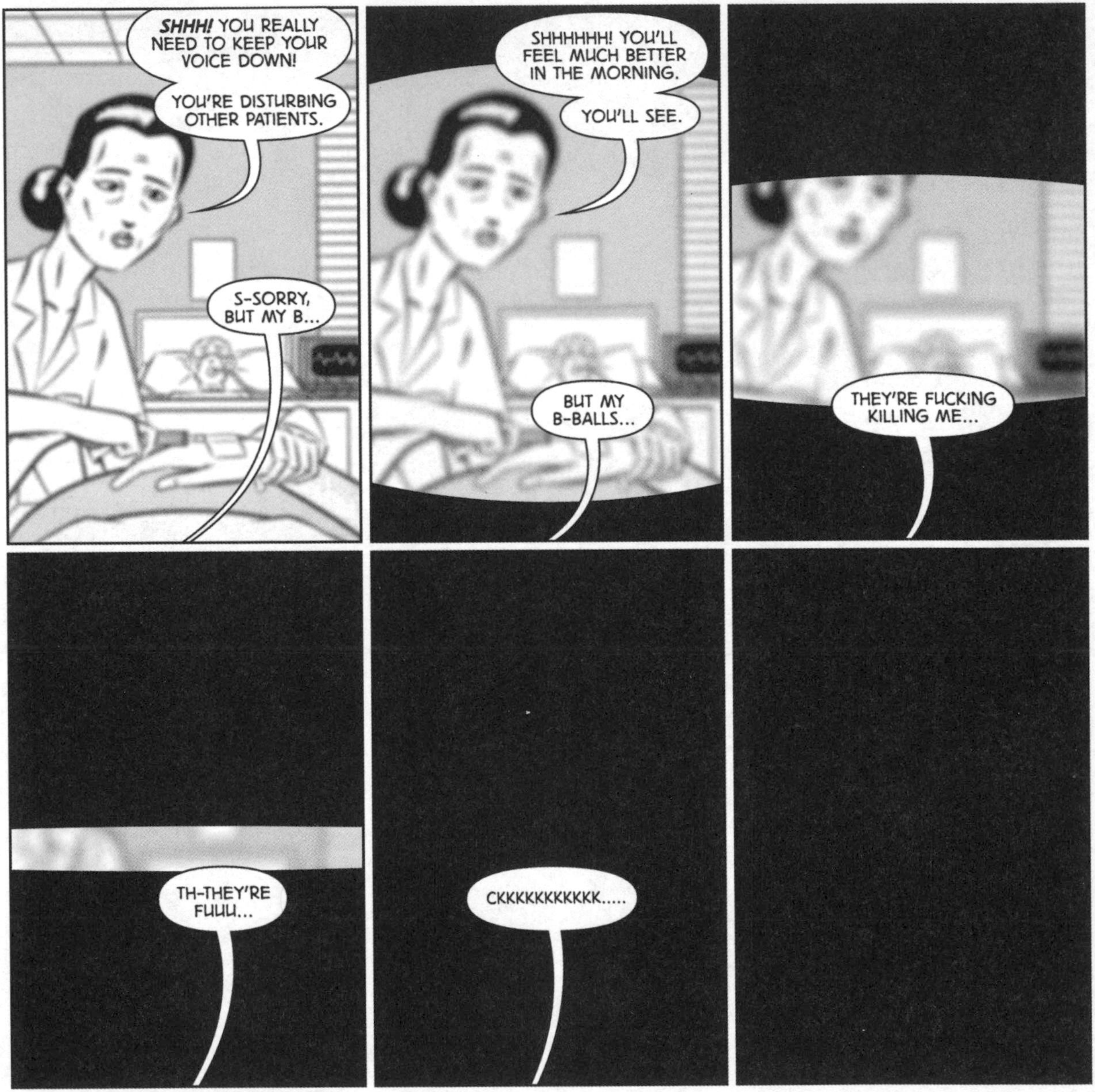
SHHH! YOU REALLY NEED TO KEEP YOUR VOICE DOWN!
YOU'RE DISTURBING OTHER PATIENTS.
S-SORRY, BUT MY B...
SHHHHHH! YOU'LL FEEL MUCH BETTER IN THE MORNING.
YOU'LL SEE.
BUT MY B-BALLS...
THEY'RE FUCKING KILLING ME...
TH-THEY'RE FUUU...
CKKKKKKKKKKK.....

4. WHATEVER YOU DO, DON'T WEAKEN

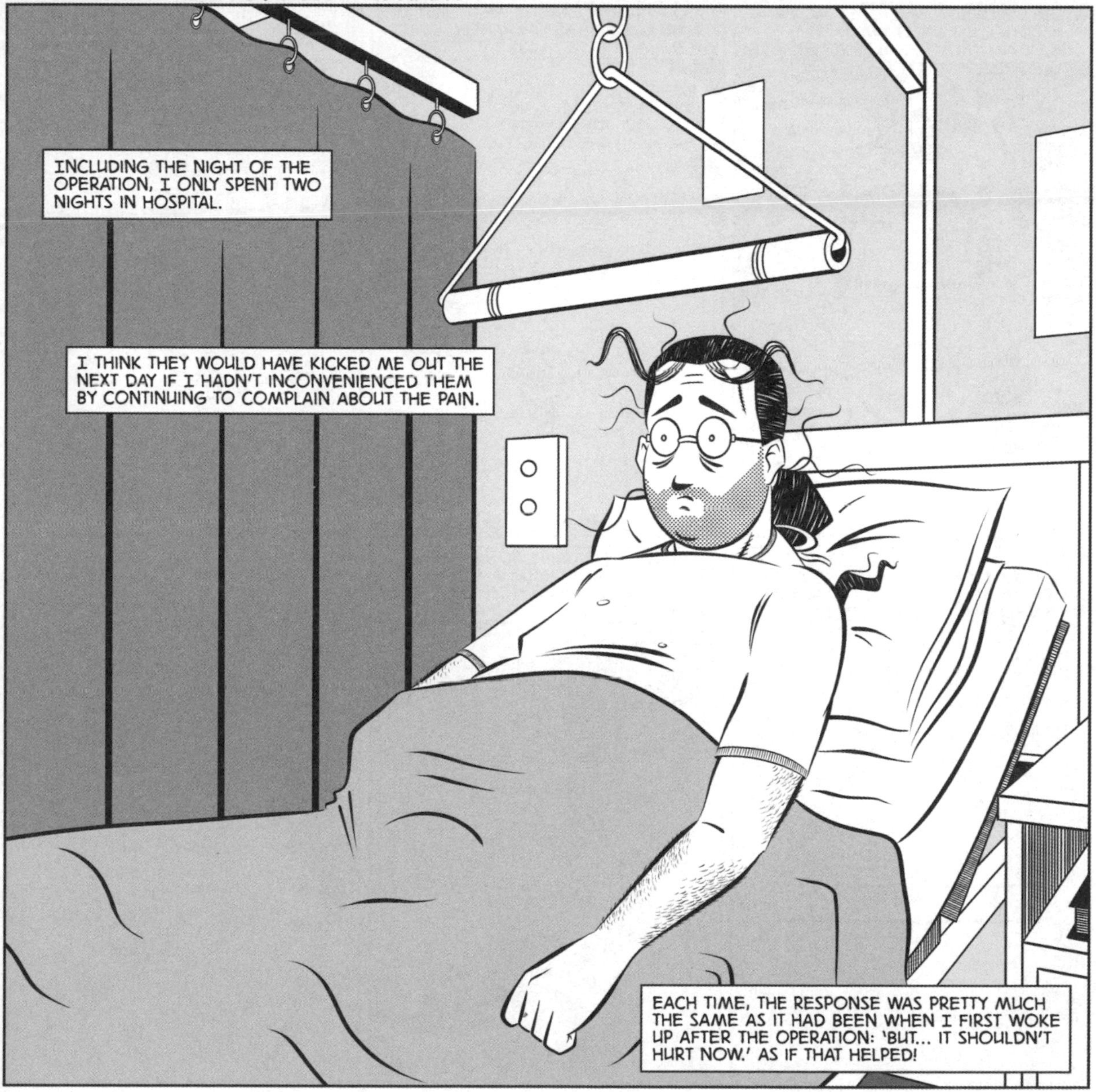

INCLUDING THE NIGHT OF THE OPERATION, I ONLY SPENT TWO NIGHTS IN HOSPITAL.
I THINK THEY WOULD HAVE KICKED ME OUT THE NEXT DAY IF I HADN'T INCONVENIENCED THEM BY CONTINUING TO COMPLAIN ABOUT THE PAIN.
EACH TIME, THE RESPONSE WAS PRETTY MUCH THE SAME AS IT HAD BEEN WHEN I FIRST WOKE UP AFTER THE OPERATION: 'BUT... IT SHOULDN'T HURT NOW.' AS IF THAT HELPED!

WHEN I WOKE UP THAT FIRST MORNING IN HOSPITAL, MY BALLS WERE STILL THROBBING WITH PAIN.

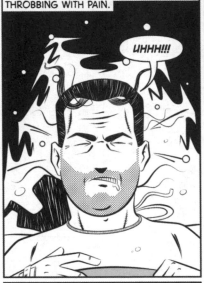

UHHH!!!

I DON'T KNOW EXACTLY WHAT THEY DID TO ME DURING THE OPERATION, BUT I KNOW WHAT IT FELT LIKE...

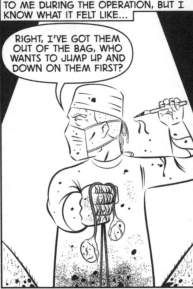

RIGHT, I'VE GOT THEM OUT OF THE BAG, WHO WANTS TO JUMP UP AND DOWN ON THEM FIRST?

I WASN'T IN QUITE AS MUCH PAIN AS I HAD BEEN THE NIGHT BEFORE, BUT I WAS ON RATHER A LOT OF PAINKILLERS.

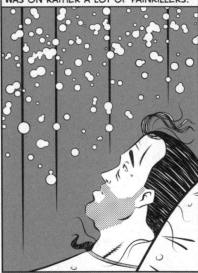

THERE WAS SOME KIND OF TRAPEZE SET UP ABOVE MY BED, TO HELP ME GET UP MORE EASILY, BUT I WAS TOO SCARED TO MOVE.

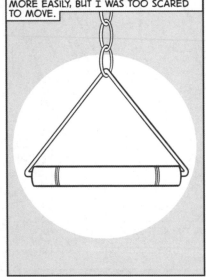

I LAY STILL FOR QUITE SOME TIME, STUNNED BY WHAT HAD HAPPENED TO ME, WATCHING A SKELETON STAFF OF DOCTORS AND NURSES GO ABOUT THEIR BUSINESS.

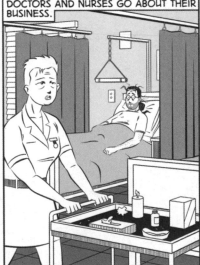

EVENTUALLY, I PLUCKED UP ENOUGH COURAGE TO LOOK UNDER THE BED-SHEETS AND INSPECT THE DAMAGE.

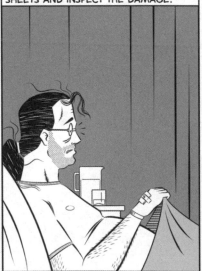

THERE WAS A LARGE, BLOODY PLASTER ON MY SCROTUM AND I WAS WEARING WHAT I ASSUME WAS SOME KIND OF TRUSS, ALTHOUGH IT LOOKED LIKE SOMEONE HAD JUST LOOSELY WRAPPED SOME BANDAGES AROUND MY WAIST AND THE TOPS OF MY THIGHS.

ALTHOUGH THE OPERATION HAD BEEN ON MY TESTICLES AND THE ONLY INCISION MADE WAS ON MY SCROTUM, I DON'T THINK ANY HAIR HAD BEEN SHAVED FROM MY SCROTUM. FOR SOME REASON, THOUGH, MY PUBIC AREA HAD BEEN PARTIALLY SHAVED AND I WAS NOW SPORTING WHAT LOOKED LIKE A REVERSE MOHAWK ABOVE MY PENIS.

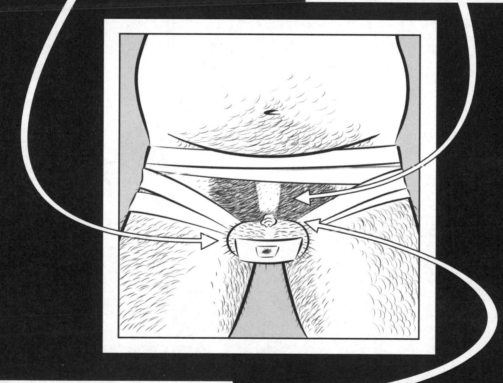

AND SPEAKING OF MY PENIS, THAT LITTLE THING HAD RETREATED SO FAR INTO MY BODY – PERHAPS AFRAID THAT IT WOULD BE NEXT FOR THE CHOP – THAT JUST ABOUT THE ONLY THING VISIBLE ON THE OUTSIDE OF MY BODY WAS A SHRIVELLED BIT OF FORESKIN, APPROXIMATELY THE SIZE OF AN ACORN.

IT WASN'T THE BIGGEST PENIS IN THE WORLD AT THE BEST OF TIMES*, BUT THIS WAS RIDICULOUS.

*IT'S A GROWER, NOT A SHOWER!

SEEING WHAT HAD BEEN DONE TO MY GENITALS MADE ME EVEN LESS INCLINED TO MOVE, BUT EVENTUALLY I NEEDED TO URINATE AND HAD TO CALL A NURSE.

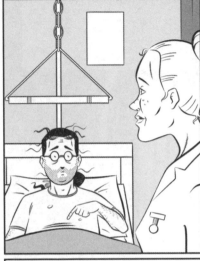

SHE BROUGHT ME A CARDBOARD URINAL I *SHOULD* HAVE BEEN ABLE TO URINATE INTO WITHOUT GETTING OUT OF BED, BUT THERE WAS A PROBLEM.

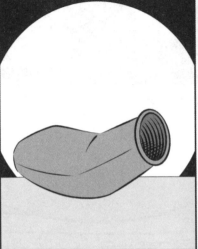

BECAUSE MY PENIS WAS SO SHRIVELLED, ALL I HAD TO BEND INTO THE URINAL WAS THE ACORN-SIZED BIT OF FORESKIN, WHICH HARDLY WENT INSIDE IT AT ALL.

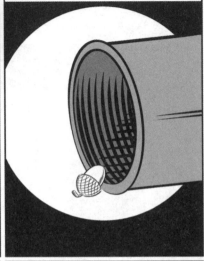

IF I TRIED TO GO LYING DOWN, I WAS HIGHLY LIKELY TO PISS ALL OVER MYSELF, SO I HAD TO GET OUT OF BED AND TRY TO GO STANDING UP...

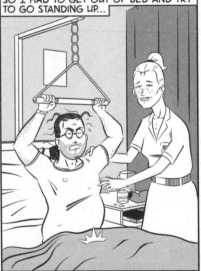

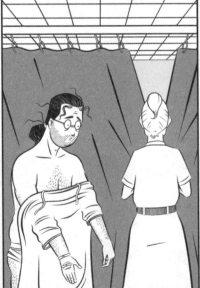

I'LL WAIT OUTSIDE. JUST LET ME KNOW WHEN YOU'VE FINISHED.

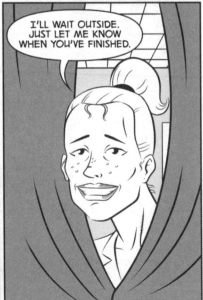

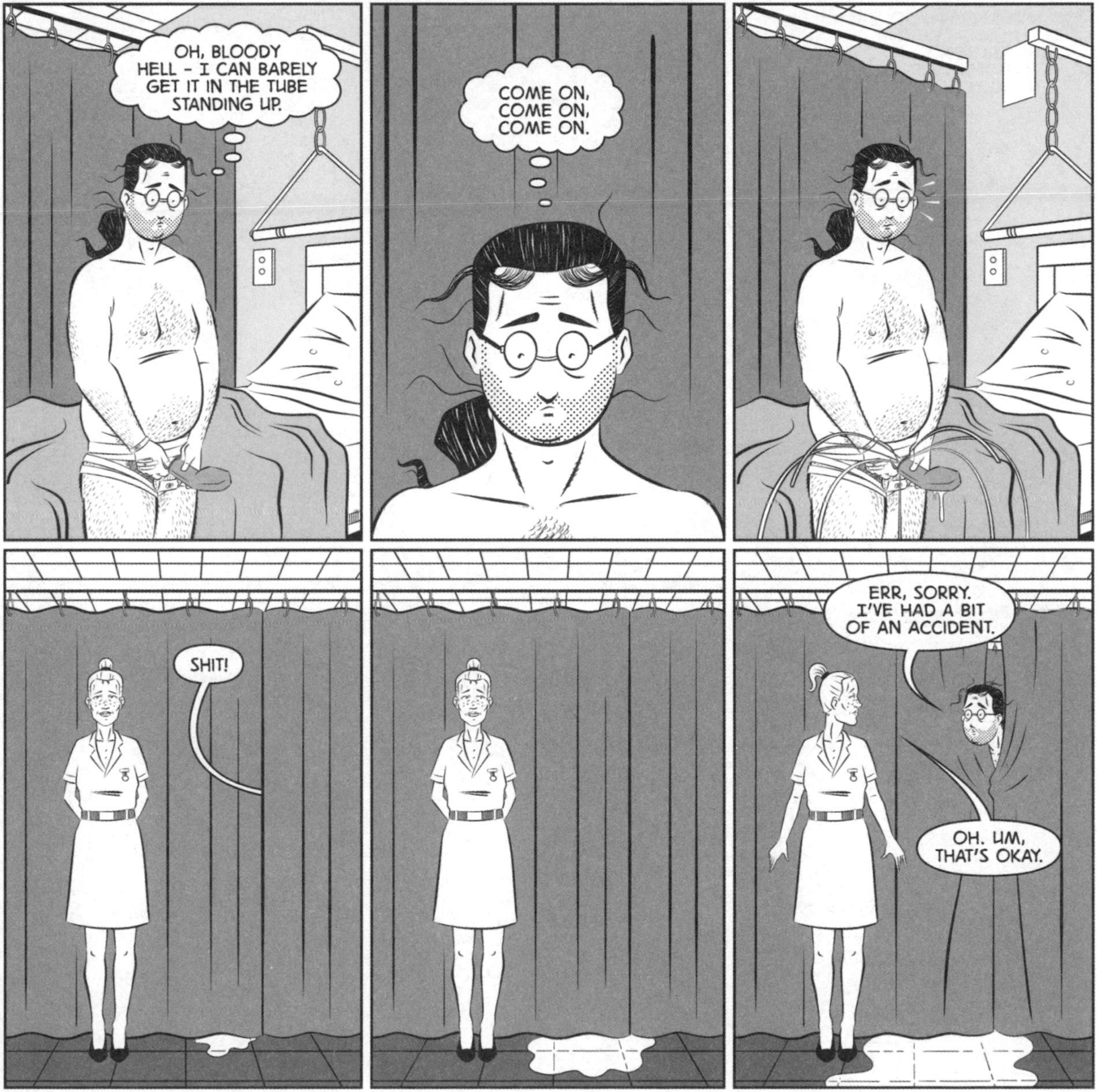
OH, BLOODY HELL - I CAN BARELY GET IT IN THE TUBE STANDING UP.
COME ON, COME ON, COME ON.
SHIT!
ERR, SORRY. I'VE HAD A BIT OF AN ACCIDENT.
OH. UM, THAT'S OKAY.

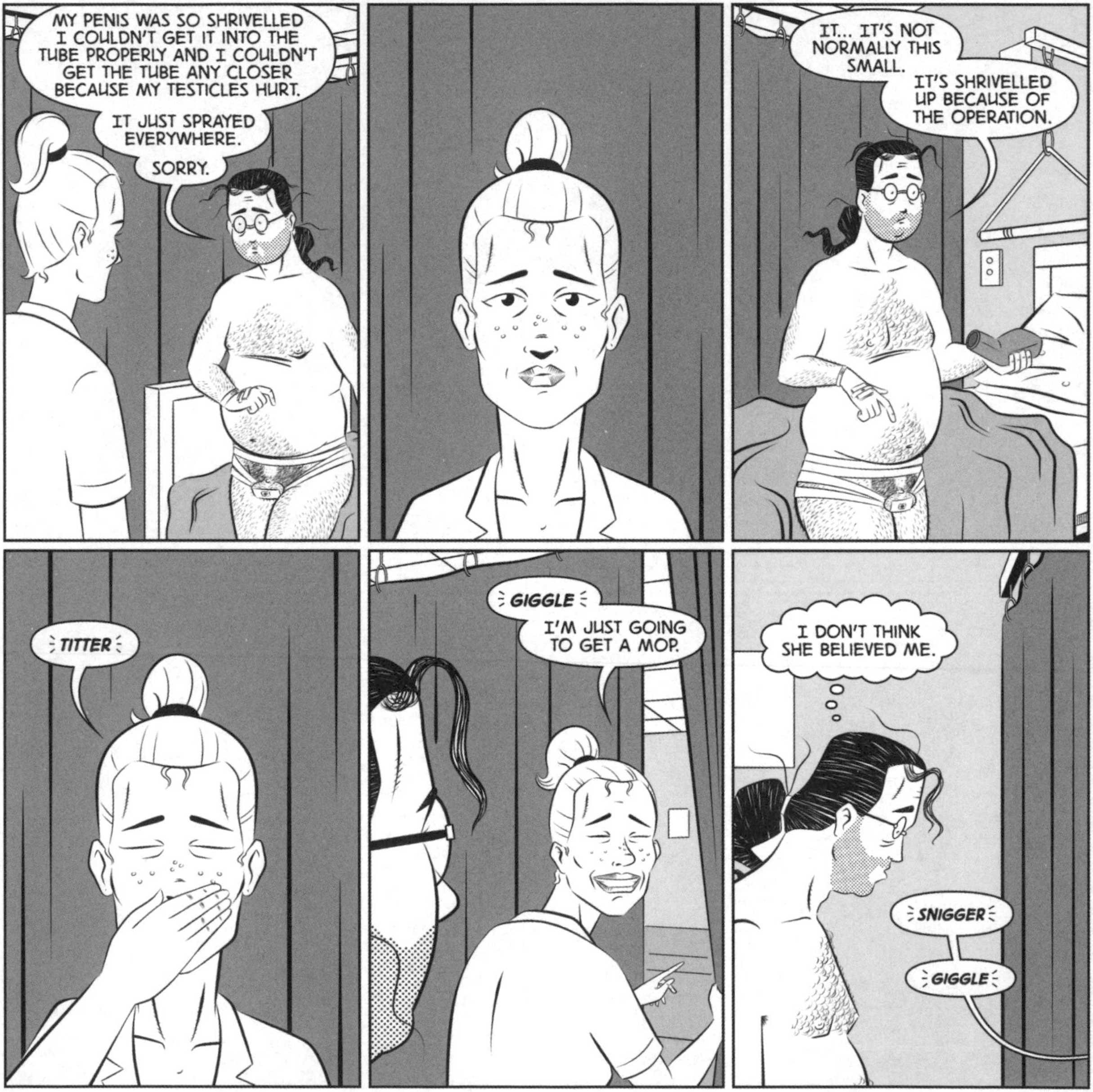
MY PENIS WAS SO SHRIVELLED I COULDN'T GET IT INTO THE TUBE PROPERLY AND I COULDN'T GET THE TUBE ANY CLOSER BECAUSE MY TESTICLES HURT.
IT JUST SPRAYED EVERYWHERE.
SORRY.
IT... IT'S NOT NORMALLY THIS SMALL.
IT'S SHRIVELLED UP BECAUSE OF THE OPERATION.
TITTER
GIGGLE
I'M JUST GOING TO GET A MOP.
I DON'T THINK SHE BELIEVED ME.
SNIGGER
GIGGLE

THE NEXT TIME I NEEDED TO PEE, I MANAGED TO GET UP AND WALK TO THE NEAREST TOILET...

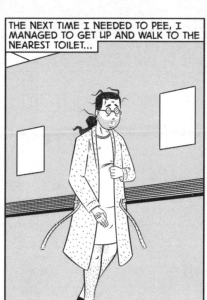

BUT WITH A SHRIVELLED PENIS AND A BIG PLASTER ON MY BALLS, I EVEN HAD TROUBLE AIMING AT A TOILET BOWL.

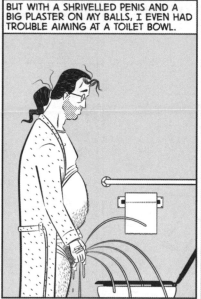

SORRY, YOU MIGHT NEED TO GET THAT MOP AGAIN.

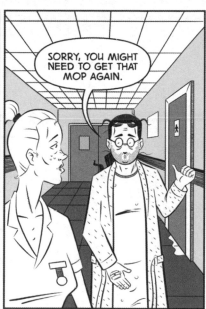

I SHARED THE HOSPITAL WARD I WAS IN WITH THREE OTHER MEN WHOSE CHRISTMASES HADN'T GONE QUITE TO PLAN:

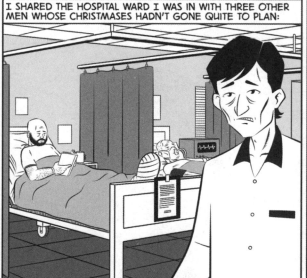

THERE WAS AN ALCOHOLIC WHOSE DRINKING HAD LED TO HIM HAVING TO HAVE SOME TOES AMPUTATED...

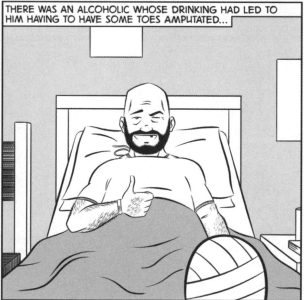

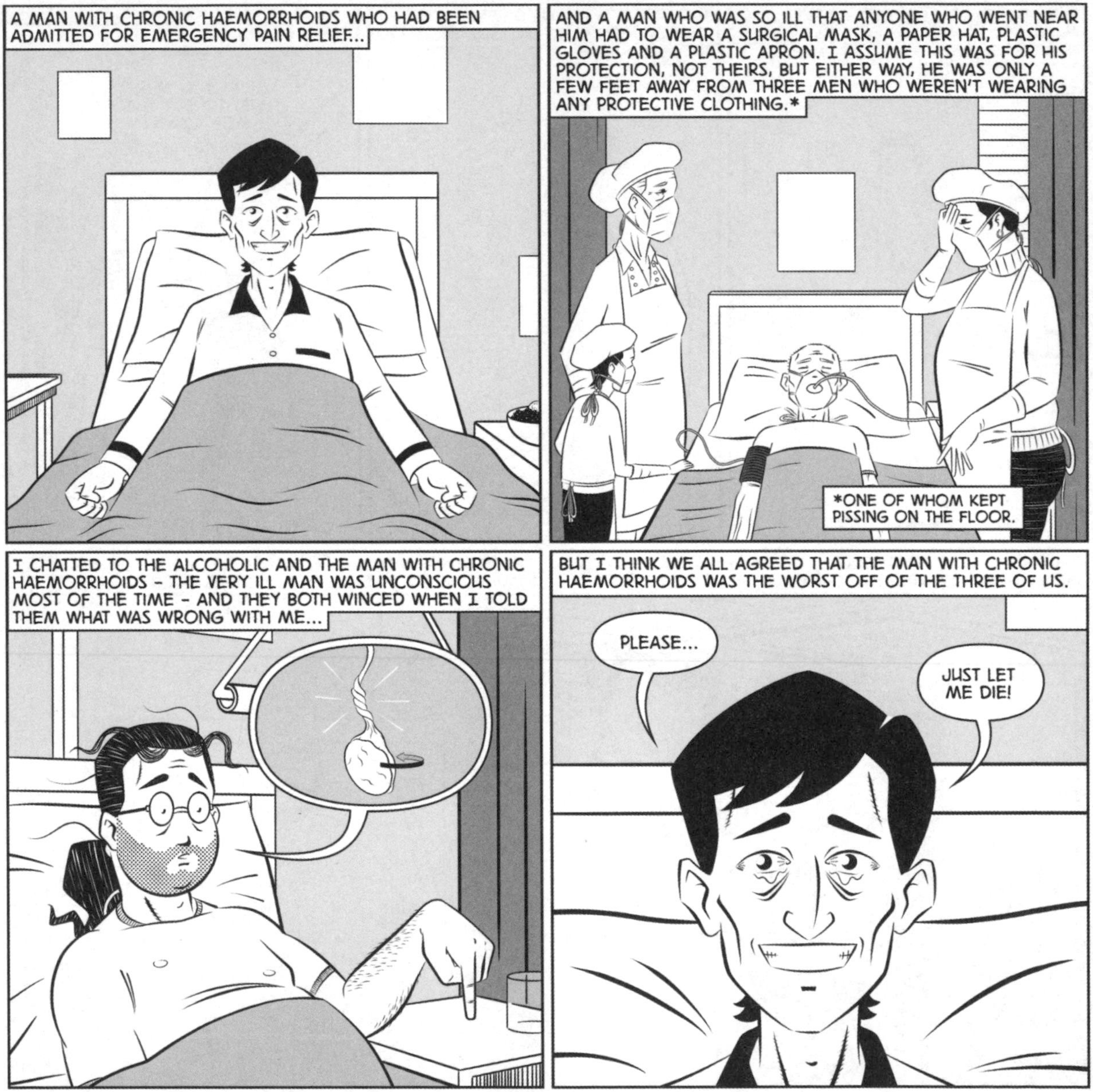
A MAN WITH CHRONIC HAEMORRHOIDS WHO HAD BEEN ADMITTED FOR EMERGENCY PAIN RELIEF...
AND A MAN WHO WAS SO ILL THAT ANYONE WHO WENT NEAR HIM HAD TO WEAR A SURGICAL MASK, A PAPER HAT, PLASTIC GLOVES AND A PLASTIC APRON. I ASSUME THIS WAS FOR HIS PROTECTION, NOT THEIRS, BUT EITHER WAY, HE WAS ONLY A FEW FEET AWAY FROM THREE MEN WHO WEREN'T WEARING ANY PROTECTIVE CLOTHING.*
*ONE OF WHOM KEPT PISSING ON THE FLOOR.
I CHATTED TO THE ALCOHOLIC AND THE MAN WITH CHRONIC HAEMORRHOIDS - THE VERY ILL MAN WAS UNCONSCIOUS MOST OF THE TIME - AND THEY BOTH WINCED WHEN I TOLD THEM WHAT WAS WRONG WITH ME...
BUT I THINK WE ALL AGREED THAT THE MAN WITH CHRONIC HAEMORRHOIDS WAS THE WORST OFF OF THE THREE OF US.
PLEASE...
JUST LET ME DIE!

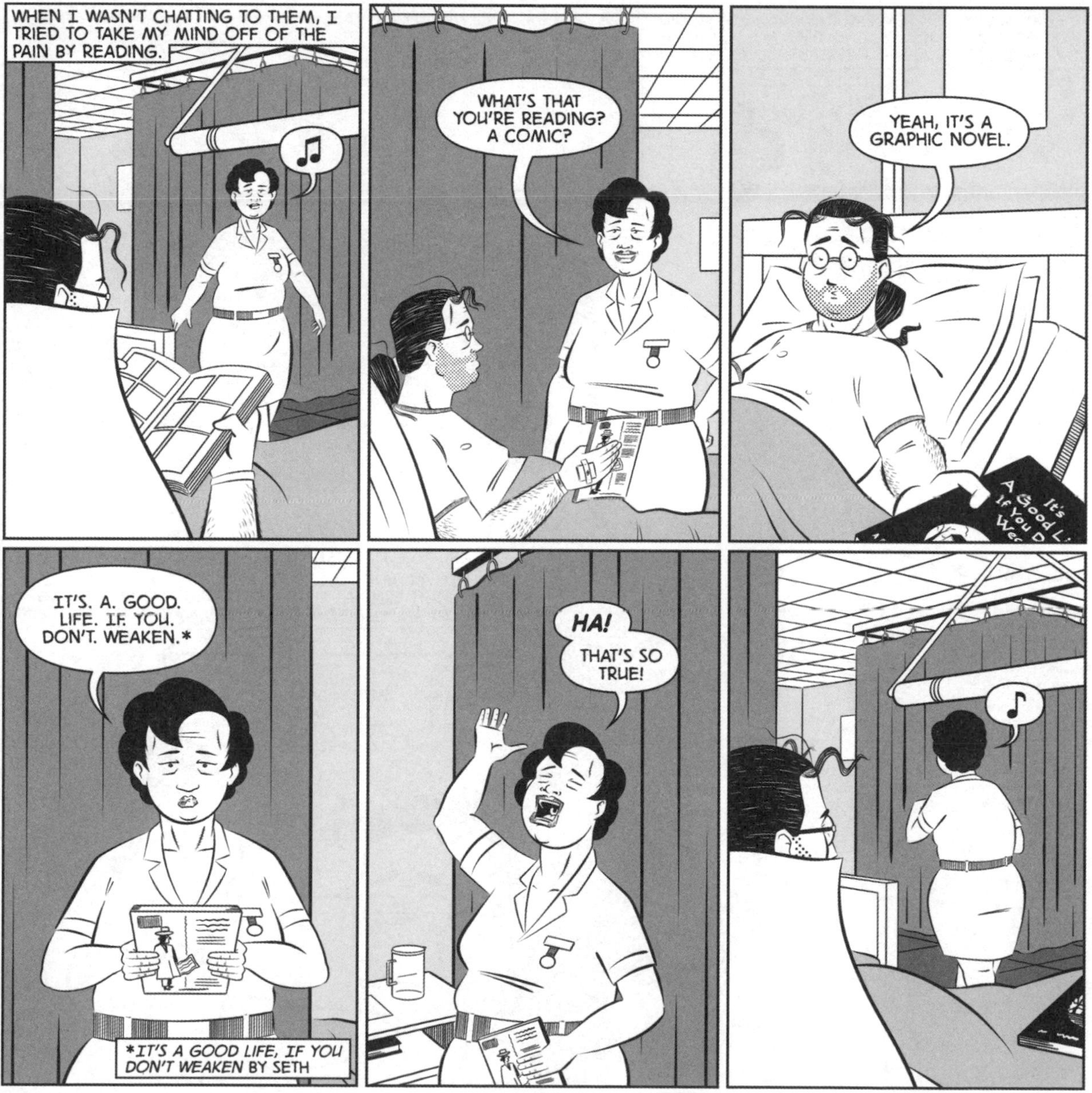
WHEN I WASN'T CHATTING TO THEM, I TRIED TO TAKE MY MIND OFF OF THE PAIN BY READING.
WHAT'S THAT YOU'RE READING? A COMIC?
YEAH, IT'S A GRAPHIC NOVEL.
IT'S. A. GOOD. LIFE. IF. YOU. DON'T. WEAKEN.*
*IT'S A GOOD LIFE, IF YOU DON'T WEAKEN BY SETH
HA!
THAT'S SO TRUE!

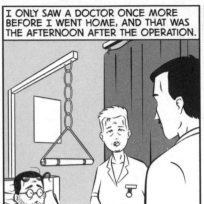

I ONLY SAW A DOCTOR ONCE MORE BEFORE I WENT HOME, AND THAT WAS THE AFTERNOON AFTER THE OPERATION.

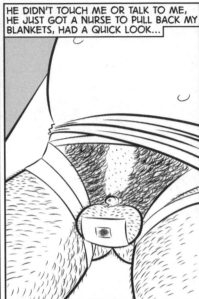

HE DIDN'T TOUCH ME OR TALK TO ME, HE JUST GOT A NURSE TO PULL BACK MY BLANKETS, HAD A QUICK LOOK...

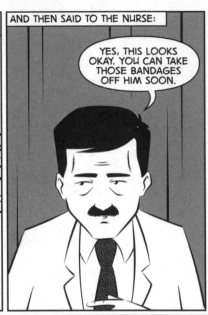

AND THEN SAID TO THE NURSE:

YES, THIS LOOKS OKAY. YOU CAN TAKE THOSE BANDAGES OFF HIM SOON.

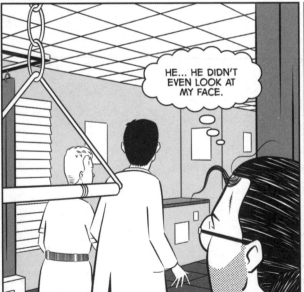

HE... HE DIDN'T EVEN LOOK AT MY FACE.

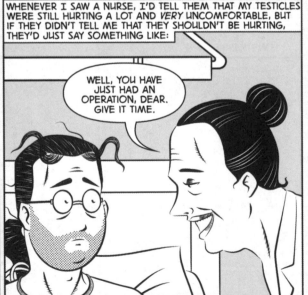

WHENEVER I SAW A NURSE, I'D TELL THEM THAT MY TESTICLES WERE STILL HURTING A LOT AND *VERY* UNCOMFORTABLE, BUT IF THEY DIDN'T TELL ME THAT THEY SHOULDN'T BE HURTING, THEY'D JUST SAY SOMETHING LIKE:

WELL, YOU HAVE JUST HAD AN OPERATION, DEAR. GIVE IT TIME.

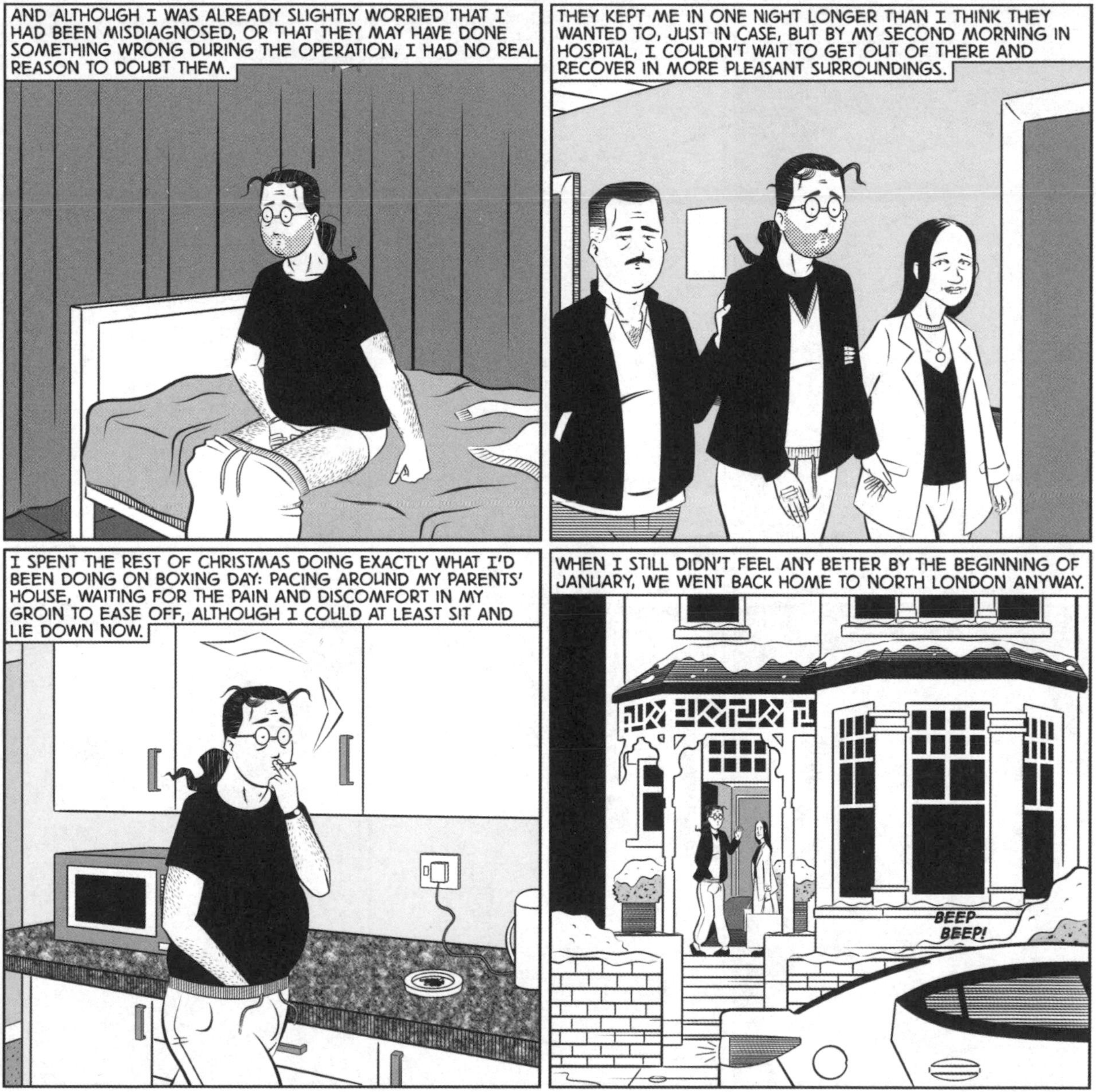
AND ALTHOUGH I WAS ALREADY SLIGHTLY WORRIED THAT I HAD BEEN MISDIAGNOSED, OR THAT THEY MAY HAVE DONE SOMETHING WRONG DURING THE OPERATION, I HAD NO REAL REASON TO DOUBT THEM.
THEY KEPT ME IN ONE NIGHT LONGER THAN I THINK THEY WANTED TO, JUST IN CASE, BUT BY MY SECOND MORNING IN HOSPITAL, I COULDN'T WAIT TO GET OUT OF THERE AND RECOVER IN MORE PLEASANT SURROUNDINGS.
I SPENT THE REST OF CHRISTMAS DOING EXACTLY WHAT I'D BEEN DOING ON BOXING DAY: PACING AROUND MY PARENTS' HOUSE, WAITING FOR THE PAIN AND DISCOMFORT IN MY GROIN TO EASE OFF, ALTHOUGH I COULD AT LEAST SIT AND LIE DOWN NOW.
WHEN I STILL DIDN'T FEEL ANY BETTER BY THE BEGINNING OF JANUARY, WE WENT BACK HOME TO NORTH LONDON ANYWAY.
BEEP BEEP!

WE WERE HOME FOR DAYS BEFORE I PLUCKED UP THE COURAGE TO TAKE THAT PLASTER OFF.

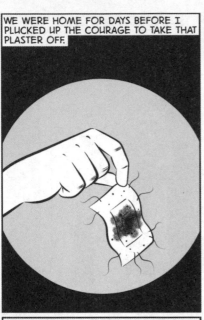

IT WAS ANOTHER FEW DAYS BEFORE I MANAGED TO PICK OFF ALL THE DRIED BLOOD TO REVEAL MY STITCHES...*

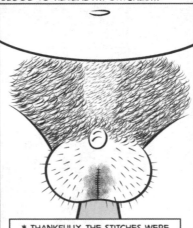

* THANKFULLY, THE STITCHES WERE THE SORT THAT DISSOLVE, SO I DIDN'T NEED TO GET THEM REMOVED.

AND IT WAS ANOTHER FEW DAYS BEFORE I MANAGED TO LOWER MYSELF INTO A HOT BATH.

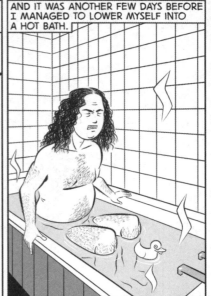

TO BE HONEST, THE PAIN DID EASE OFF FAIRLY QUICKLY, BUT THE DISCOMFORT DIDN'T.

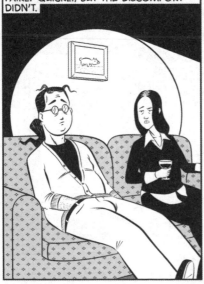

MY TESTICLES FELT LIKE THEY WERE TOO HIGH UP AND MY GROIN WAS EXTREMELY UNCOMFORTABLE, NO MATTER WHAT I WAS DOING.

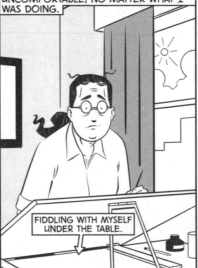

FIDDLING WITH MYSELF UNDER THE TABLE.

EVEN BEING NAKED FELT UNPLEASANT, SO I'D GET DRESSED AS QUICKLY AS I COULD AND STARTED TO SLEEP IN MY UNDERWEAR.

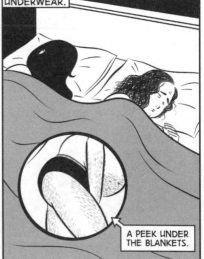

A PEEK UNDER THE BLANKETS.

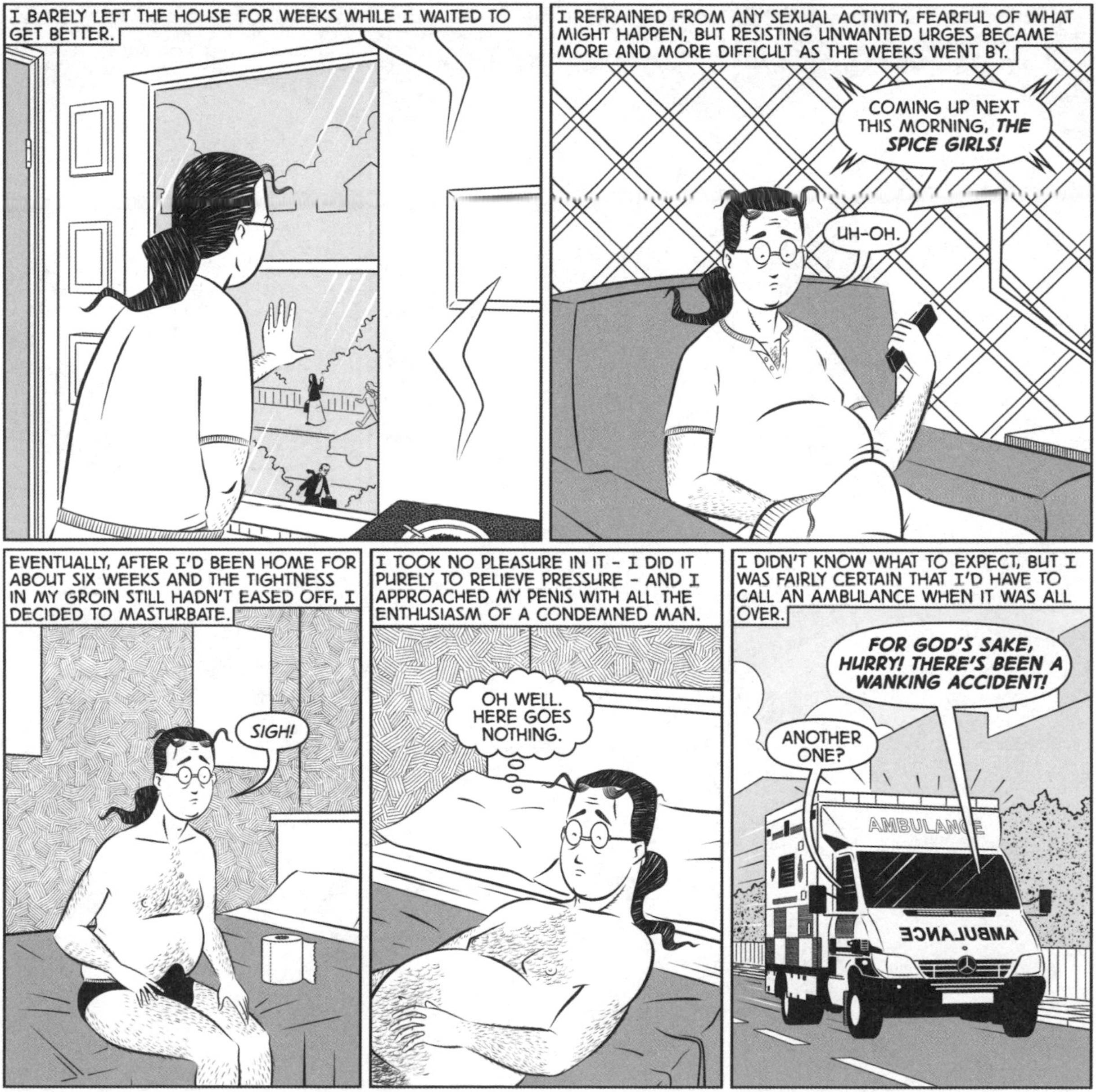

I BARELY LEFT THE HOUSE FOR WEEKS WHILE I WAITED TO GET BETTER.
I REFRAINED FROM ANY SEXUAL ACTIVITY, FEARFUL OF WHAT MIGHT HAPPEN, BUT RESISTING UNWANTED URGES BECAME MORE AND MORE DIFFICULT AS THE WEEKS WENT BY.
COMING UP NEXT THIS MORNING, ***THE SPICE GIRLS!***
UH-OH.
EVENTUALLY, AFTER I'D BEEN HOME FOR ABOUT SIX WEEKS AND THE TIGHTNESS IN MY GROIN STILL HADN'T EASED OFF, I DECIDED TO MASTURBATE.
SIGH!
I TOOK NO PLEASURE IN IT - I DID IT PURELY TO RELIEVE PRESSURE - AND I APPROACHED MY PENIS WITH ALL THE ENTHUSIASM OF A CONDEMNED MAN.
OH WELL. HERE GOES NOTHING.
I DIDN'T KNOW WHAT TO EXPECT, BUT I WAS FAIRLY CERTAIN THAT I'D HAVE TO CALL AN AMBULANCE WHEN IT WAS ALL OVER.
FOR GOD'S SAKE, HURRY! THERE'S BEEN A WANKING ACCIDENT!
ANOTHER ONE?
AMBULANCE

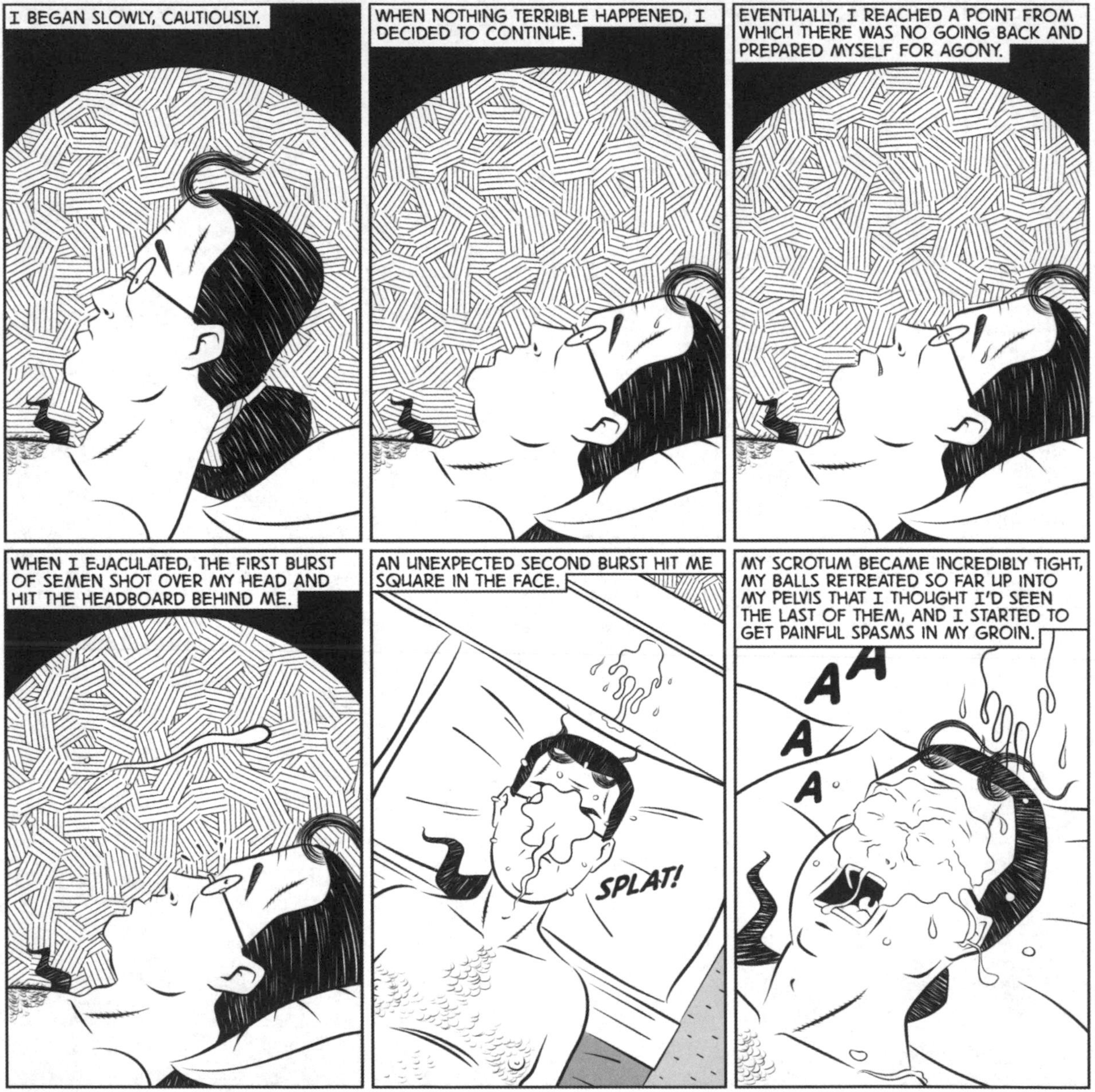
I BEGAN SLOWLY, CAUTIOUSLY.
WHEN NOTHING TERRIBLE HAPPENED, I DECIDED TO CONTINUE.
EVENTUALLY, I REACHED A POINT FROM WHICH THERE WAS NO GOING BACK AND PREPARED MYSELF FOR AGONY.
WHEN I EJACULATED, THE FIRST BURST OF SEMEN SHOT OVER MY HEAD AND HIT THE HEADBOARD BEHIND ME.
AN UNEXPECTED SECOND BURST HIT ME SQUARE IN THE FACE.
SPLAT!
MY SCROTUM BECAME INCREDIBLY TIGHT, MY BALLS RETREATED SO FAR UP INTO MY PELVIS THAT I THOUGHT I'D SEEN THE LAST OF THEM, AND I STARTED TO GET PAINFUL SPASMS IN MY GROIN.
AAAAA

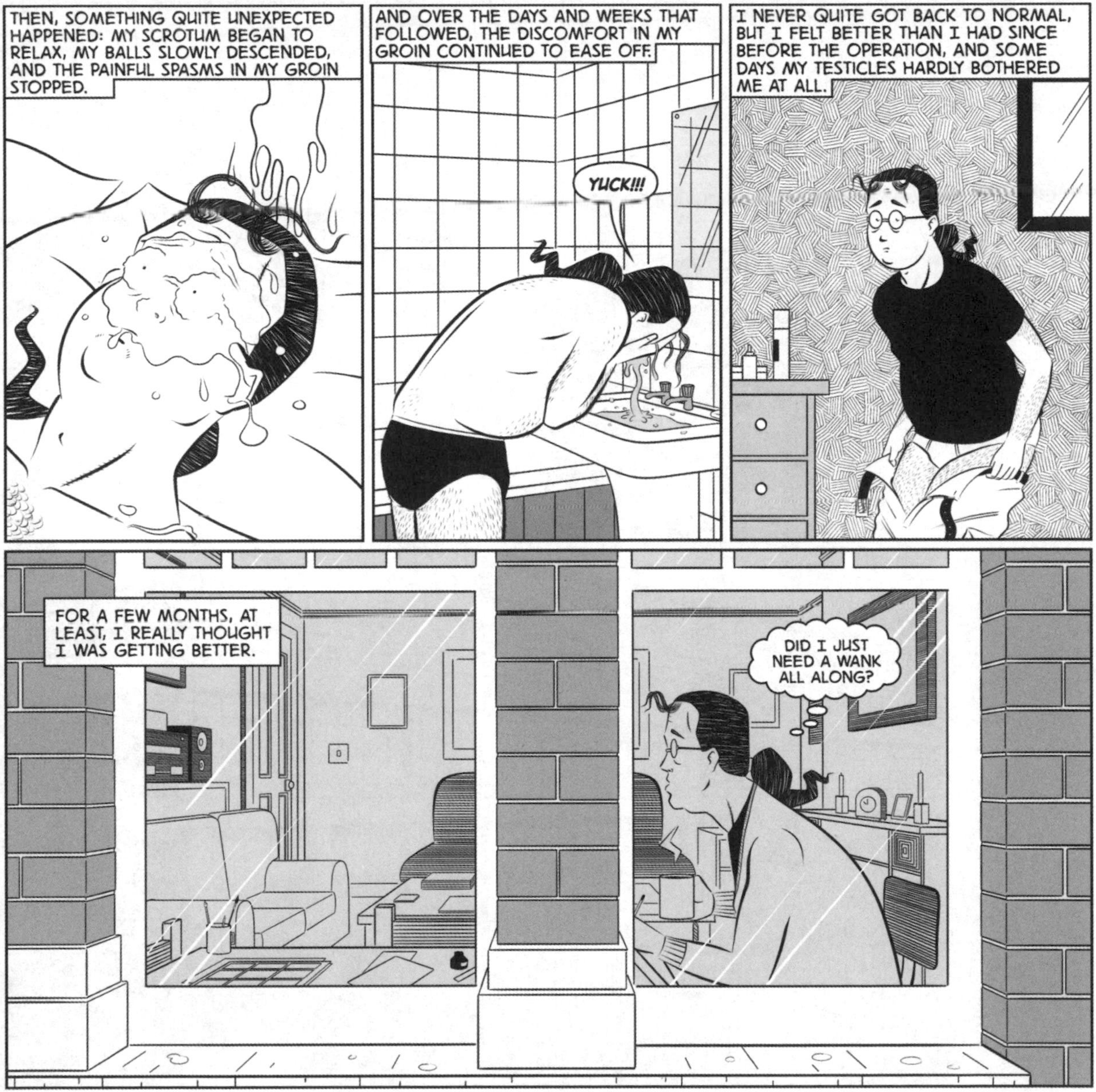
THEN, SOMETHING QUITE UNEXPECTED HAPPENED: MY SCROTUM BEGAN TO RELAX, MY BALLS SLOWLY DESCENDED, AND THE PAINFUL SPASMS IN MY GROIN STOPPED.
AND OVER THE DAYS AND WEEKS THAT FOLLOWED, THE DISCOMFORT IN MY GROIN CONTINUED TO EASE OFF.
YUCK!!!
I NEVER QUITE GOT BACK TO NORMAL, BUT I FELT BETTER THAN I HAD SINCE BEFORE THE OPERATION, AND SOME DAYS MY TESTICLES HARDLY BOTHERED ME AT ALL.
FOR A FEW MONTHS, AT LEAST, I REALLY THOUGHT I WAS GETTING BETTER.
DID I JUST NEED A WANK ALL ALONG?

5. UROLOGY FOR BEGINNERS

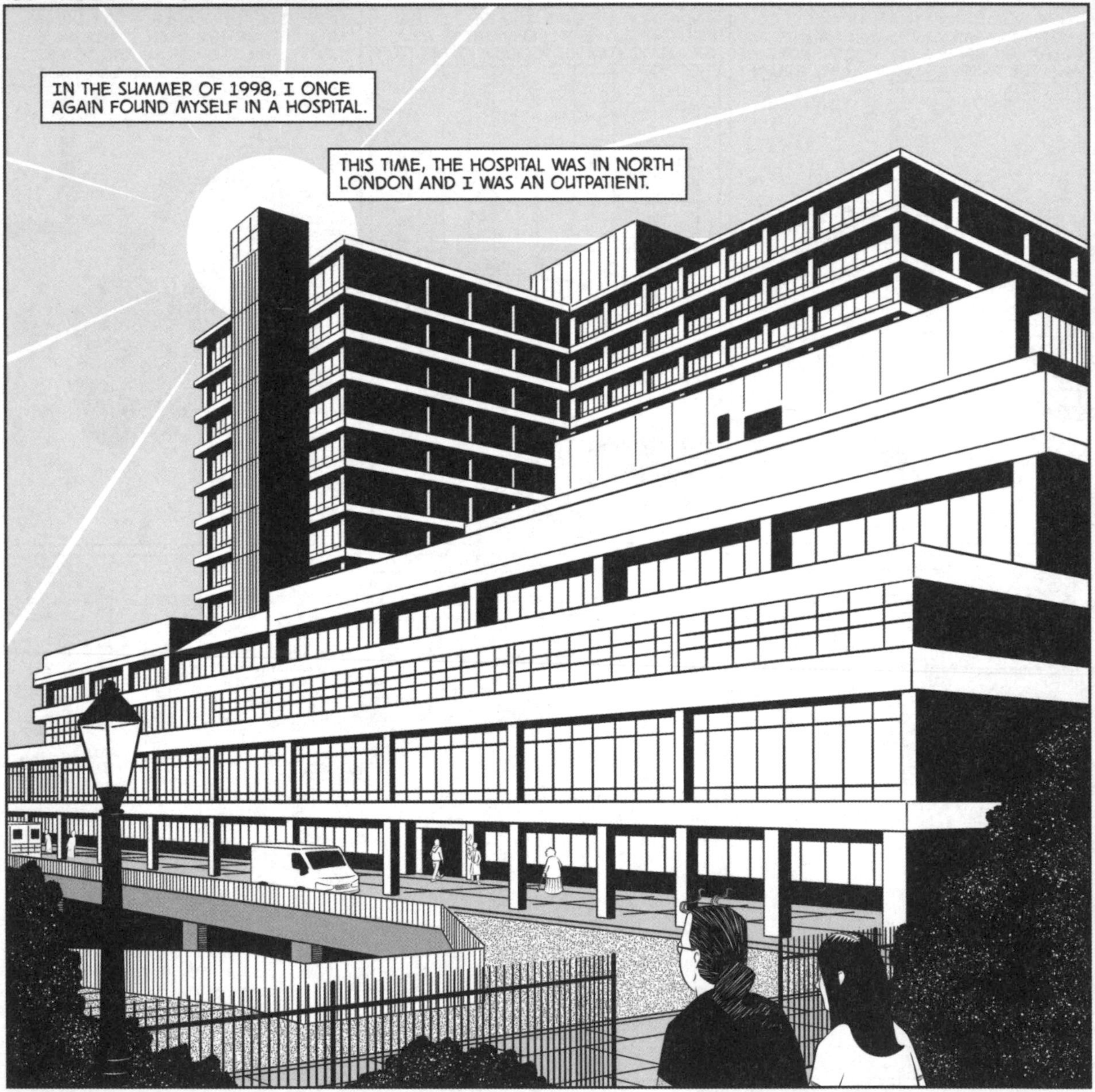
IN THE SUMMER OF 1998, I ONCE AGAIN FOUND MYSELF IN A HOSPITAL.
THIS TIME, THE HOSPITAL WAS IN NORTH LONDON AND I WAS AN OUTPATIENT.

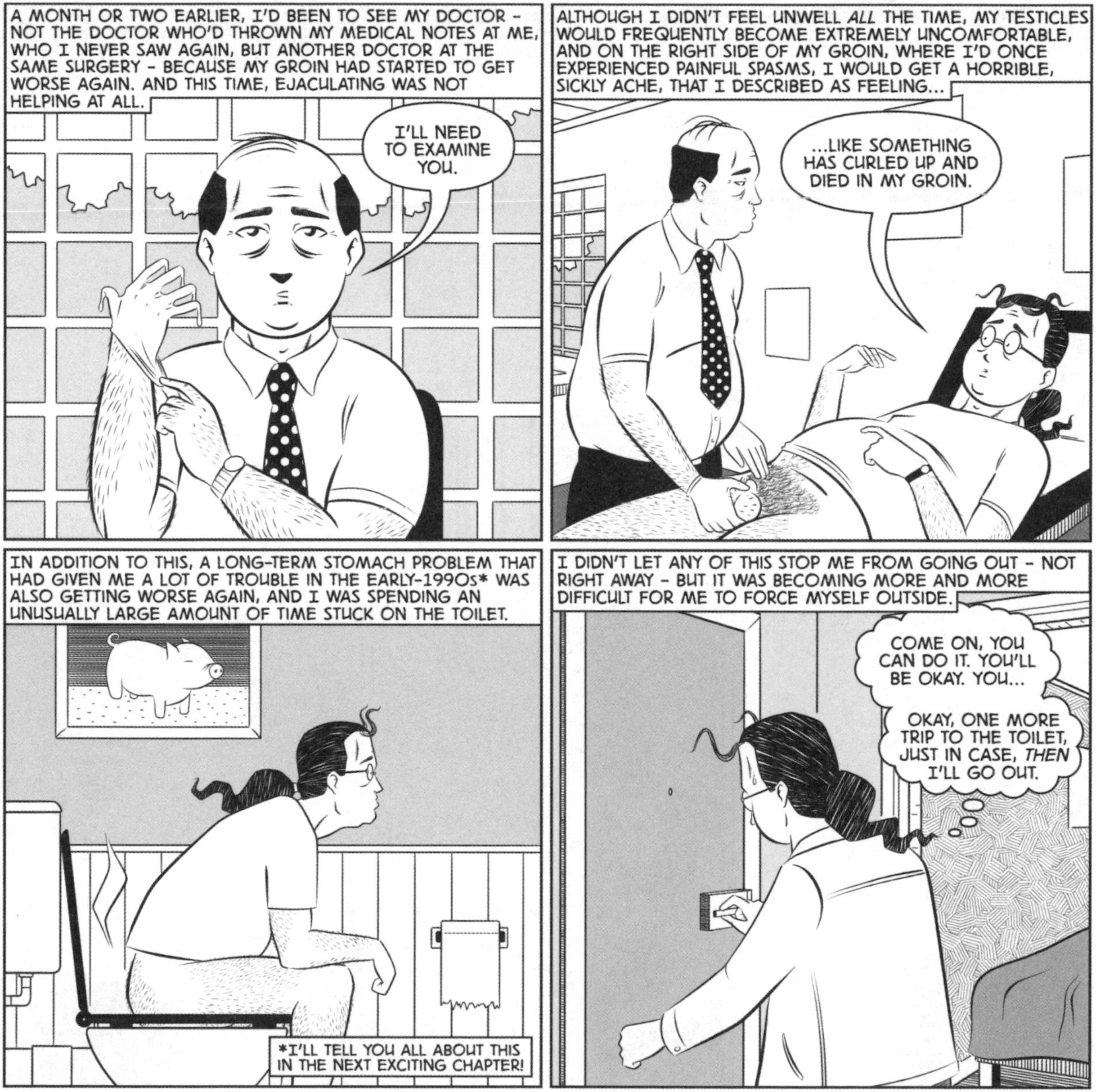
A MONTH OR TWO EARLIER, I'D BEEN TO SEE MY DOCTOR - NOT THE DOCTOR WHO'D THROWN MY MEDICAL NOTES AT ME, WHO I NEVER SAW AGAIN, BUT ANOTHER DOCTOR AT THE SAME SURGERY - BECAUSE MY GROIN HAD STARTED TO GET WORSE AGAIN. AND THIS TIME, EJACULATING WAS NOT HELPING AT ALL.
I'LL NEED TO EXAMINE YOU.
ALTHOUGH I DIDN'T FEEL UNWELL *ALL* THE TIME, MY TESTICLES WOULD FREQUENTLY BECOME EXTREMELY UNCOMFORTABLE, AND ON THE RIGHT SIDE OF MY GROIN, WHERE I'D ONCE EXPERIENCED PAINFUL SPASMS, I WOULD GET A HORRIBLE, SICKLY ACHE, THAT I DESCRIBED AS FEELING...
...LIKE SOMETHING HAS CURLED UP AND DIED IN MY GROIN.
IN ADDITION TO THIS, A LONG-TERM STOMACH PROBLEM THAT HAD GIVEN ME A LOT OF TROUBLE IN THE EARLY-1990s* WAS ALSO GETTING WORSE AGAIN, AND I WAS SPENDING AN UNUSUALLY LARGE AMOUNT OF TIME STUCK ON THE TOILET.
*I'LL TELL YOU ALL ABOUT THIS IN THE NEXT EXCITING CHAPTER!
I DIDN'T LET ANY OF THIS STOP ME FROM GOING OUT - NOT RIGHT AWAY - BUT IT WAS BECOMING MORE AND MORE DIFFICULT FOR ME TO FORCE MYSELF OUTSIDE.
COME ON, YOU CAN DO IT. YOU'LL BE OKAY. YOU...
OKAY, ONE MORE TRIP TO THE TOILET, JUST IN CASE, *THEN* I'LL GO OUT.

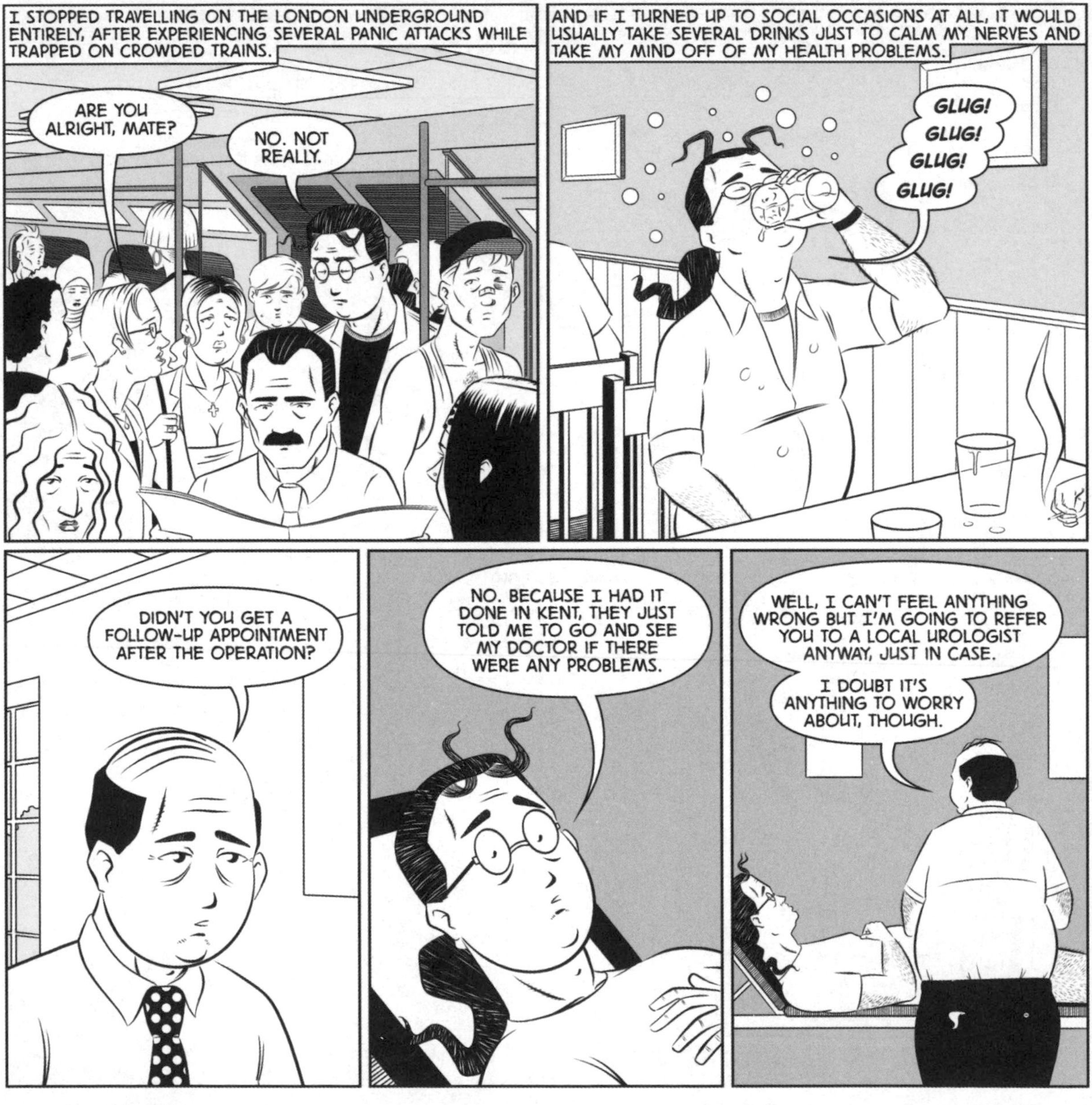
I STOPPED TRAVELLING ON THE LONDON UNDERGROUND ENTIRELY, AFTER EXPERIENCING SEVERAL PANIC ATTACKS WHILE TRAPPED ON CROWDED TRAINS.
ARE YOU ALRIGHT, MATE?
NO. NOT REALLY.
AND IF I TURNED UP TO SOCIAL OCCASIONS AT ALL, IT WOULD USUALLY TAKE SEVERAL DRINKS JUST TO CALM MY NERVES AND TAKE MY MIND OFF OF MY HEALTH PROBLEMS.
GLUG! GLUG! GLUG! GLUG!
DIDN'T YOU GET A FOLLOW-UP APPOINTMENT AFTER THE OPERATION?
NO. BECAUSE I HAD IT DONE IN KENT, THEY JUST TOLD ME TO GO AND SEE MY DOCTOR IF THERE WERE ANY PROBLEMS.
WELL, I CAN'T FEEL ANYTHING WRONG BUT I'M GOING TO REFER YOU TO A LOCAL UROLOGIST ANYWAY, JUST IN CASE.
I DOUBT IT'S ANYTHING TO WORRY ABOUT, THOUGH.

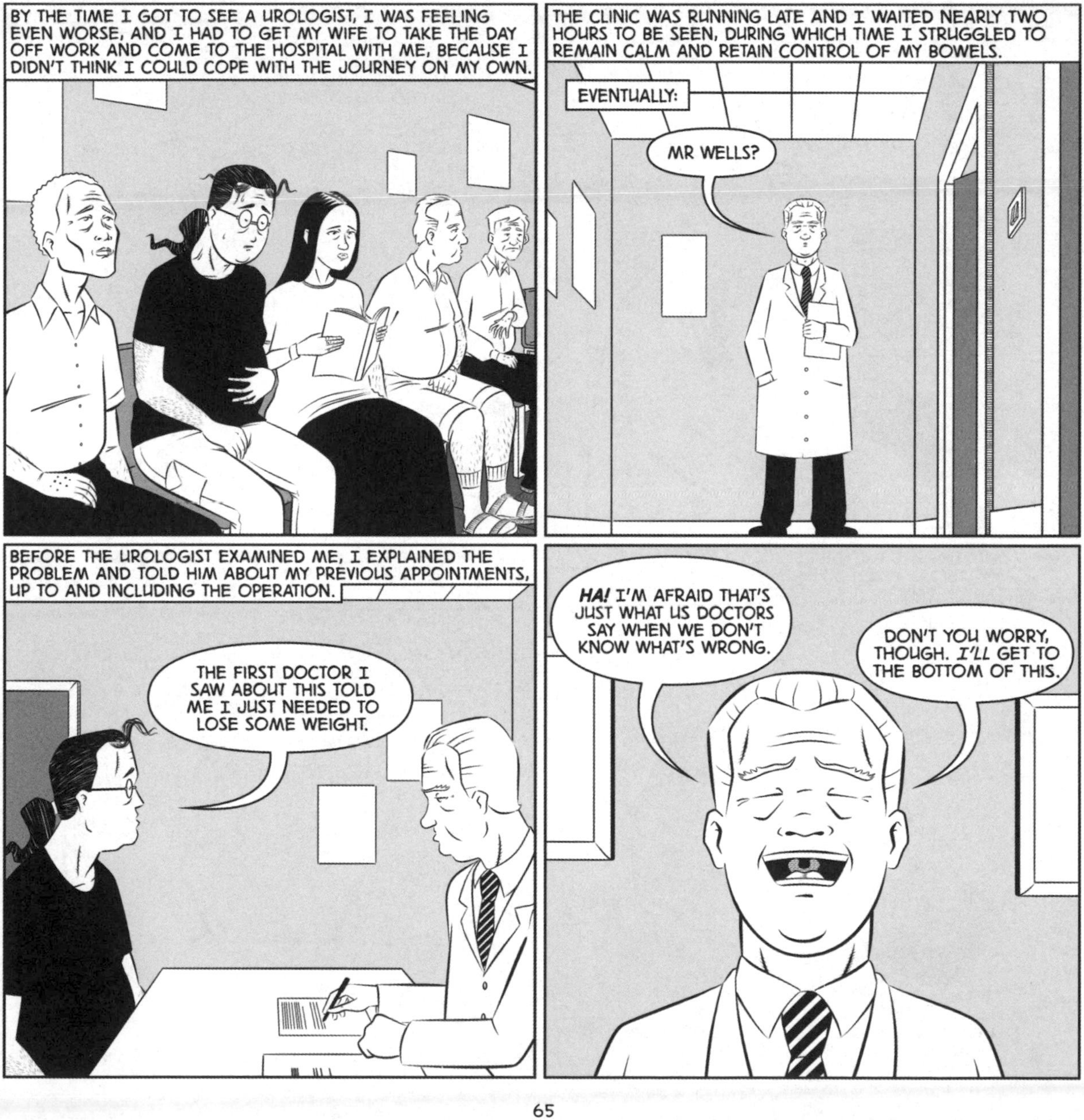
BY THE TIME I GOT TO SEE A UROLOGIST, I WAS FEELING EVEN WORSE, AND I HAD TO GET MY WIFE TO TAKE THE DAY OFF WORK AND COME TO THE HOSPITAL WITH ME, BECAUSE I DIDN'T THINK I COULD COPE WITH THE JOURNEY ON MY OWN.
THE CLINIC WAS RUNNING LATE AND I WAITED NEARLY TWO HOURS TO BE SEEN, DURING WHICH TIME I STRUGGLED TO REMAIN CALM AND RETAIN CONTROL OF MY BOWELS.
EVENTUALLY:
MR WELLS?
BEFORE THE UROLOGIST EXAMINED ME, I EXPLAINED THE PROBLEM AND TOLD HIM ABOUT MY PREVIOUS APPOINTMENTS, UP TO AND INCLUDING THE OPERATION.
THE FIRST DOCTOR I SAW ABOUT THIS TOLD ME I JUST NEEDED TO LOSE SOME WEIGHT.
HA! I'M AFRAID THAT'S JUST WHAT US DOCTORS SAY WHEN WE DON'T KNOW WHAT'S WRONG.
DON'T YOU WORRY, THOUGH. *I'LL* GET TO THE BOTTOM OF THIS.

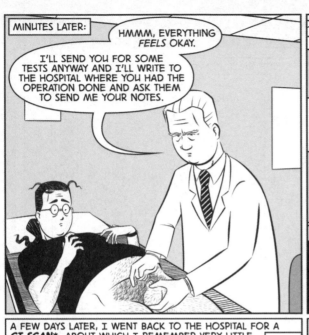

MINUTES LATER:

HMMM, EVERYTHING *FEELS* OKAY.

I'LL SEND YOU FOR SOME TESTS ANYWAY AND I'LL WRITE TO THE HOSPITAL WHERE YOU HAD THE OPERATION DONE AND ASK THEM TO SEND ME YOUR NOTES.

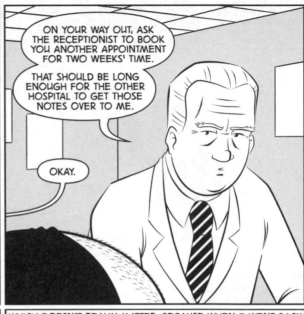

ON YOUR WAY OUT, ASK THE RECEPTIONIST TO BOOK YOU ANOTHER APPOINTMENT FOR TWO WEEKS' TIME.

THAT SHOULD BE LONG ENOUGH FOR THE OTHER HOSPITAL TO GET THOSE NOTES OVER TO ME.

OKAY.

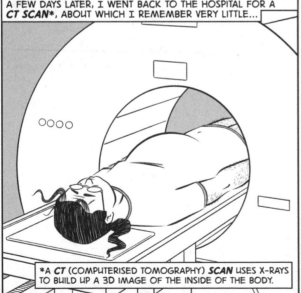

A FEW DAYS LATER, I WENT BACK TO THE HOSPITAL FOR A *CT SCAN**, ABOUT WHICH I REMEMBER VERY LITTLE...

*A *CT* (COMPUTERISED TOMOGRAPHY) *SCAN* USES X-RAYS TO BUILD UP A 3D IMAGE OF THE INSIDE OF THE BODY.

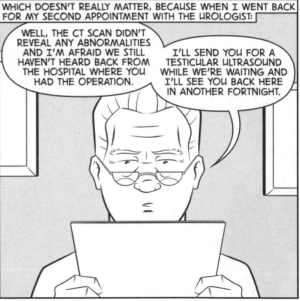

WHICH DOESN'T REALLY MATTER, BECAUSE WHEN I WENT BACK FOR MY SECOND APPOINTMENT WITH THE UROLOGIST:

WELL, THE CT SCAN DIDN'T REVEAL ANY ABNORMALITIES AND I'M AFRAID WE STILL HAVEN'T HEARD BACK FROM THE HOSPITAL WHERE YOU HAD THE OPERATION.

I'LL SEND YOU FOR A TESTICULAR ULTRASOUND WHILE WE'RE WAITING AND I'LL SEE YOU BACK HERE IN ANOTHER FORTNIGHT.

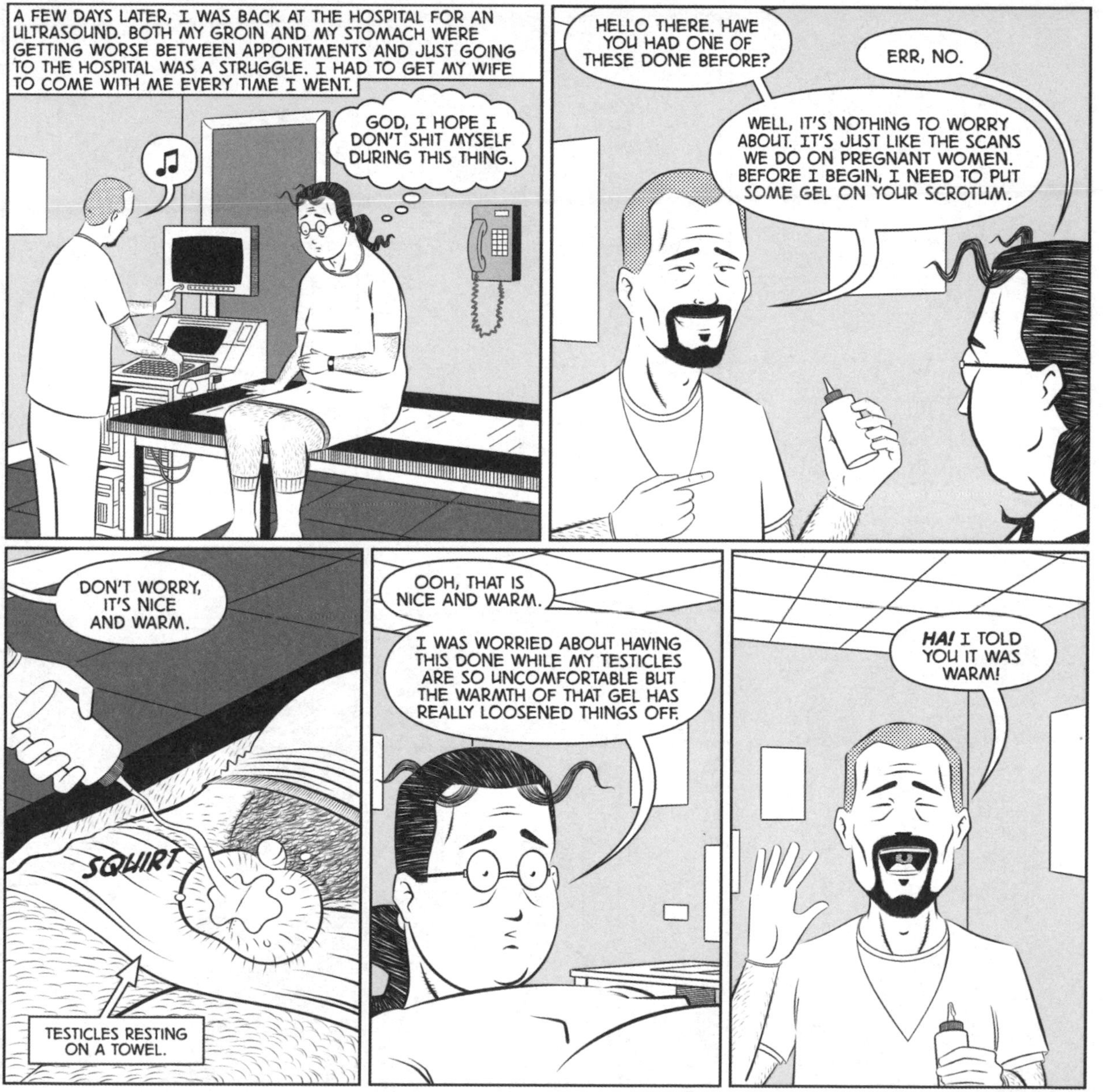
A FEW DAYS LATER, I WAS BACK AT THE HOSPITAL FOR AN ULTRASOUND. BOTH MY GROIN AND MY STOMACH WERE GETTING WORSE BETWEEN APPOINTMENTS AND JUST GOING TO THE HOSPITAL WAS A STRUGGLE. I HAD TO GET MY WIFE TO COME WITH ME EVERY TIME I WENT.
♫
GOD, I HOPE I DON'T SHIT MYSELF DURING THIS THING.
HELLO THERE. HAVE YOU HAD ONE OF THESE DONE BEFORE?
ERR, NO.
WELL, IT'S NOTHING TO WORRY ABOUT. IT'S JUST LIKE THE SCANS WE DO ON PREGNANT WOMEN. BEFORE I BEGIN, I NEED TO PUT SOME GEL ON YOUR SCROTUM.
DON'T WORRY, IT'S NICE AND WARM.
SQUIRT
TESTICLES RESTING ON A TOWEL.
OOH, THAT IS NICE AND WARM.
I WAS WORRIED ABOUT HAVING THIS DONE WHILE MY TESTICLES ARE SO UNCOMFORTABLE BUT THE WARMTH OF THAT GEL HAS REALLY LOOSENED THINGS OFF.
HA! I TOLD YOU IT WAS WARM!

RIGHT, LET'S GET ON WITH IT, SHALL WE?
TUM-DE-DUM...
RING RING
RING RING
RING RING
RING RING
SORRY, DO YOU MIND IF I JUST ANSWER THAT?
RING RING
RING RING
UM, NO. THAT'S OKAY.

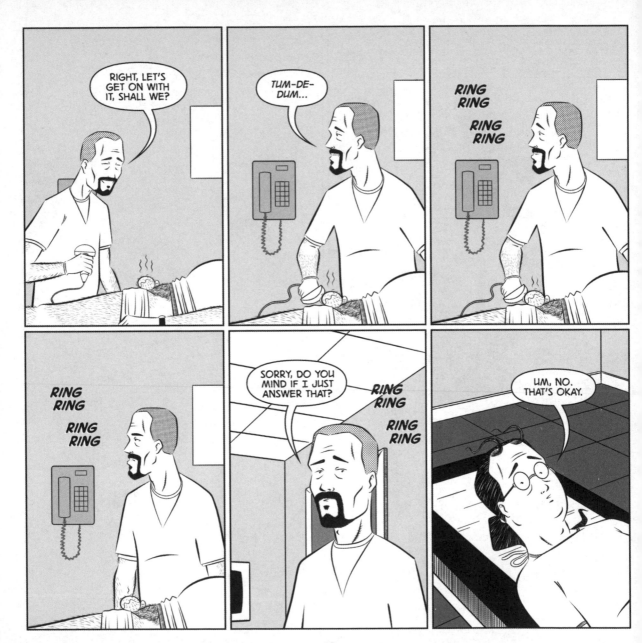

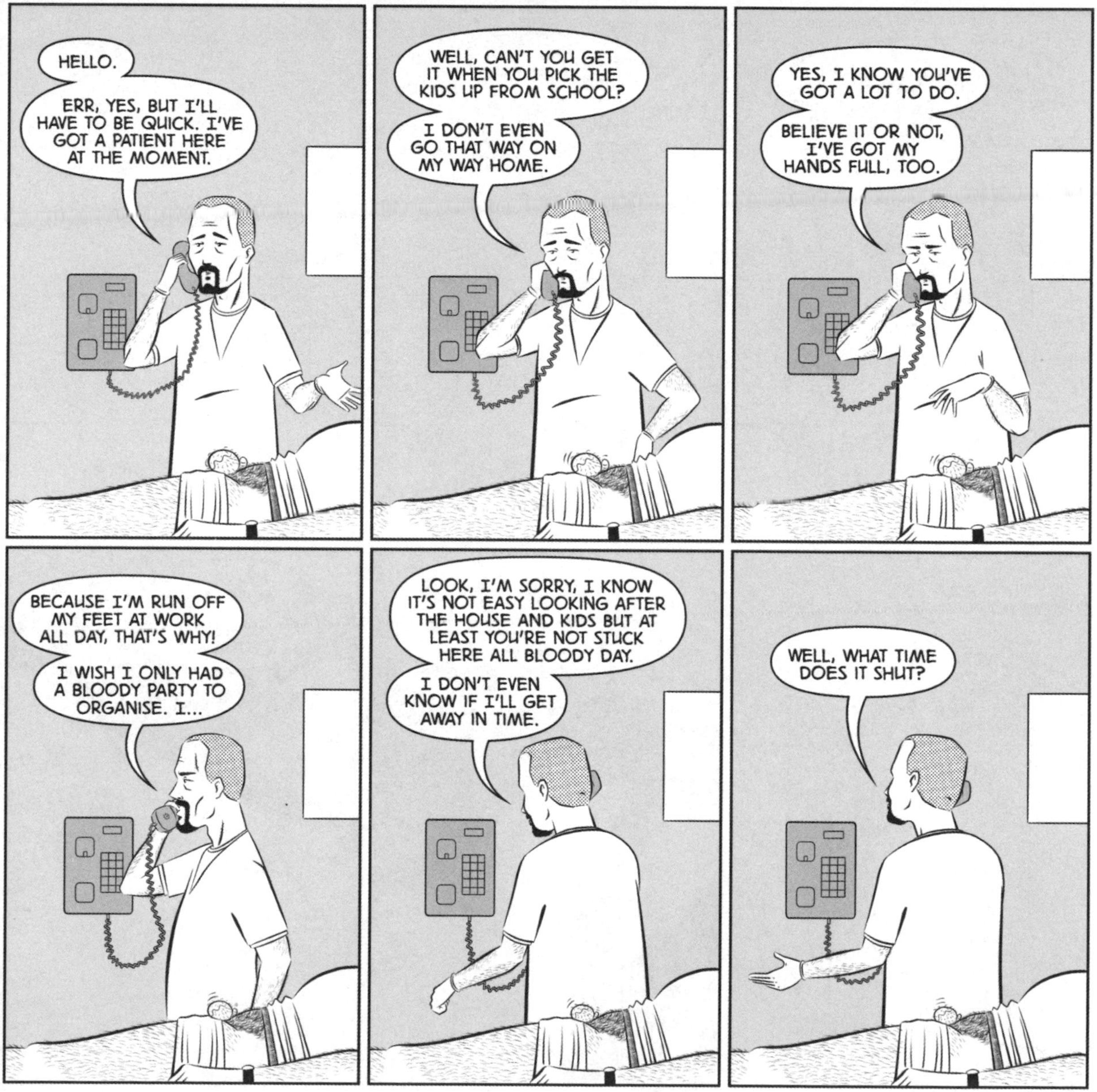
HELLO.
ERR, YES, BUT I'LL HAVE TO BE QUICK. I'VE GOT A PATIENT HERE AT THE MOMENT.
WELL, CAN'T YOU GET IT WHEN YOU PICK THE KIDS UP FROM SCHOOL?
I DON'T EVEN GO THAT WAY ON MY WAY HOME.
YES, I KNOW YOU'VE GOT A LOT TO DO.
BELIEVE IT OR NOT, I'VE GOT MY HANDS FULL, TOO.
BECAUSE I'M RUN OFF MY FEET AT WORK ALL DAY, THAT'S WHY!
I WISH I ONLY HAD A BLOODY PARTY TO ORGANISE. I...
LOOK, I'M SORRY, I KNOW IT'S NOT EASY LOOKING AFTER THE HOUSE AND KIDS BUT AT LEAST YOU'RE NOT STUCK HERE ALL BLOODY DAY.
I DON'T EVEN KNOW IF I'LL GET AWAY IN TIME.
WELL, WHAT TIME DOES IT SHUT?

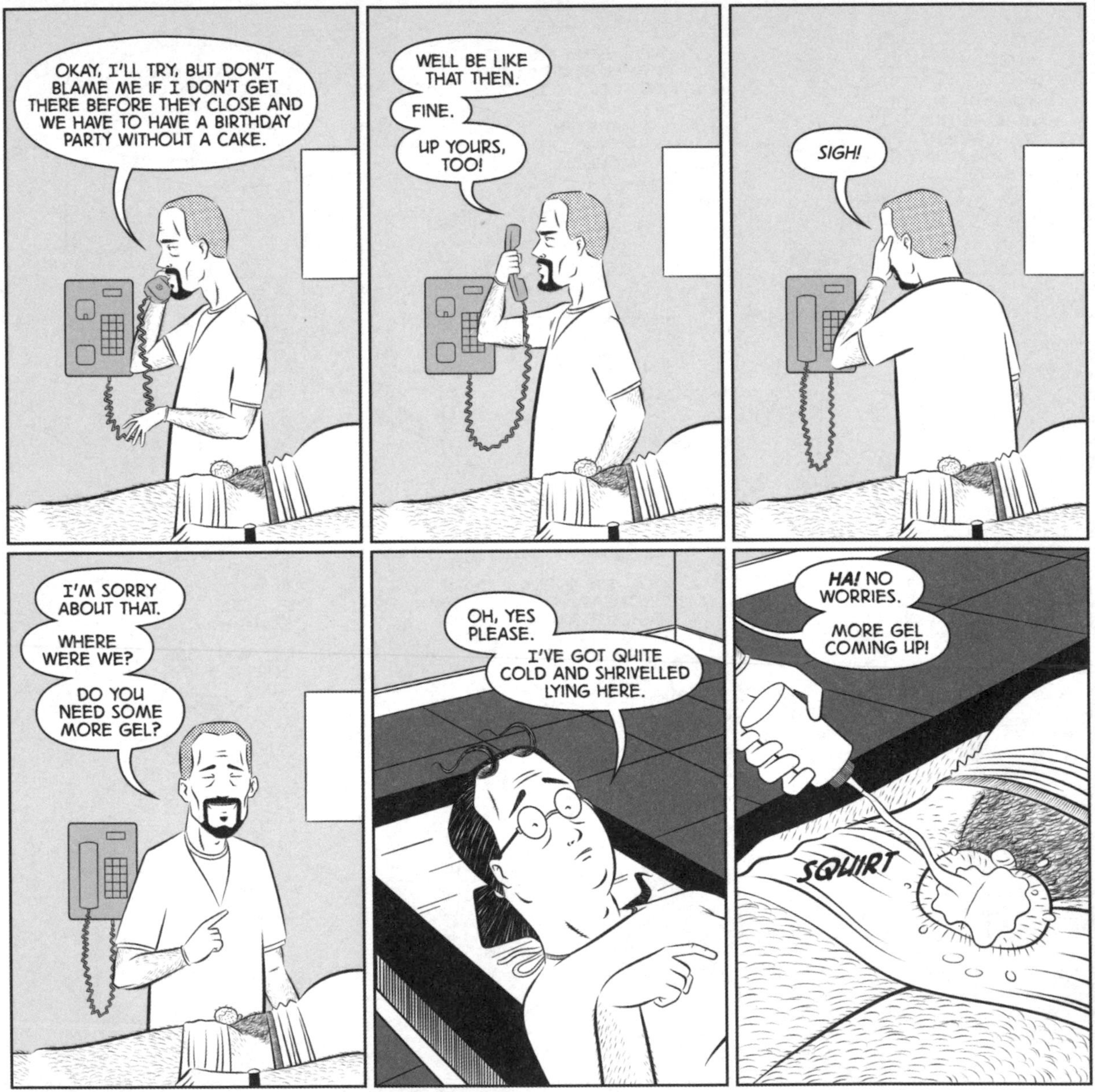
OKAY, I'LL TRY, BUT DON'T BLAME ME IF I DON'T GET THERE BEFORE THEY CLOSE AND WE HAVE TO HAVE A BIRTHDAY PARTY WITHOUT A CAKE.
WELL BE LIKE THAT THEN.
FINE.
UP YOURS, TOO!
SIGH!
I'M SORRY ABOUT THAT.
WHERE WERE WE?
DO YOU NEED SOME MORE GEL?
OH, YES PLEASE.
I'VE GOT QUITE COLD AND SHRIVELLED LYING HERE.
HA! NO WORRIES.
MORE GEL COMING UP!
SQUIRT

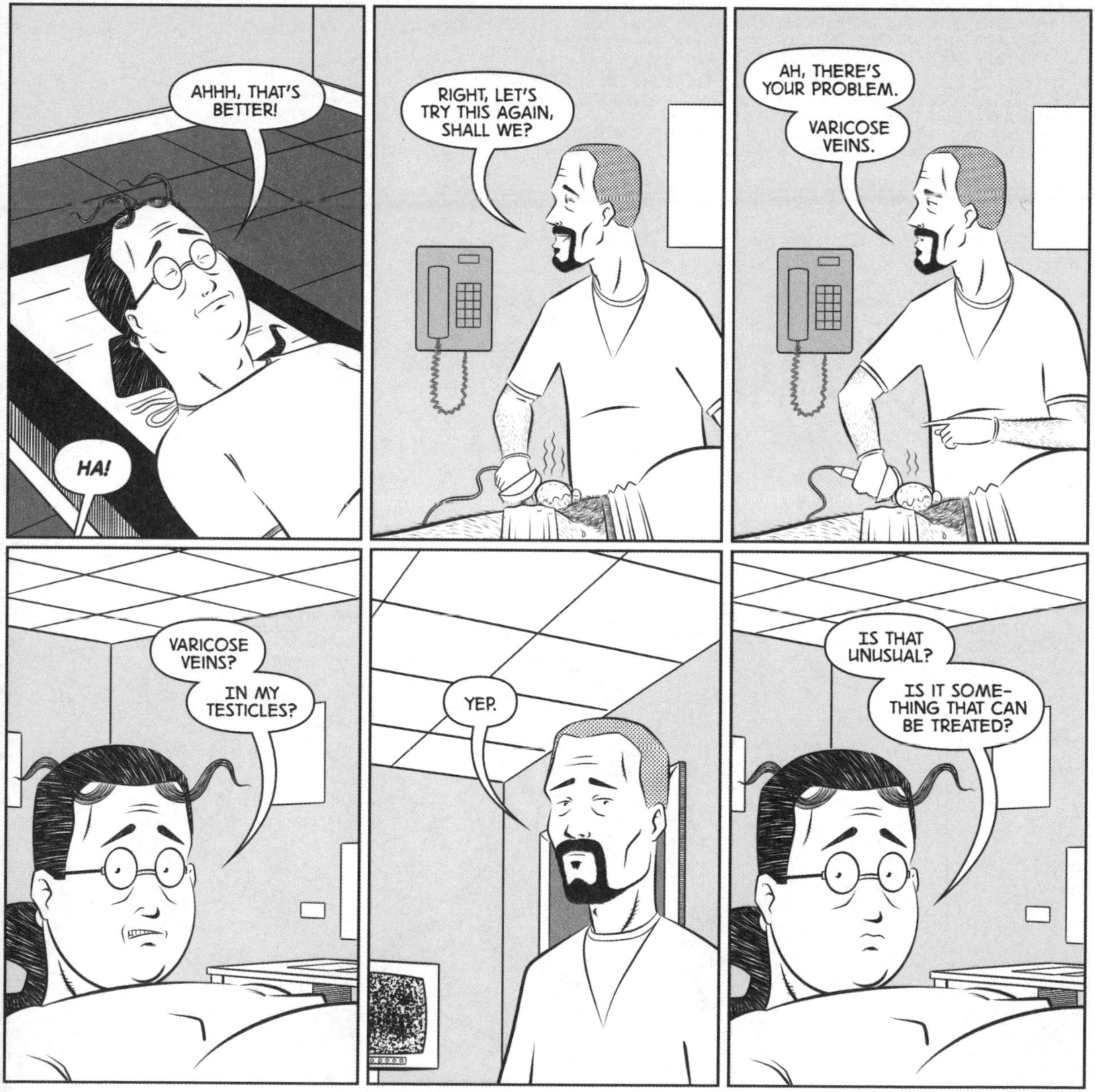
AHHH, THAT'S BETTER!
HA!
RIGHT, LET'S TRY THIS AGAIN, SHALL WE?
AH, THERE'S YOUR PROBLEM.
VARICOSE VEINS.
VARICOSE VEINS?
IN MY TESTICLES?
YEP.
IS THAT UNUSUAL?
IS IT SOMETHING THAT CAN BE TREATED?

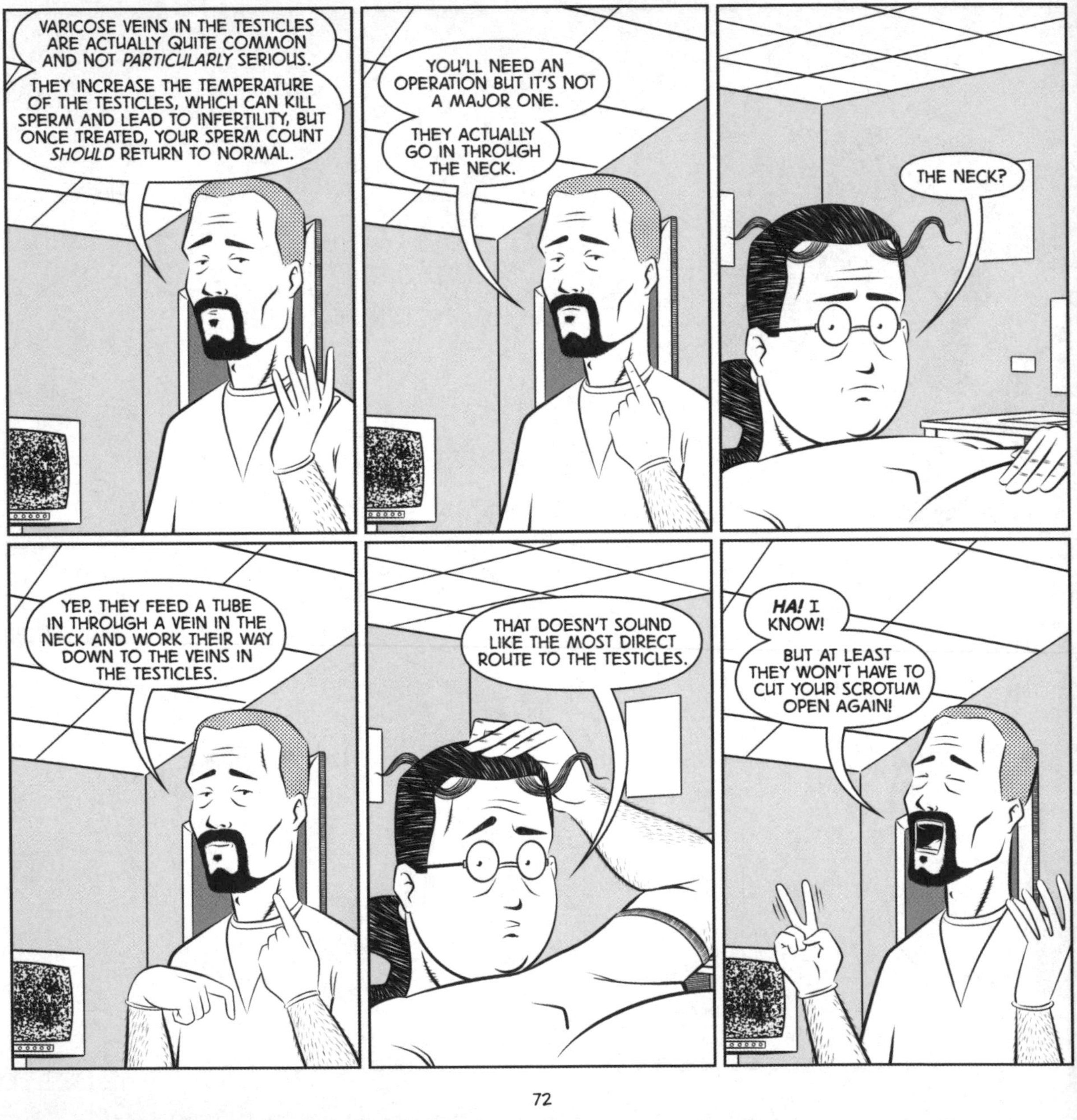
VARICOSE VEINS IN THE TESTICLES ARE ACTUALLY QUITE COMMON AND NOT *PARTICULARLY* SERIOUS.
THEY INCREASE THE TEMPERATURE OF THE TESTICLES, WHICH CAN KILL SPERM AND LEAD TO INFERTILITY, BUT ONCE TREATED, YOUR SPERM COUNT *SHOULD* RETURN TO NORMAL.
YOU'LL NEED AN OPERATION BUT IT'S NOT A MAJOR ONE.
THEY ACTUALLY GO IN THROUGH THE NECK.
THE NECK?
YEP. THEY FEED A TUBE IN THROUGH A VEIN IN THE NECK AND WORK THEIR WAY DOWN TO THE VEINS IN THE TESTICLES.
THAT DOESN'T SOUND LIKE THE MOST DIRECT ROUTE TO THE TESTICLES.
HA! I KNOW!
BUT AT LEAST THEY WON'T HAVE TO CUT YOUR SCROTUM OPEN AGAIN!

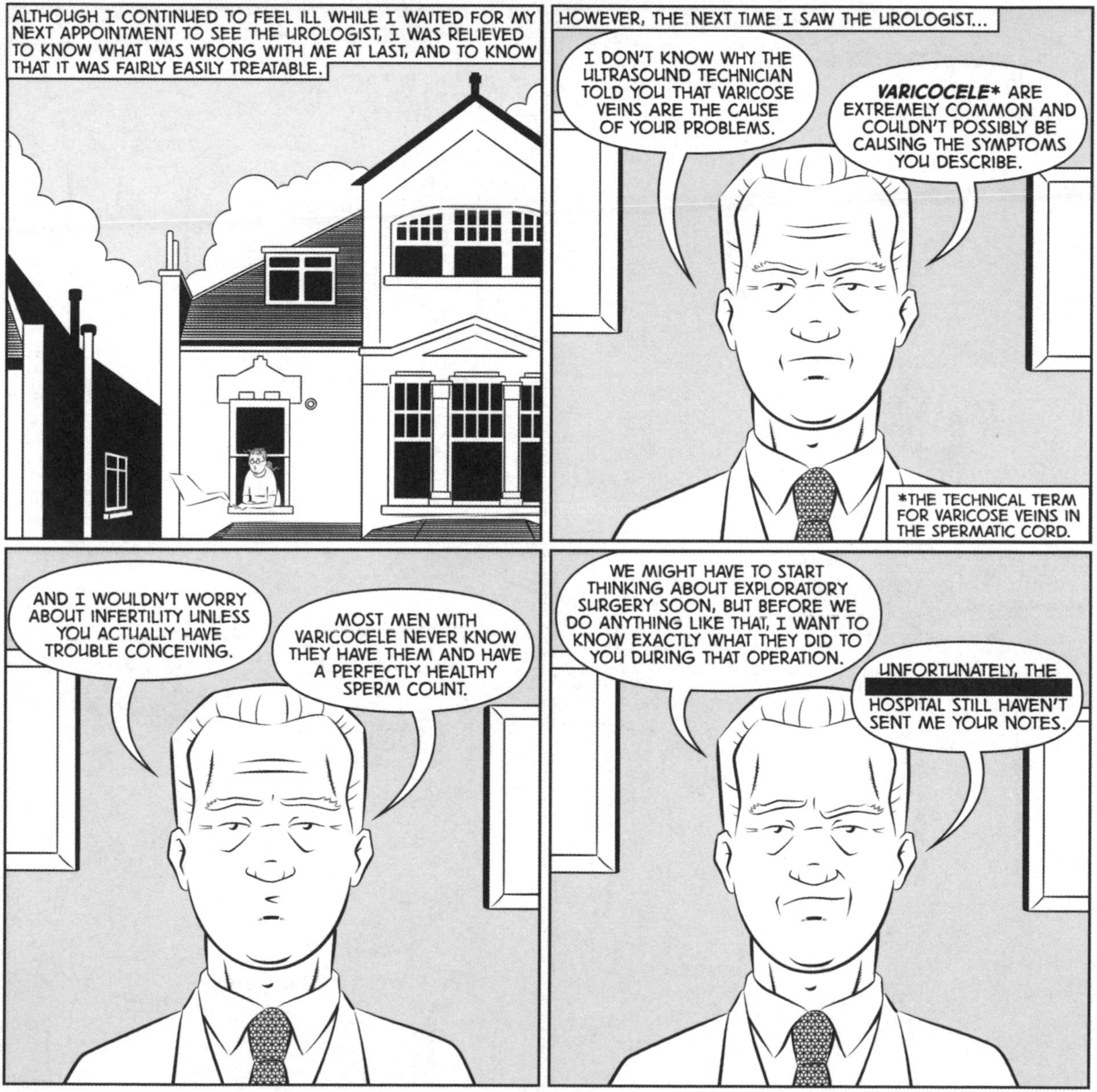
ALTHOUGH I CONTINUED TO FEEL ILL WHILE I WAITED FOR MY NEXT APPOINTMENT TO SEE THE UROLOGIST, I WAS RELIEVED TO KNOW WHAT WAS WRONG WITH ME AT LAST, AND TO KNOW THAT IT WAS FAIRLY EASILY TREATABLE.
HOWEVER, THE NEXT TIME I SAW THE UROLOGIST...
I DON'T KNOW WHY THE ULTRASOUND TECHNICIAN TOLD YOU THAT VARICOSE VEINS ARE THE CAUSE OF YOUR PROBLEMS.
*VARICOCELE** ARE EXTREMELY COMMON AND COULDN'T POSSIBLY BE CAUSING THE SYMPTOMS YOU DESCRIBE.
*THE TECHNICAL TERM FOR VARICOSE VEINS IN THE SPERMATIC CORD.
AND I WOULDN'T WORRY ABOUT INFERTILITY UNLESS YOU ACTUALLY HAVE TROUBLE CONCEIVING.
MOST MEN WITH VARICOCELE NEVER KNOW THEY HAVE THEM AND HAVE A PERFECTLY HEALTHY SPERM COUNT.
WE MIGHT HAVE TO START THINKING ABOUT EXPLORATORY SURGERY SOON, BUT BEFORE WE DO ANYTHING LIKE THAT, I WANT TO KNOW EXACTLY WHAT THEY DID TO YOU DURING THAT OPERATION.
UNFORTUNATELY, THE [redacted] HOSPITAL STILL HAVEN'T SENT ME YOUR NOTES.

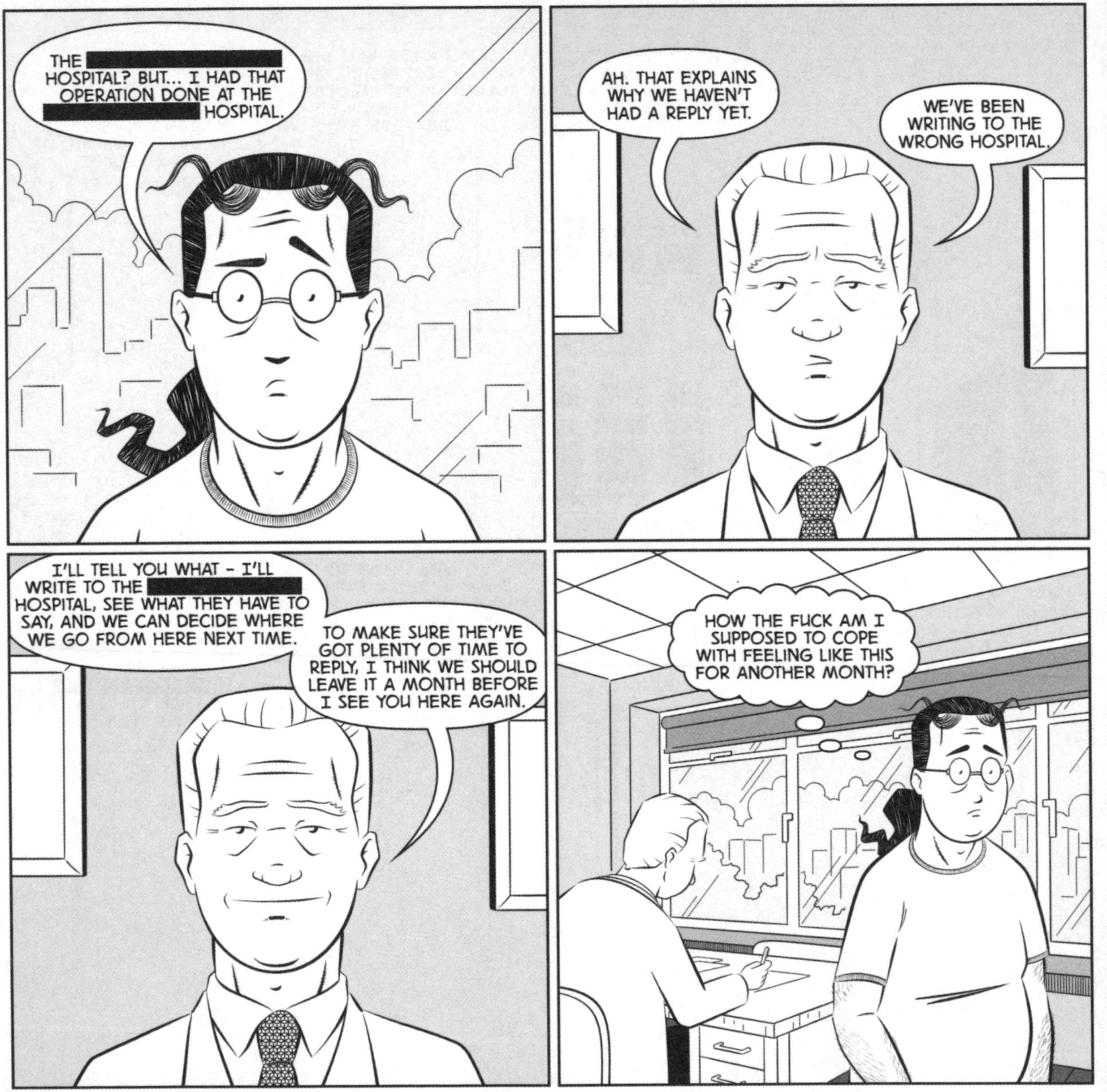
THE [redacted] HOSPITAL? BUT... I HAD THAT OPERATION DONE AT THE [redacted] HOSPITAL.
AH. THAT EXPLAINS WHY WE HAVEN'T HAD A REPLY YET.
WE'VE BEEN WRITING TO THE WRONG HOSPITAL.
I'LL TELL YOU WHAT - I'LL WRITE TO THE [redacted] HOSPITAL, SEE WHAT THEY HAVE TO SAY, AND WE CAN DECIDE WHERE WE GO FROM HERE NEXT TIME.
TO MAKE SURE THEY'VE GOT PLENTY OF TIME TO REPLY, I THINK WE SHOULD LEAVE IT A MONTH BEFORE I SEE YOU HERE AGAIN.
HOW THE FUCK AM I SUPPOSED TO COPE WITH FEELING LIKE THIS FOR ANOTHER MONTH?

THAT MONTH BETWEEN HOSPITAL APPOINTMENTS REALLY DRAGGED, AND NOW THAT I WAS BACK TO HAVING NO IDEA WHAT WAS WRONG WITH ME, I *REALLY* STARTED TO WORRY.

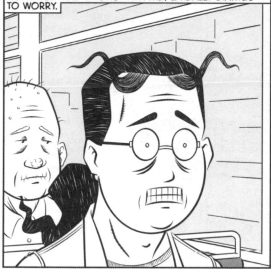

I WAS NEVER WORRIED THAT I MIGHT HAVE SOMETHING LIFE-THREATENING, LIKE CANCER - I FIGURED THAT WOULD HAVE BEEN SPOTTED FAIRLY QUICKLY. INSTEAD, WHAT WORRIED ME WAS THE WORSENING SYMPTOMS OF WHATEVER WAS WRONG WITH ME, AND NOT KNOWING WHAT MIGHT HAPPEN NEXT.

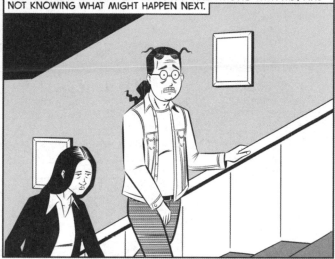

MY SCROTUM WAS OFTEN SO TIGHT AND UNCOMFORTABLE THAT I COULD ONLY JUST FEEL MY TESTICLES - PARTICULARLY MY RIGHT TESTICLE - ON THE OUTSIDE OF MY BODY. I STILL THOUGHT IT WAS POSSIBLE FOR MY TESTICLES TO RETREAT UP INTO MY PELVIS ENTIRELY AND I USUALLY HAD ONE HAND HOVERING OVER MY GROIN, MAKING SURE EVERYTHING WAS (JUST ABOUT) WHERE IT SHOULD BE.

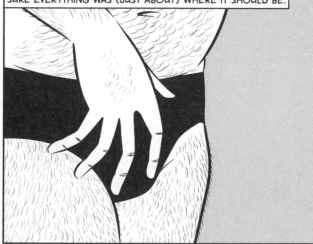

IF I FELT THIS BAD WHEN MY TESTICLES WERE JUST UNUSUALLY HIGH UP, HOW WOULD I FEEL WHEN THEY DISAPPEARED ENTIRELY? WORSE STILL, WHAT IF THIS HAPPENED WHEN I WAS OUT IN PUBLIC?

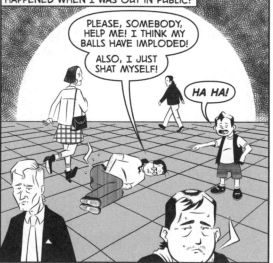

PLEASE, SOMEBODY, HELP ME! I THINK MY BALLS HAVE IMPLODED!

ALSO, I JUST SHAT MYSELF!

HA HA!

A WEEK OR SO INTO THAT MONTH BETWEEN UROLOGY APPOINTMENTS, MY WIFE AND I GOT IN A TAXI AND WENT TO THE A&E DEPARTMENT OF ANOTHER NEARBY HOSPITAL.

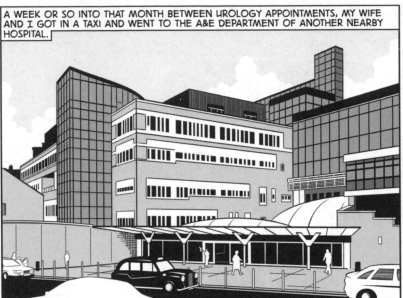

AFTER I'D DESCRIBED MY SYMPTOMS TO A RECEPTIONIST, I WAS RUSHED IN TO SEE A DOCTOR RIGHT AWAY.

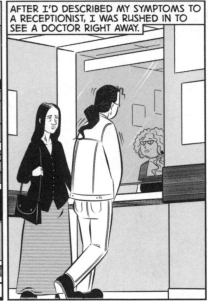

THIS DOCTOR – WHO MAY OR MAY NOT HAVE BEEN A UROLOGIST – EXAMINED ME THOROUGHLY...

EEK!

SQUEAK SQUEAK

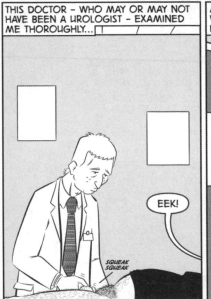

AND THEN *SEEMED* TO TAKE NOTES WHILE I TOLD HIM MY RECENT MEDICAL HISTORY.

MMM-HMM.

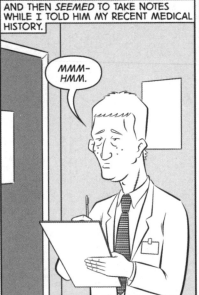

THEN, HE SAID:

WELL, I CAN'T FEEL ANY-THING WRONG AT ALL AND I REALLY DON'T KNOW WHY YOU CAME HERE WHEN YOU'RE ALREADY SEEING A UROLOGIST ELSEWHERE.

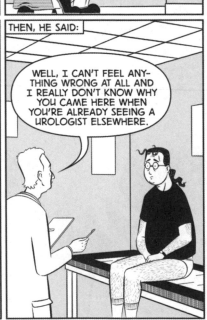

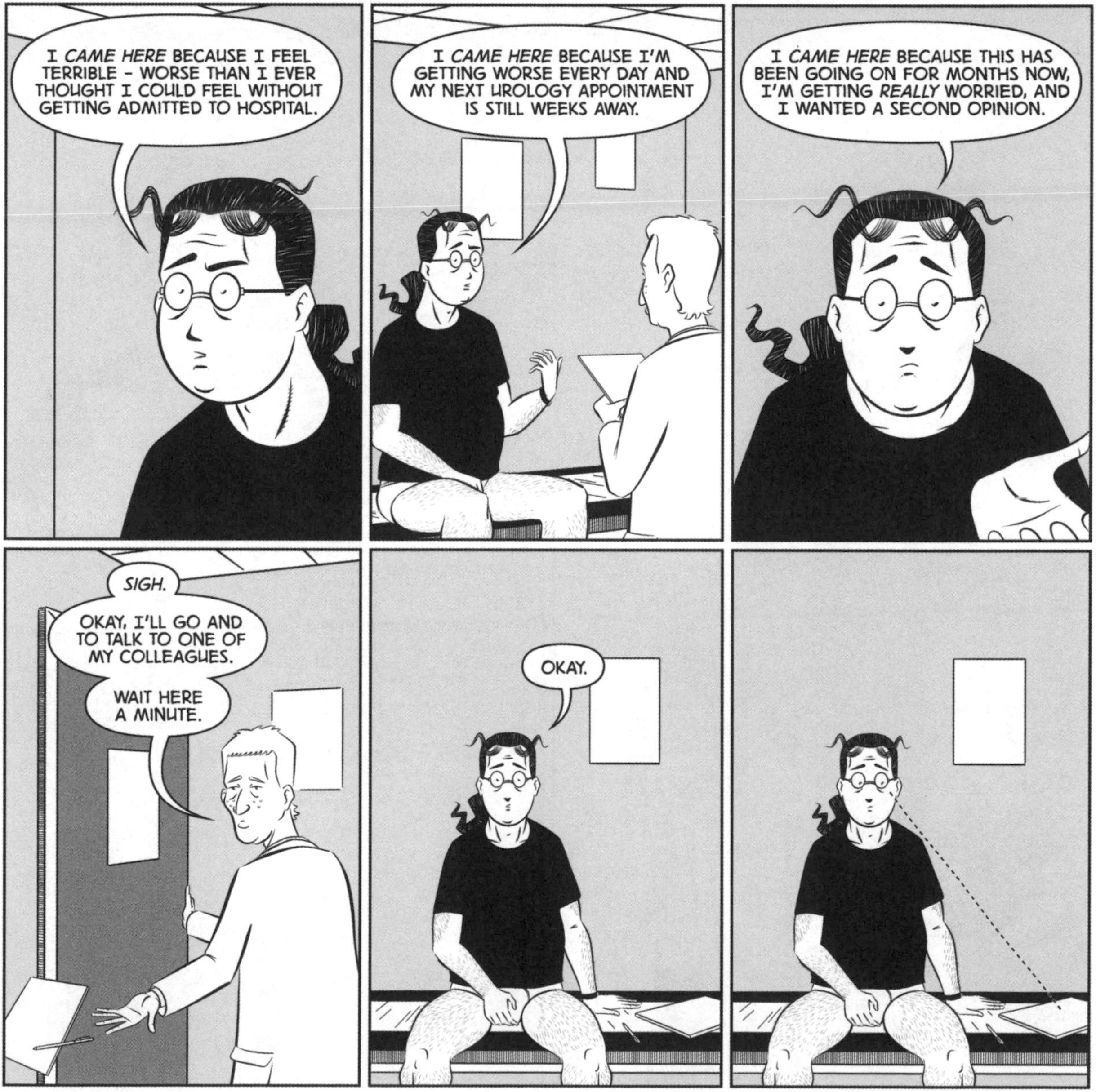
I *CAME HERE* BECAUSE I FEEL TERRIBLE - WORSE THAN I EVER THOUGHT I COULD FEEL WITHOUT GETTING ADMITTED TO HOSPITAL.
I *CAME HERE* BECAUSE I'M GETTING WORSE EVERY DAY AND MY NEXT UROLOGY APPOINTMENT IS STILL WEEKS AWAY.
I *CAME HERE* BECAUSE THIS HAS BEEN GOING ON FOR MONTHS NOW, I'M GETTING *REALLY* WORRIED, AND I WANTED A SECOND OPINION.
SIGH.
OKAY, I'LL GO AND TO TALK TO ONE OF MY COLLEAGUES.
WAIT HERE A MINUTE.
OKAY.

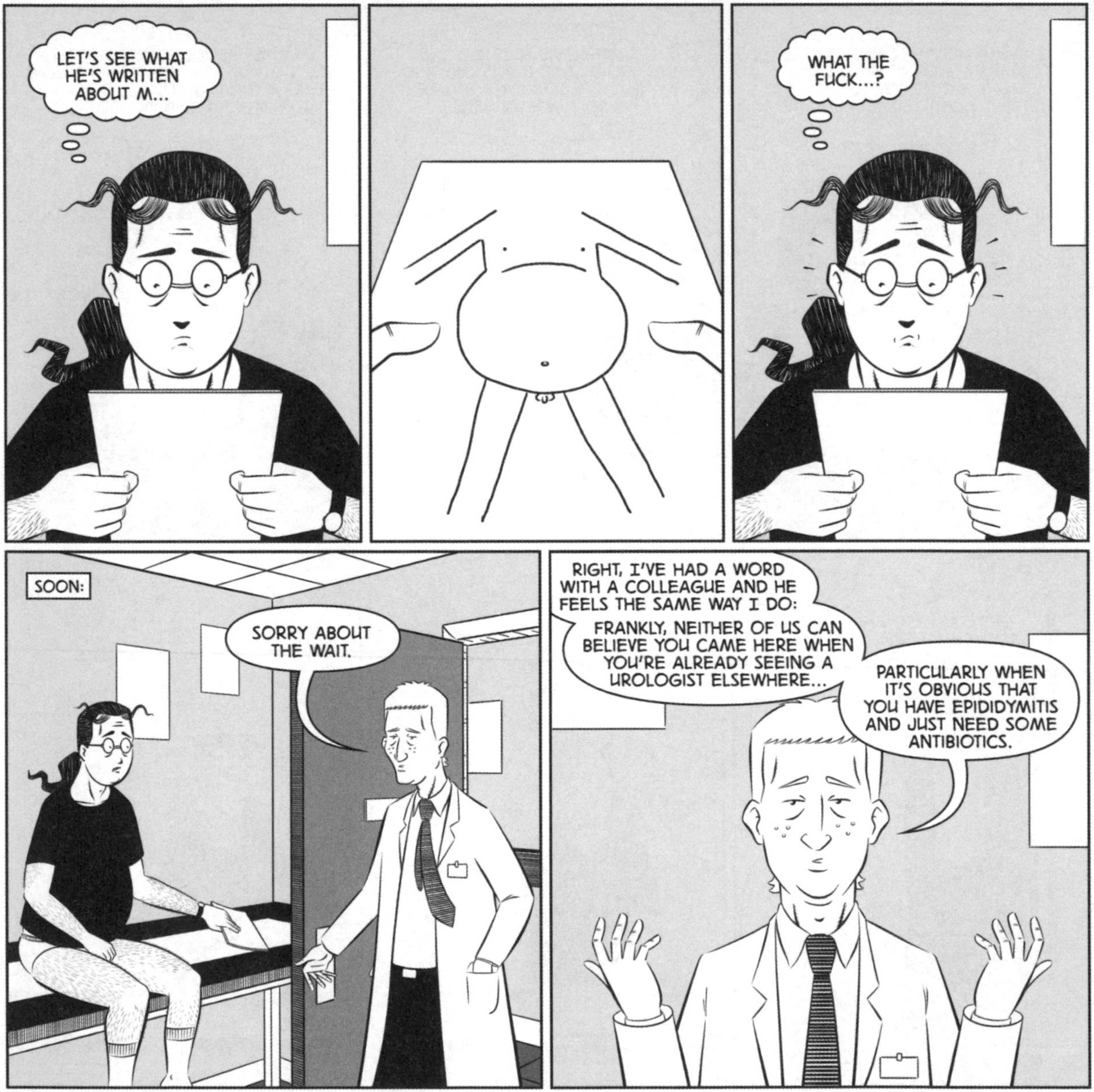
LET'S SEE WHAT HE'S WRITTEN ABOUT M...
WHAT THE FUCK...?
SOON:
SORRY ABOUT THE WAIT.
RIGHT, I'VE HAD A WORD WITH A COLLEAGUE AND HE FEELS THE SAME WAY I DO:
FRANKLY, NEITHER OF US CAN BELIEVE YOU CAME HERE WHEN YOU'RE ALREADY SEEING A UROLOGIST ELSEWHERE...
PARTICULARLY WHEN IT'S OBVIOUS THAT YOU HAVE EPIDIDYMITIS AND JUST NEED SOME ANTIBIOTICS.

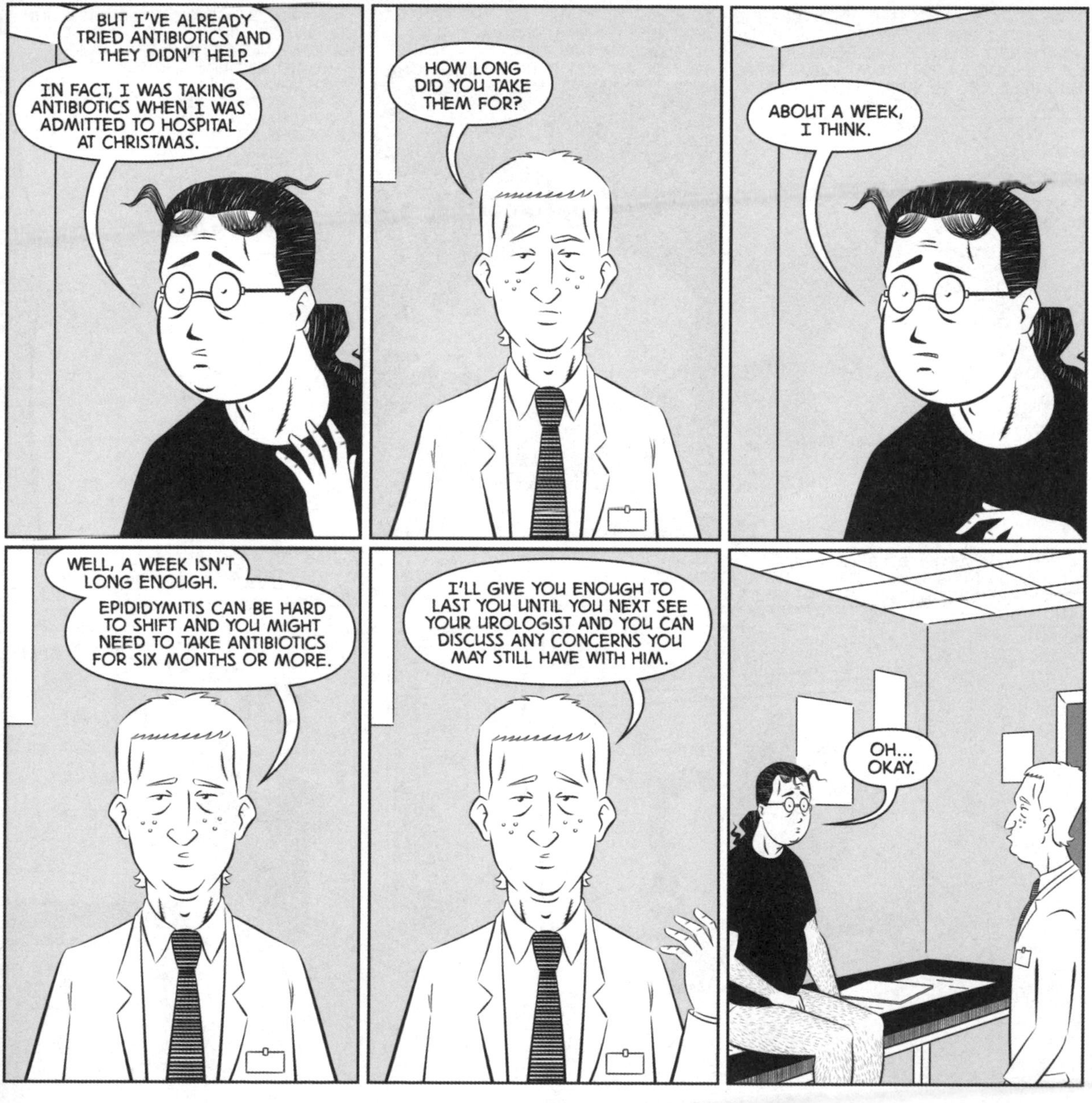
BUT I'VE ALREADY TRIED ANTIBIOTICS AND THEY DIDN'T HELP.
IN FACT, I WAS TAKING ANTIBIOTICS WHEN I WAS ADMITTED TO HOSPITAL AT CHRISTMAS.
HOW LONG DID YOU TAKE THEM FOR?
ABOUT A WEEK, I THINK.
WELL, A WEEK ISN'T LONG ENOUGH.
EPIDIDYMITIS CAN BE HARD TO SHIFT AND YOU MIGHT NEED TO TAKE ANTIBIOTICS FOR SIX MONTHS OR MORE.
I'LL GIVE YOU ENOUGH TO LAST YOU UNTIL YOU NEXT SEE YOUR UROLOGIST AND YOU CAN DISCUSS ANY CONCERNS YOU MAY STILL HAVE WITH HIM.
OH... OKAY.

I WENT HOME AND STARTED TAKING THE ANTIBIOTICS BUT MY SYMPTOMS QUICKLY WORSENED. UP UNTIL THIS POINT, MOST OF THE DISCOMFORT IN MY PUBIC AREA HAD BEEN ON THE RIGHT SIDE, BUT NOW I HAD IT ON THE LEFT SIDE, TOO.

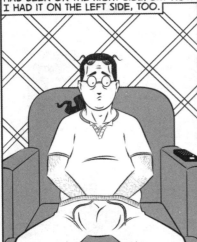

IN ADDITION TO THIS AND THE GENERAL TIGHTNESS OF MY SCROTUM, I ALSO DEVELOPED A THROBBING PAIN AT THE BACK OF MY LEFT TESTICLE.

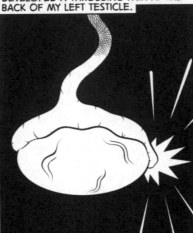

I HAD ALREADY BEEN FINDING IT QUITE UNCOMFORTABLE TO WALK, BUT NOW WALKING WAS GETTING *REALLY* UN-PLEASANT, BECAUSE THE TOP OF MY THIGH WAS RUBBING AGAINST THE BACK OF MY PAINFUL TESTICLE, AGGRAVATING THE PAIN AND CAUSING MY TESTICLES TO RETREAT EVEN FURTHER INTO THE SAFETY OF MY PELVIS.

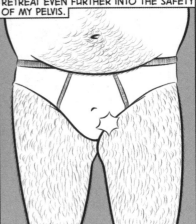

A FEW DAYS AFTER I'D BEGUN TAKING THE ANTIBIOTICS, I CRAWLED INTO BED AND STAYED THERE FOR MOST OF THE NEXT TWO WEEKS, ONLY GETTING UP TO USE THE TOILET, EAT AND SMOKE.

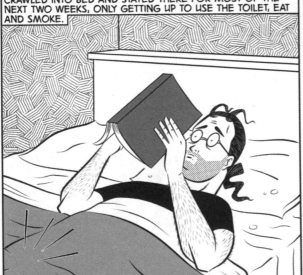

EVERY TIME I TOOK A PUFF ON A CIGARETTE, I WOULD GET SHOOTING PAINS IN MY TESTICLES, WHICH SEEMED TO BE GETTING WORSE BY THE DAY.

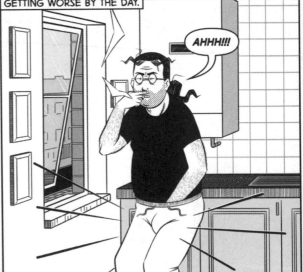

AHHH!!!

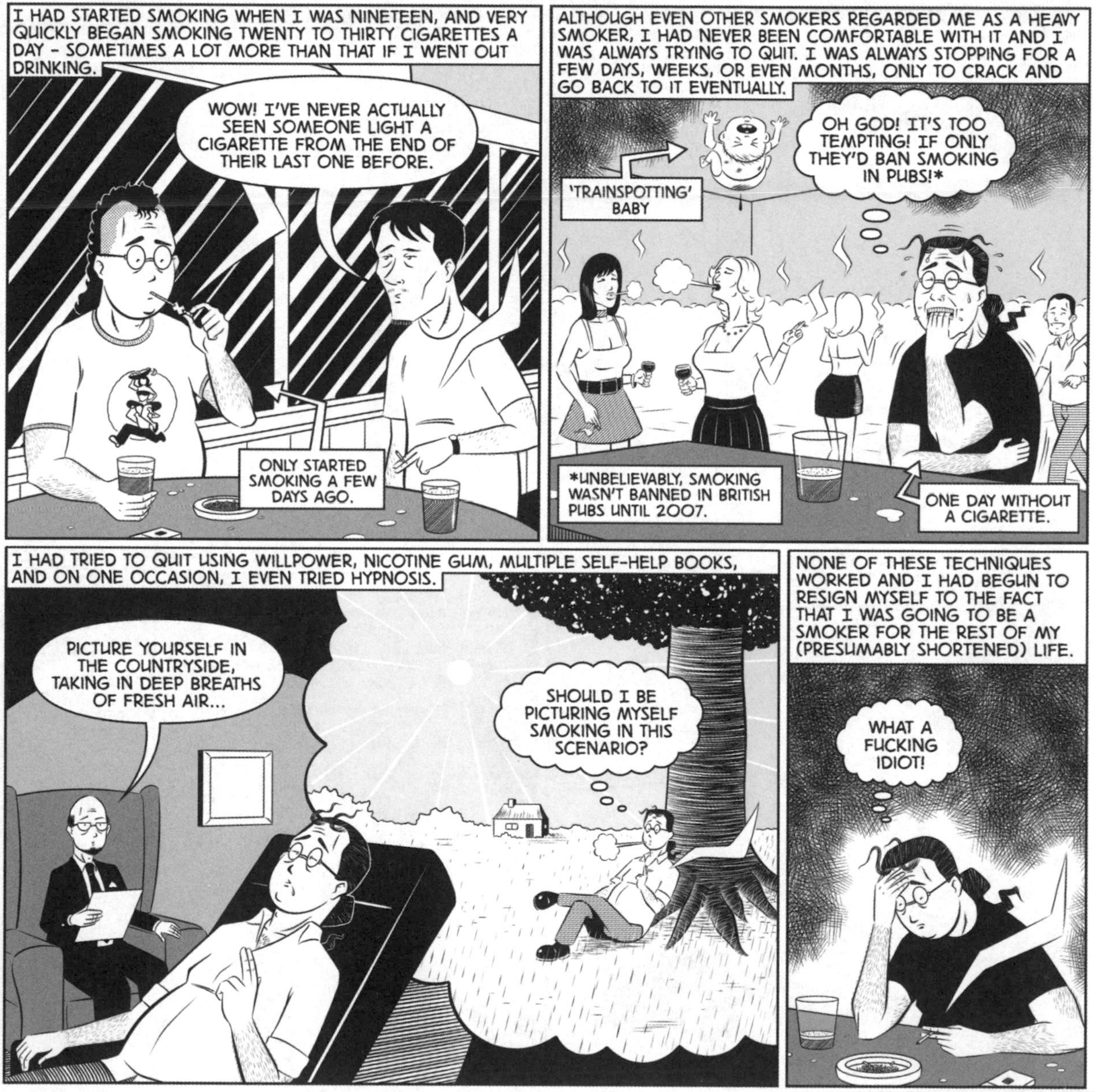
I HAD STARTED SMOKING WHEN I WAS NINETEEN, AND VERY QUICKLY BEGAN SMOKING TWENTY TO THIRTY CIGARETTES A DAY - SOMETIMES A LOT MORE THAN THAT IF I WENT OUT DRINKING.
WOW! I'VE NEVER ACTUALLY SEEN SOMEONE LIGHT A CIGARETTE FROM THE END OF THEIR LAST ONE BEFORE.
ONLY STARTED SMOKING A FEW DAYS AGO.
ALTHOUGH EVEN OTHER SMOKERS REGARDED ME AS A HEAVY SMOKER, I HAD NEVER BEEN COMFORTABLE WITH IT AND I WAS ALWAYS TRYING TO QUIT. I WAS ALWAYS STOPPING FOR A FEW DAYS, WEEKS, OR EVEN MONTHS, ONLY TO CRACK AND GO BACK TO IT EVENTUALLY.
'TRAINSPOTTING' BABY
OH GOD! IT'S TOO TEMPTING! IF ONLY THEY'D BAN SMOKING IN PUBS!*
*UNBELIEVABLY, SMOKING WASN'T BANNED IN BRITISH PUBS UNTIL 2007.
ONE DAY WITHOUT A CIGARETTE.
I HAD TRIED TO QUIT USING WILLPOWER, NICOTINE GUM, MULTIPLE SELF-HELP BOOKS, AND ON ONE OCCASION, I EVEN TRIED HYPNOSIS.
PICTURE YOURSELF IN THE COUNTRYSIDE, TAKING IN DEEP BREATHS OF FRESH AIR...
SHOULD I BE PICTURING MYSELF SMOKING IN THIS SCENARIO?
NONE OF THESE TECHNIQUES WORKED AND I HAD BEGUN TO RESIGN MYSELF TO THE FACT THAT I WAS GOING TO BE A SMOKER FOR THE REST OF MY (PRESUMABLY SHORTENED) LIFE.
WHAT A FUCKING IDIOT!

HOWEVER, IN SEPTEMBER 1998, A LITTLE UNDER SIX MONTHS BEFORE MY THIRTIETH BIRTHDAY, I FINALLY FOUND THE METHOD THAT WORKED FOR ME.

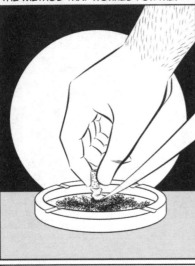

TERRIFIED BY THE TESTICLE PAINS I WAS EXPERIENCING, I DECIDED TO HAVE YET ANOTHER GO AT QUITTING. I PUT OUT ANOTHER IN A VERY LONG LINE OF CIGARETTES, SEMI-CONVINCED THAT I WOULD BE SMOKING AGAIN WITHIN A FEW DAYS, CRAWLED BACK INTO BED...

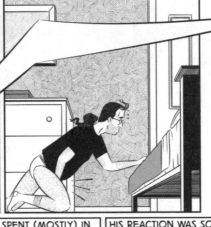

AND I HAVEN'T SMOKED SINCE.

TOWARDS THE END OF THAT FORTNIGHT I SPENT (MOSTLY) IN BED, JUST A FEW DAYS INTO MY NEW LIFE AS A NON-SMOKER, I CALLED MY DOCTOR AND CONVINCED HIM TO COME OUT FOR A HOME VISIT, BECAUSE I FELT TOO ILL TO WALK TO THE SURGERY.

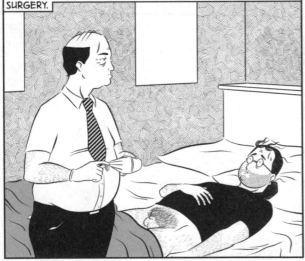

HIS REACTION WAS SOMEWHAT FAMILIAR:

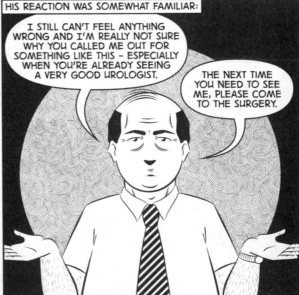

I STILL CAN'T FEEL ANYTHING WRONG AND I'M REALLY NOT SURE WHY YOU CALLED ME OUT FOR SOMETHING LIKE THIS – ESPECIALLY WHEN YOU'RE ALREADY SEEING A VERY GOOD UROLOGIST.

THE NEXT TIME YOU NEED TO SEE ME, PLEASE COME TO THE SURGERY.

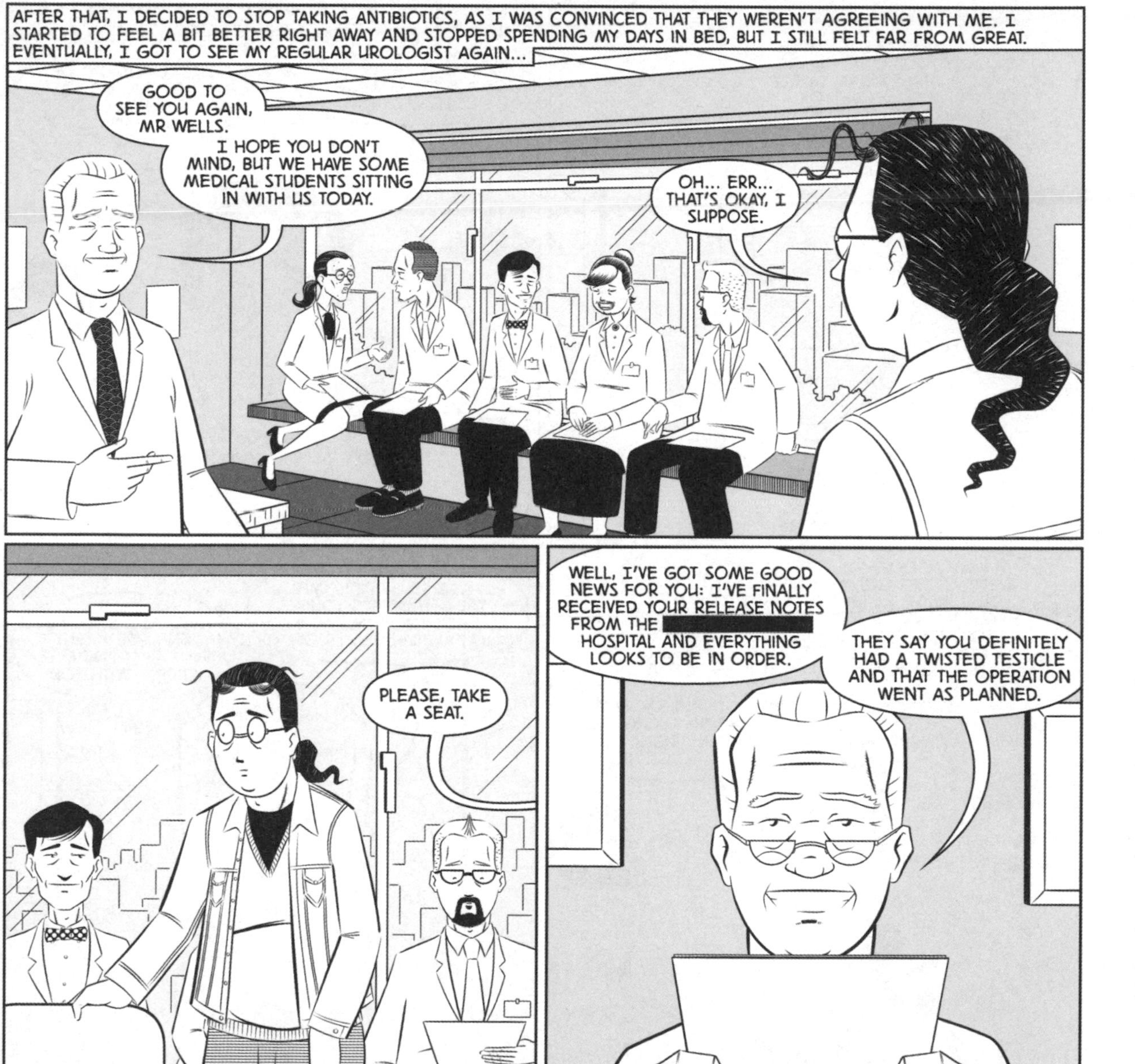
AFTER THAT, I DECIDED TO STOP TAKING ANTIBIOTICS, AS I WAS CONVINCED THAT THEY WEREN'T AGREEING WITH ME. I STARTED TO FEEL A BIT BETTER RIGHT AWAY AND STOPPED SPENDING MY DAYS IN BED, BUT I STILL FELT FAR FROM GREAT. EVENTUALLY, I GOT TO SEE MY REGULAR UROLOGIST AGAIN...
GOOD TO SEE YOU AGAIN, MR WELLS.
I HOPE YOU DON'T MIND, BUT WE HAVE SOME MEDICAL STUDENTS SITTING IN WITH US TODAY.
OH... ERR... THAT'S OKAY, I SUPPOSE.
PLEASE, TAKE A SEAT.
WELL, I'VE GOT SOME GOOD NEWS FOR YOU: I'VE FINALLY RECEIVED YOUR RELEASE NOTES FROM THE [redacted] HOSPITAL AND EVERYTHING LOOKS TO BE IN ORDER.
THEY SAY YOU DEFINITELY HAD A TWISTED TESTICLE AND THAT THE OPERATION WENT AS PLANNED.

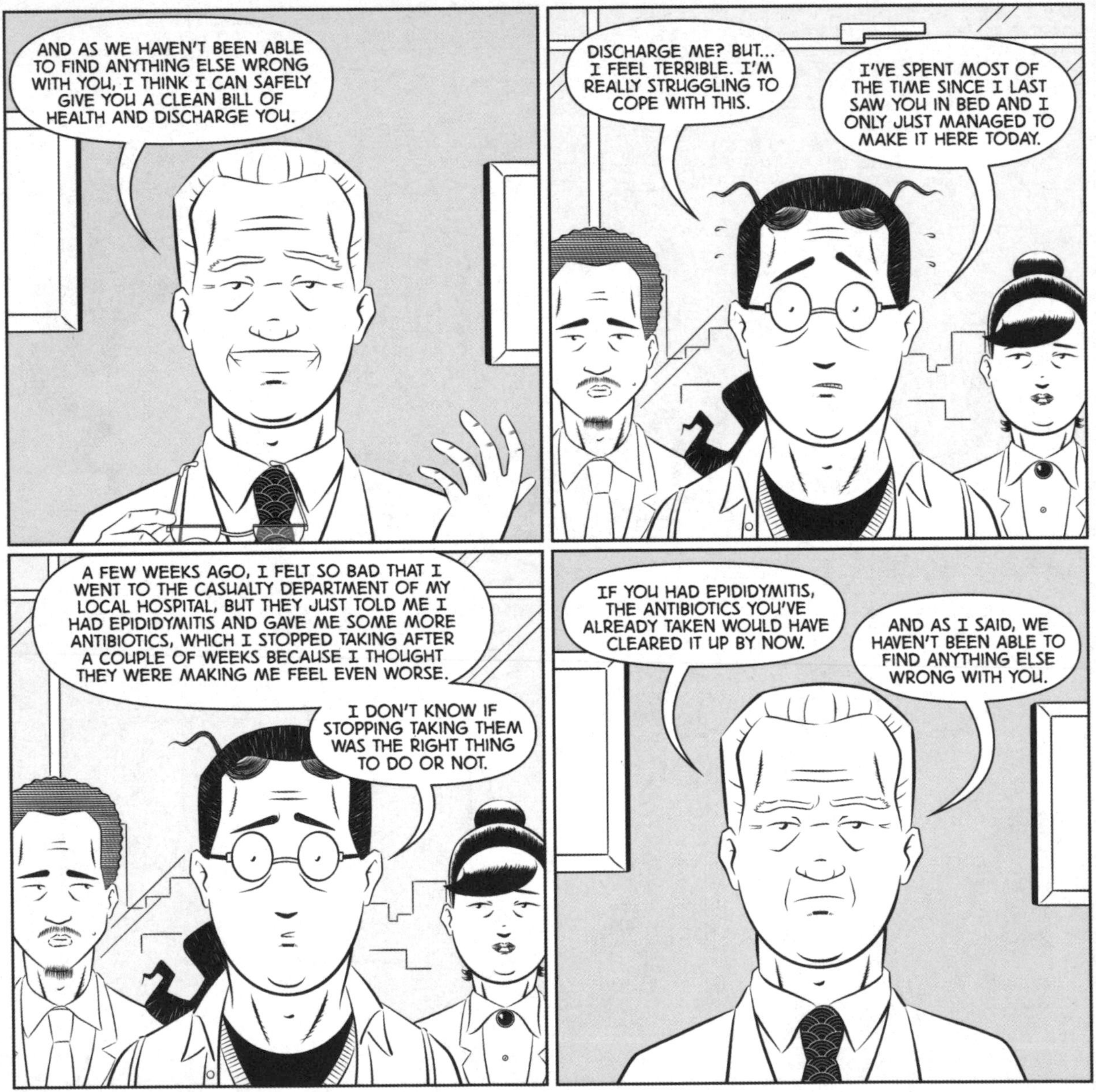
AND AS WE HAVEN'T BEEN ABLE TO FIND ANYTHING ELSE WRONG WITH YOU, I THINK I CAN SAFELY GIVE YOU A CLEAN BILL OF HEALTH AND DISCHARGE YOU.
DISCHARGE ME? BUT... I FEEL TERRIBLE. I'M REALLY STRUGGLING TO COPE WITH THIS.
I'VE SPENT MOST OF THE TIME SINCE I LAST SAW YOU IN BED AND I ONLY JUST MANAGED TO MAKE IT HERE TODAY.
A FEW WEEKS AGO, I FELT SO BAD THAT I WENT TO THE CASUALTY DEPARTMENT OF MY LOCAL HOSPITAL, BUT THEY JUST TOLD ME I HAD EPIDIDYMITIS AND GAVE ME SOME MORE ANTIBIOTICS, WHICH I STOPPED TAKING AFTER A COUPLE OF WEEKS BECAUSE I THOUGHT THEY WERE MAKING ME FEEL EVEN WORSE.
I DON'T KNOW IF STOPPING TAKING THEM WAS THE RIGHT THING TO DO OR NOT.
IF YOU HAD EPIDIDYMITIS, THE ANTIBIOTICS YOU'VE ALREADY TAKEN WOULD HAVE CLEARED IT UP BY NOW.
AND AS I SAID, WE HAVEN'T BEEN ABLE TO FIND ANYTHING ELSE WRONG WITH YOU.

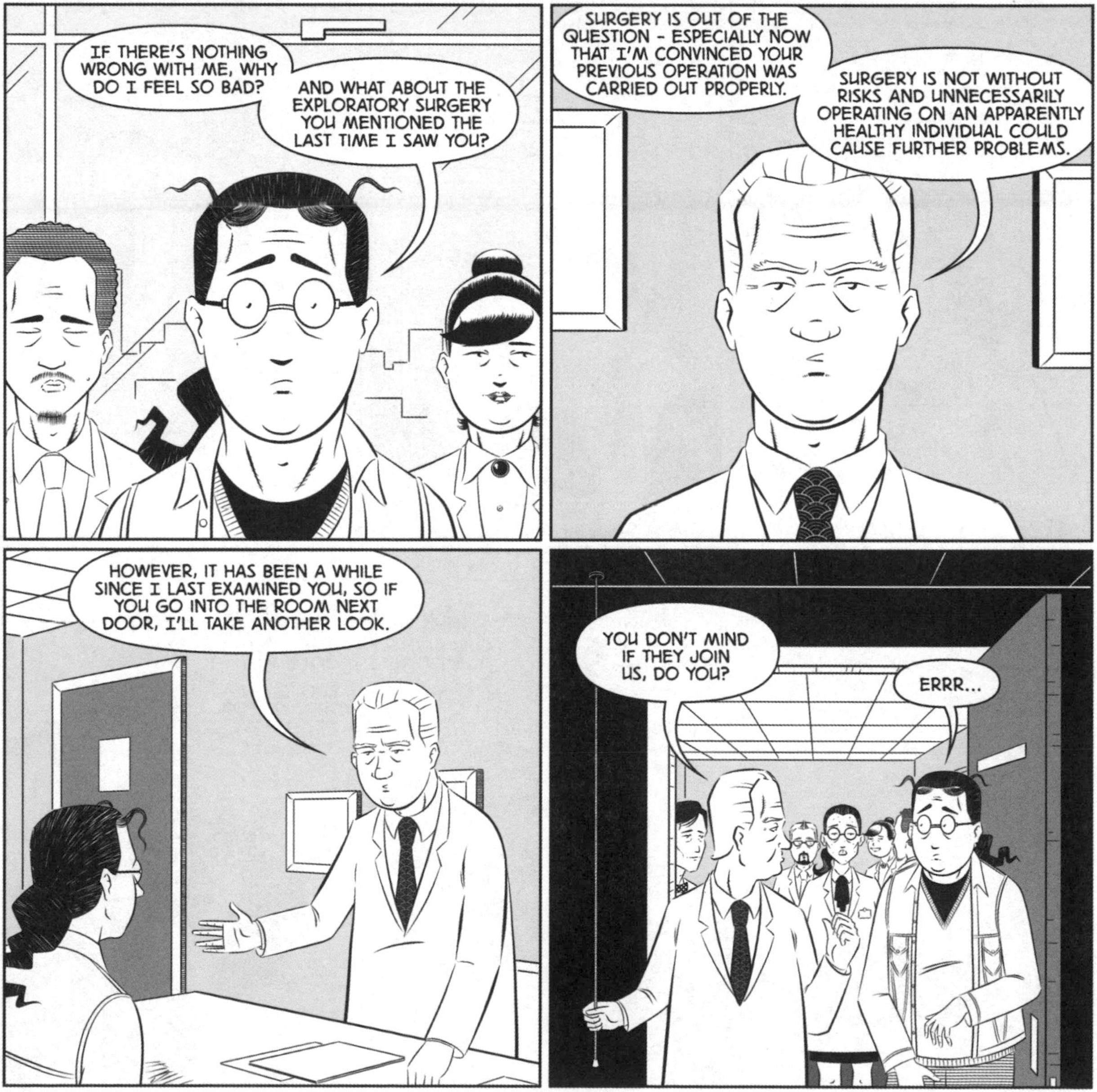
IF THERE'S NOTHING WRONG WITH ME, WHY DO I FEEL SO BAD?
AND WHAT ABOUT THE EXPLORATORY SURGERY YOU MENTIONED THE LAST TIME I SAW YOU?
SURGERY IS OUT OF THE QUESTION - ESPECIALLY NOW THAT I'M CONVINCED YOUR PREVIOUS OPERATION WAS CARRIED OUT PROPERLY.
SURGERY IS NOT WITHOUT RISKS AND UNNECESSARILY OPERATING ON AN APPARENTLY HEALTHY INDIVIDUAL COULD CAUSE FURTHER PROBLEMS.
HOWEVER, IT HAS BEEN A WHILE SINCE I LAST EXAMINED YOU, SO IF YOU GO INTO THE ROOM NEXT DOOR, I'LL TAKE ANOTHER LOOK.
YOU DON'T MIND IF THEY JOIN US, DO YOU?
ERRR...

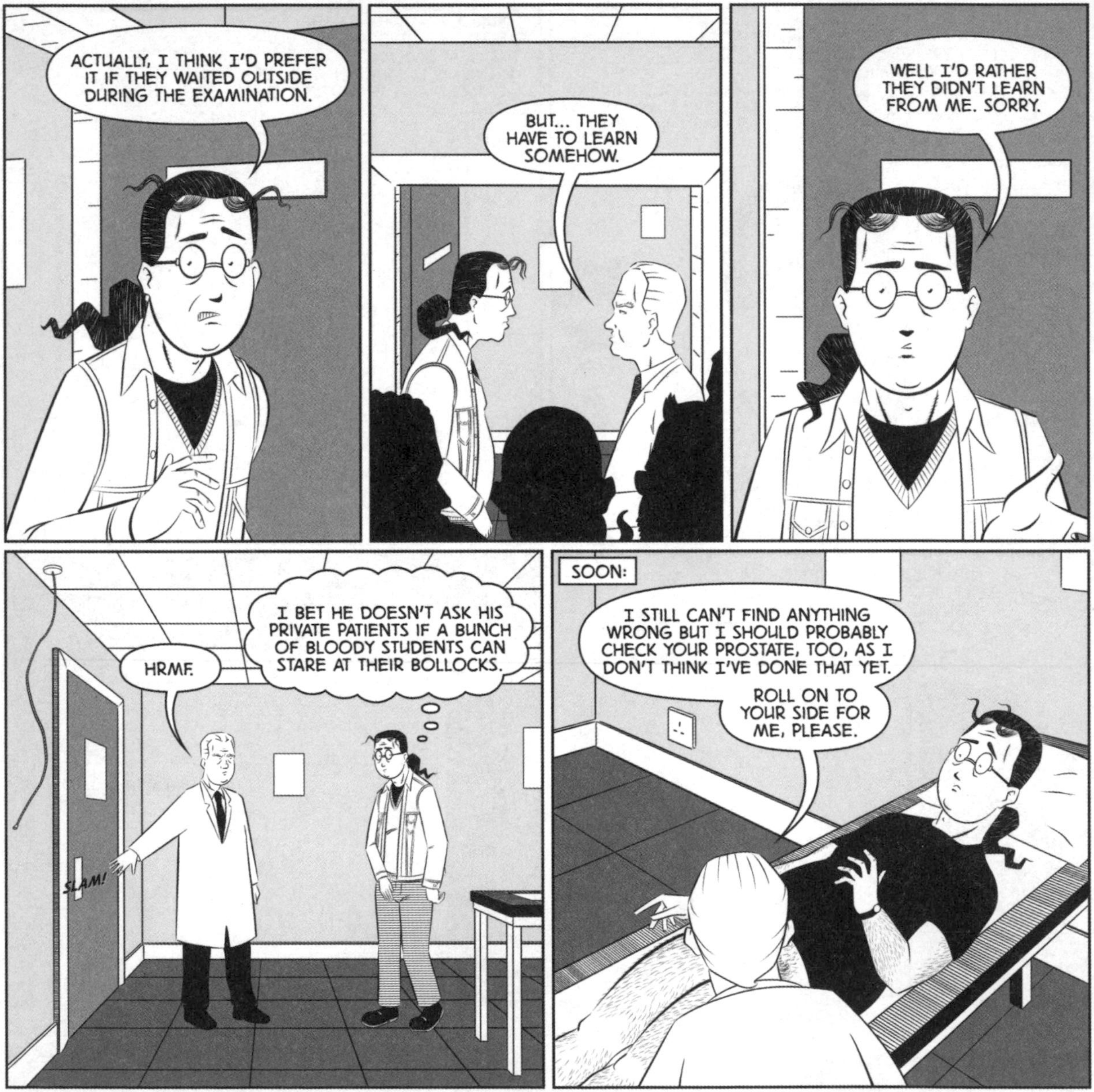
ACTUALLY, I THINK I'D PREFER IT IF THEY WAITED OUTSIDE DURING THE EXAMINATION.
BUT... THEY HAVE TO LEARN SOMEHOW.
WELL I'D RATHER THEY DIDN'T LEARN FROM ME. SORRY.
HRMF.
SLAM!
I BET HE DOESN'T ASK HIS PRIVATE PATIENTS IF A BUNCH OF BLOODY STUDENTS CAN STARE AT THEIR BOLLOCKS.
SOON:
I STILL CAN'T FIND ANYTHING WRONG BUT I SHOULD PROBABLY CHECK YOUR PROSTATE, TOO, AS I DON'T THINK I'VE DONE THAT YET.
ROLL ON TO YOUR SIDE FOR ME, PLEASE.

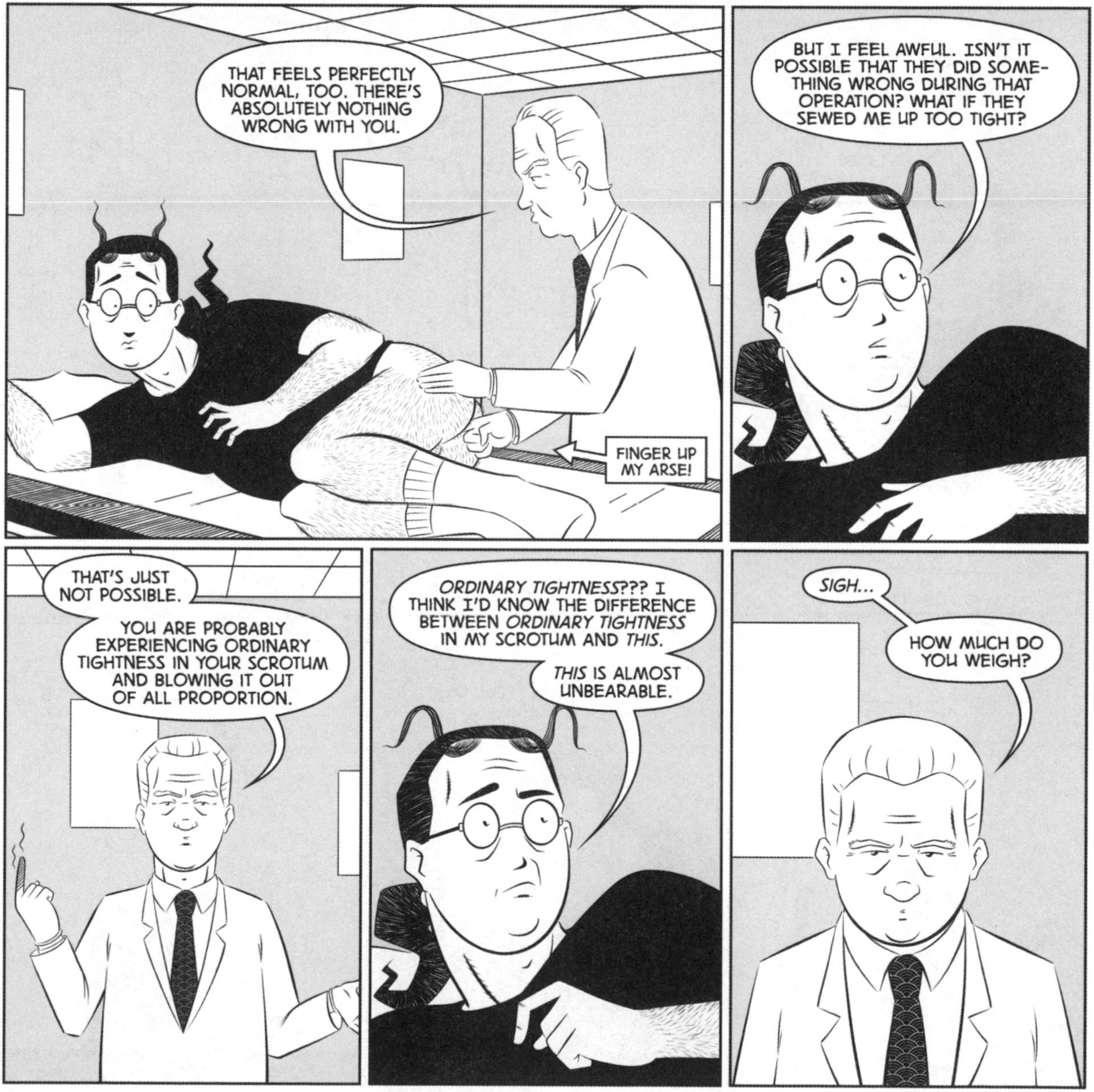
THAT FEELS PERFECTLY NORMAL, TOO. THERE'S ABSOLUTELY NOTHING WRONG WITH YOU.
FINGER UP MY ARSE!
BUT I FEEL AWFUL. ISN'T IT POSSIBLE THAT THEY DID SOME-THING WRONG DURING THAT OPERATION? WHAT IF THEY SEWED ME UP TOO TIGHT?
THAT'S JUST NOT POSSIBLE.
YOU ARE PROBABLY EXPERIENCING ORDINARY TIGHTNESS IN YOUR SCROTUM AND BLOWING IT OUT OF ALL PROPORTION.
ORDINARY TIGHTNESS??? I THINK I'D KNOW THE DIFFERENCE BETWEEN ORDINARY TIGHTNESS IN MY SCROTUM AND THIS.
THIS IS ALMOST UNBEARABLE.
SIGH...
HOW MUCH DO YOU WEIGH?

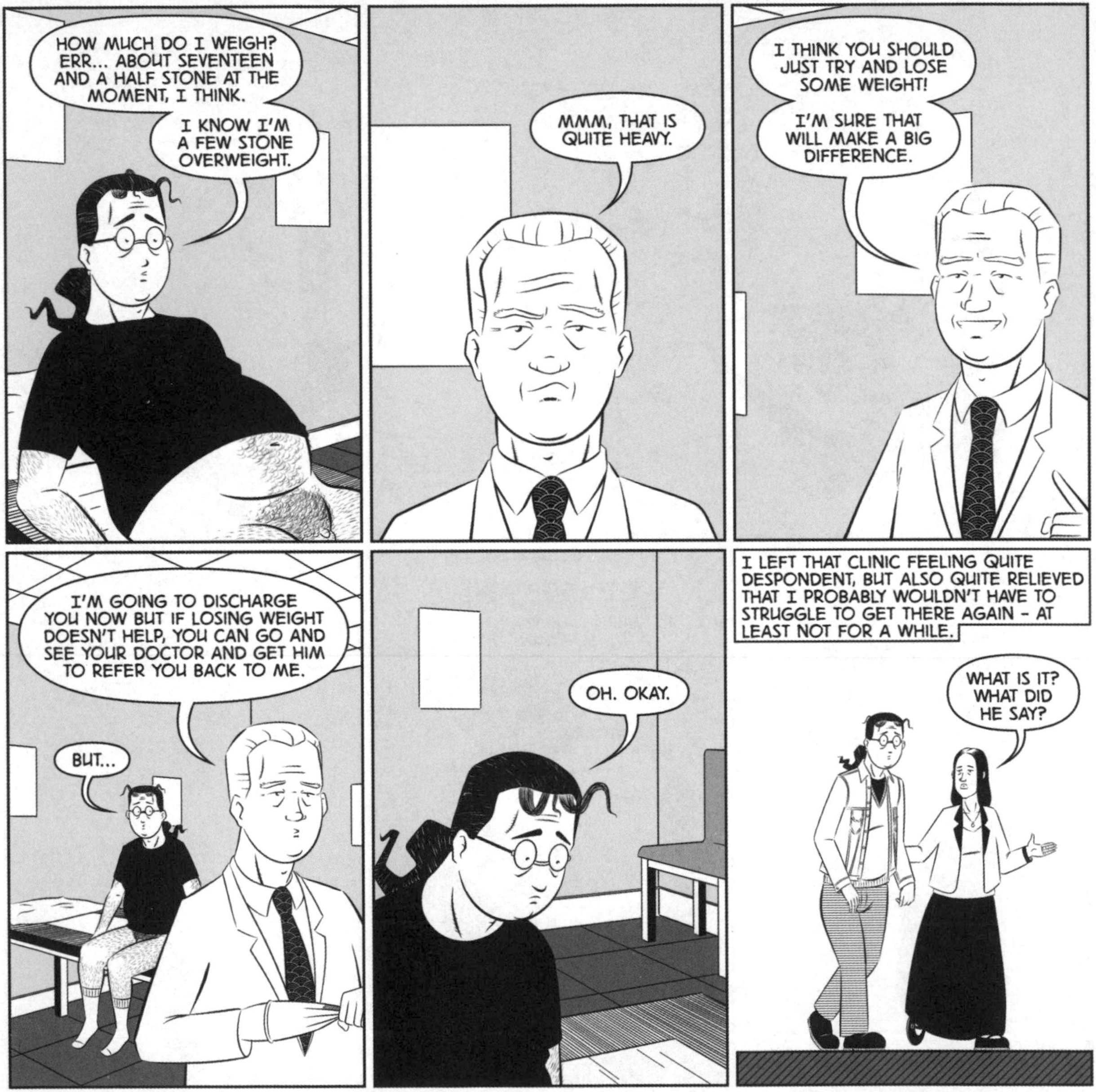
HOW MUCH DO I WEIGH? ERR... ABOUT SEVENTEEN AND A HALF STONE AT THE MOMENT, I THINK.
I KNOW I'M A FEW STONE OVERWEIGHT.
MMM, THAT IS QUITE HEAVY.
I THINK YOU SHOULD JUST TRY AND LOSE SOME WEIGHT!
I'M SURE THAT WILL MAKE A BIG DIFFERENCE.
I'M GOING TO DISCHARGE YOU NOW BUT IF LOSING WEIGHT DOESN'T HELP, YOU CAN GO AND SEE YOUR DOCTOR AND GET HIM TO REFER YOU BACK TO ME.
BUT...
OH. OKAY.
I LEFT THAT CLINIC FEELING QUITE DESPONDENT, BUT ALSO QUITE RELIEVED THAT I PROBABLY WOULDN'T HAVE TO STRUGGLE TO GET THERE AGAIN - AT LEAST NOT FOR A WHILE.
WHAT IS IT? WHAT DID HE SAY?

JUST BEFORE I LEFT THE HOSPITAL, I NEEDED TO URINATE URGENTLY. AFTER I'D BEEN, THE TIGHTNESS IN MY GROIN EASED OFF A LOT AND I FELT MUCH BETTER FOR THE REST OF THAT DAY.
BLOODY HELL - LOOSE BALLS!
HAVING MY PROSTATE PRODDED SEEMED TO HAVE DONE ME SOME GOOD.
BLADDER
PROSTATE
CLENCHED ANUS
BEFORE WE HEADED HOME, MY WIFE AND I STOPPED FOR LUNCH IN A NEARBY PUB AND THE DESPAIR I'D BEEN FEELING SLOWLY EASED OFF, TOO. I DECIDED THAT I WASN'T GOING TO WASTE ANY MORE TIME GOING TO SEE DOCTORS.
I MEAN, IF THINGS GOT *REALLY* BAD, THEN AT SOME POINT I'D HAVE TO GO BACK TO A HOSPITAL AND THEY'D FIND SOMETHING WRONG WITH ME EVENTUALLY, WOULDN'T THEY? FOR NOW, THOUGH, I WAS GOING TO TRY AND SORT MY OWN HEALTH OUT BY DIETING.
SELF-HELP
ASTROLOGY
AFTER ALL, DIETING HAD WORKED THE LAST TIME I'D BEEN ILL, HADN'T IT?

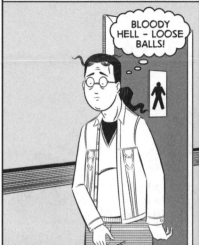

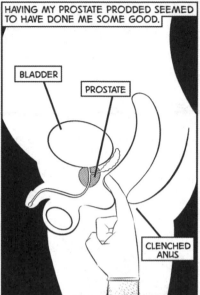

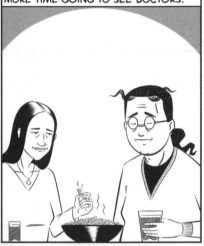

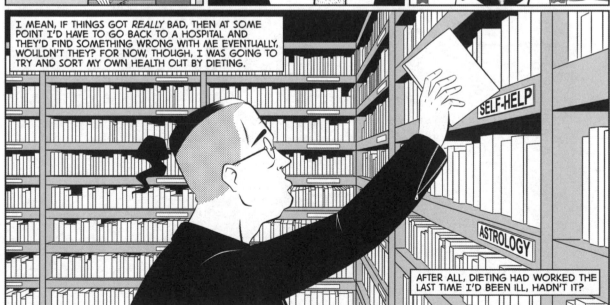

6. FLASHBACK (OR: HOW I LEARNED TO HATE MY COLON)

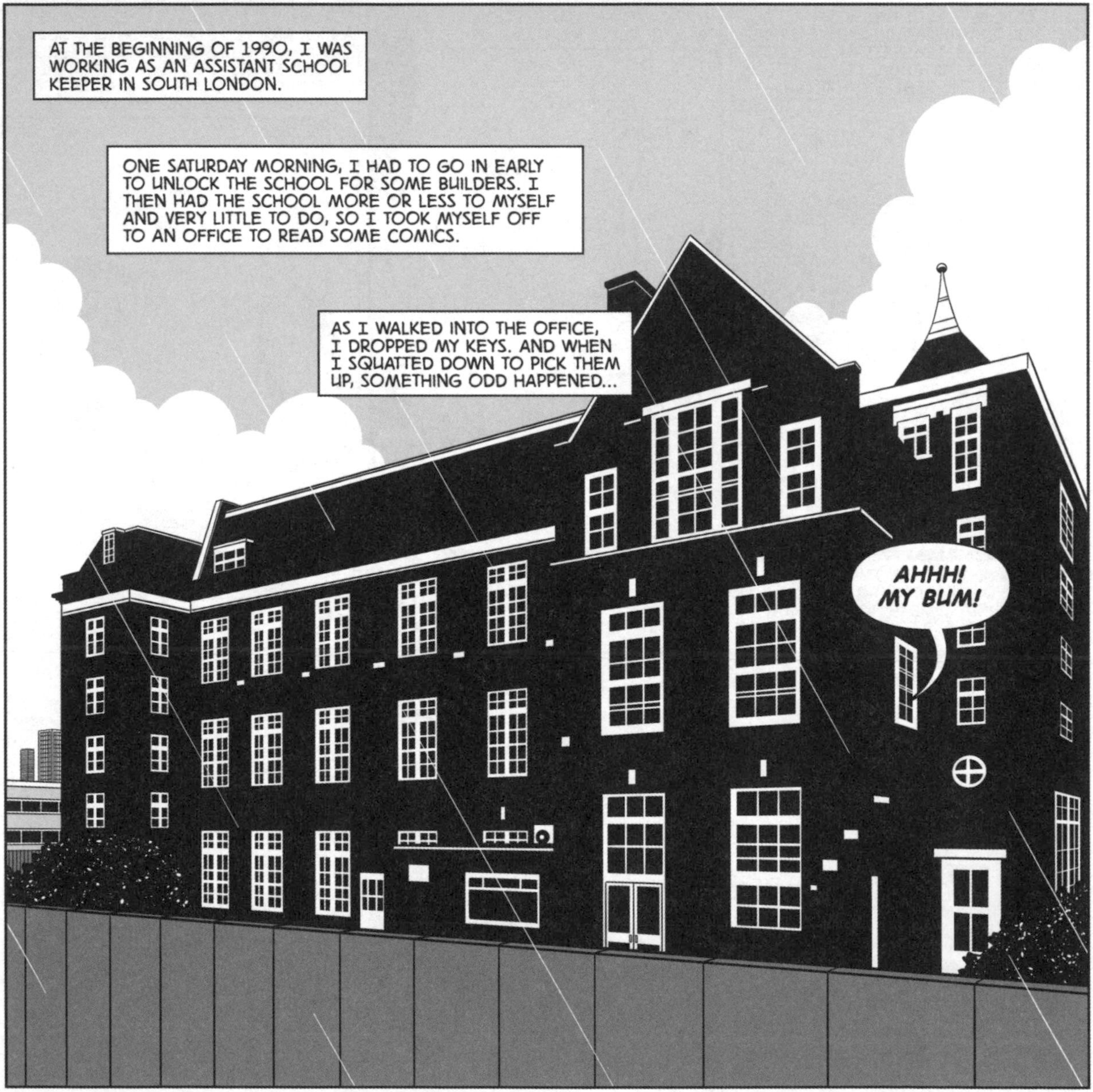
AT THE BEGINNING OF 1990, I WAS WORKING AS AN ASSISTANT SCHOOL KEEPER IN SOUTH LONDON.
ONE SATURDAY MORNING, I HAD TO GO IN EARLY TO UNLOCK THE SCHOOL FOR SOME BUILDERS. I THEN HAD THE SCHOOL MORE OR LESS TO MYSELF AND VERY LITTLE TO DO, SO I TOOK MYSELF OFF TO AN OFFICE TO READ SOME COMICS.
AS I WALKED INTO THE OFFICE, I DROPPED MY KEYS. AND WHEN I SQUATTED DOWN TO PICK THEM UP, SOMETHING ODD HAPPENED...
AHHH! MY BUM!

IN THE COUPLE OF YEARS BEFORE THIS, LIKE A LOT OF PEOPLE IN THEIR LATE-TEENS, I HAD: A) DISCOVERED THE JOYS OF ALCOHOL (AND DODGY LATE-NIGHT EATING ESTABLISHMENTS)...

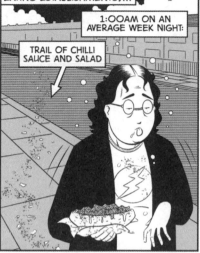

1:OOAM ON AN AVERAGE WEEK NIGHT:

TRAIL OF CHILLI SAUCE AND SALAD

AND B) STARTED SMOKING.

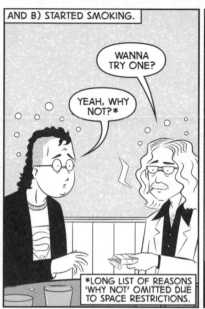

WANNA TRY ONE?

YEAH, WHY NOT?*

*LONG LIST OF REASONS 'WHY NOT' OMITTED DUE TO SPACE RESTRICTIONS.

THIS HAD BEEN FUN FOR A WHILE, BUT MY UNHEALTHY LIFESTYLE SOON CAUGHT UP WITH ME.

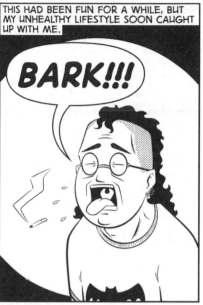

BARK!!!

I PUT ON A LOT OF WEIGHT, DEVELOPED A PERSISTENT CHEST INFECTION, WHICH REQUIRED SEVERAL COURSES OF ANTIBIOTICS, AND I BEGAN TO FEEL *EXTREMELY* RUN DOWN.

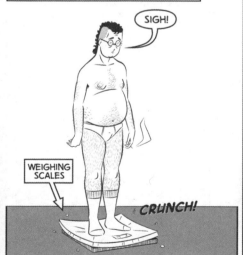

SIGH!

WEIGHING SCALES

CRUNCH!

BY THE BEGINNING OF 1990, SHORTLY BEFORE MY TWENTY-FIRST BIRTHDAY, I WEIGHED ABOUT EIGHTEEN-AND-A-HALF STONE - THE MOST THAT I HAVE EVER WEIGHED - AND HAD ALMOST NO ENERGY AT ALL.

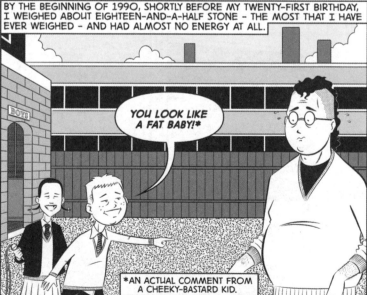

YOU LOOK LIKE A FAT BABY!*

BOYS

*AN ACTUAL COMMENT FROM A CHEEKY-BASTARD KID.

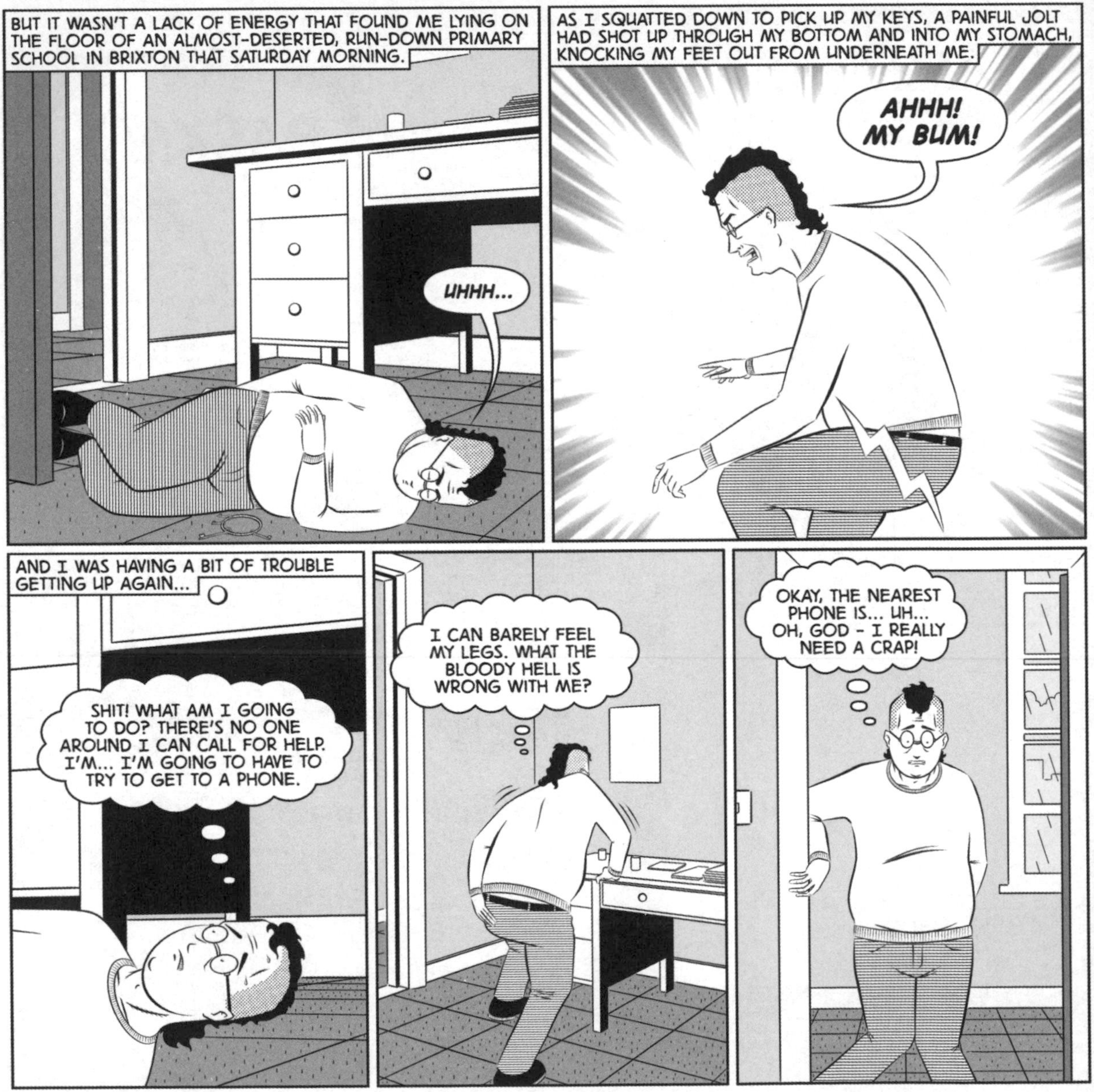
BUT IT WASN'T A LACK OF ENERGY THAT FOUND ME LYING ON THE FLOOR OF AN ALMOST-DESERTED, RUN-DOWN PRIMARY SCHOOL IN BRIXTON THAT SATURDAY MORNING.
UHHH...
AS I SQUATTED DOWN TO PICK UP MY KEYS, A PAINFUL JOLT HAD SHOT UP THROUGH MY BOTTOM AND INTO MY STOMACH, KNOCKING MY FEET OUT FROM UNDERNEATH ME.
AHHH! MY BUM!
AND I WAS HAVING A BIT OF TROUBLE GETTING UP AGAIN...
SHIT! WHAT AM I GOING TO DO? THERE'S NO ONE AROUND I CAN CALL FOR HELP. I'M... I'M GOING TO HAVE TO TRY TO GET TO A PHONE.
I CAN BARELY FEEL MY LEGS. WHAT THE BLOODY HELL IS WRONG WITH ME?
OKAY, THE NEAREST PHONE IS... UH... OH, GOD - I REALLY NEED A CRAP!

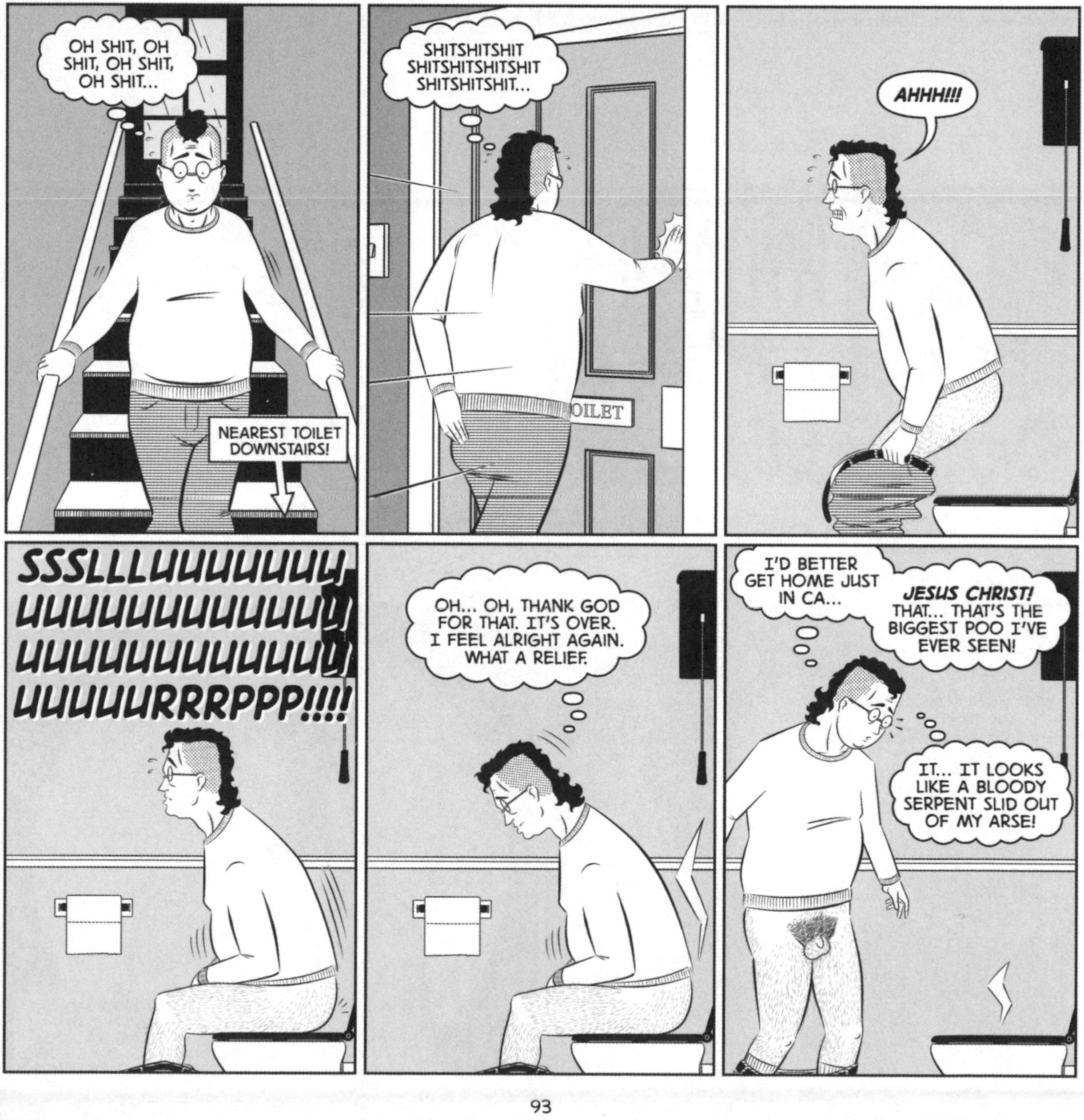
OH SHIT, OH SHIT, OH SHIT, OH SHIT...
NEAREST TOILET DOWNSTAIRS!
SHITSHITSHIT SHITSHITSHITSHIT SHITSHITSHIT...
OILET
AHHH!!!
SSSLLLUUUUUUUU UUUUUUUUUUUUUU UUUUUUUUUUUUUU UUUUURRRPPP!!!!
OH... OH, THANK GOD FOR THAT. IT'S OVER. I FEEL ALRIGHT AGAIN. WHAT A RELIEF.
I'D BETTER GET HOME JUST IN CA...
JESUS CHRIST! THAT... THAT'S THE BIGGEST POO I'VE EVER SEEN!
IT... IT LOOKS LIKE A BLOODY SERPENT SLID OUT OF MY ARSE!

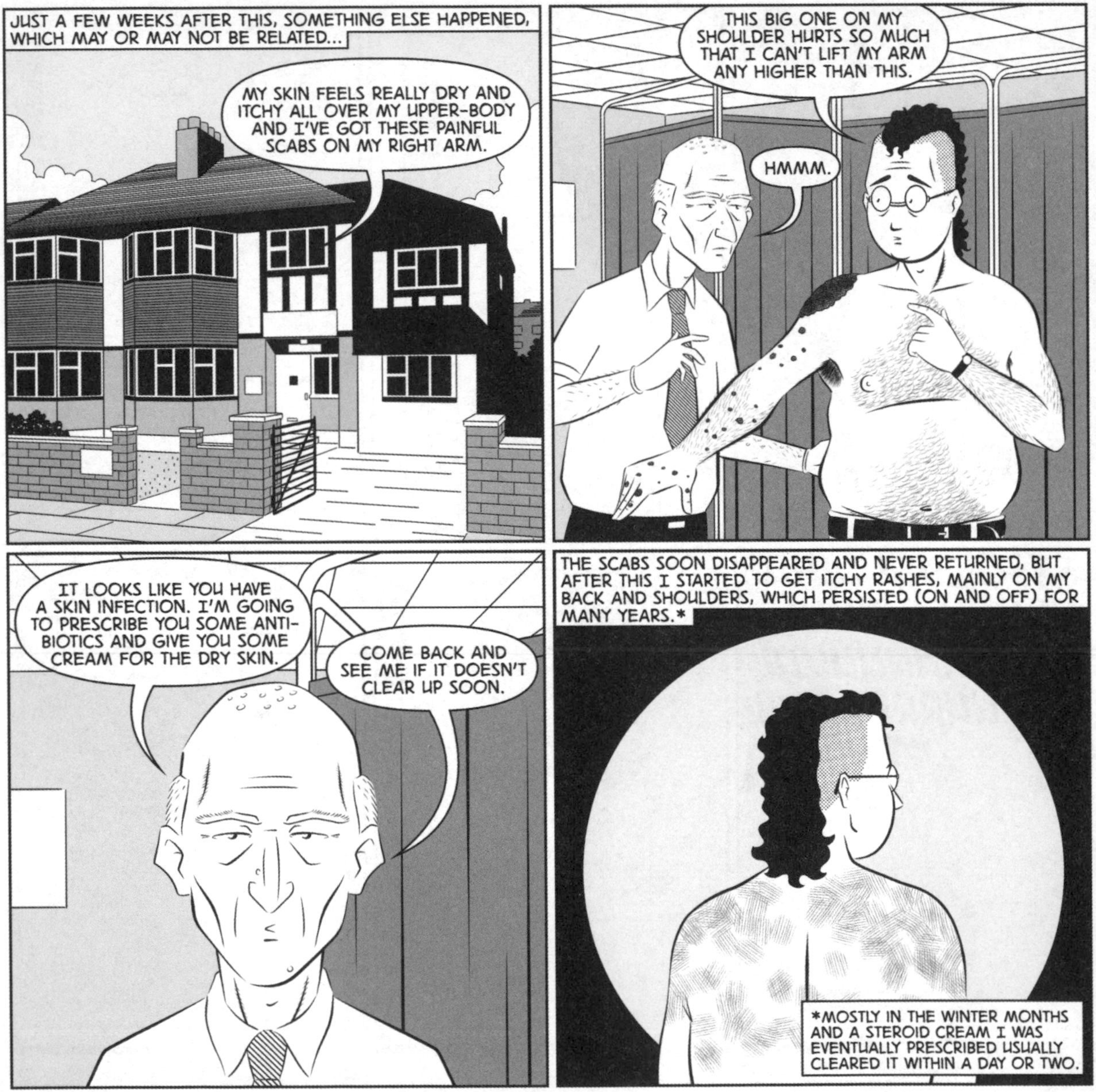
JUST A FEW WEEKS AFTER THIS, SOMETHING ELSE HAPPENED, WHICH MAY OR MAY NOT BE RELATED...
MY SKIN FEELS REALLY DRY AND ITCHY ALL OVER MY UPPER-BODY AND I'VE GOT THESE PAINFUL SCABS ON MY RIGHT ARM.
THIS BIG ONE ON MY SHOULDER HURTS SO MUCH THAT I CAN'T LIFT MY ARM ANY HIGHER THAN THIS.
HMMM.
IT LOOKS LIKE YOU HAVE A SKIN INFECTION. I'M GOING TO PRESCRIBE YOU SOME ANTI-BIOTICS AND GIVE YOU SOME CREAM FOR THE DRY SKIN.
COME BACK AND SEE ME IF IT DOESN'T CLEAR UP SOON.
THE SCABS SOON DISAPPEARED AND NEVER RETURNED, BUT AFTER THIS I STARTED TO GET ITCHY RASHES, MAINLY ON MY BACK AND SHOULDERS, WHICH PERSISTED (ON AND OFF) FOR MANY YEARS.*
*MOSTLY IN THE WINTER MONTHS AND A STEROID CREAM I WAS EVENTUALLY PRESCRIBED USUALLY CLEARED IT WITHIN A DAY OR TWO.

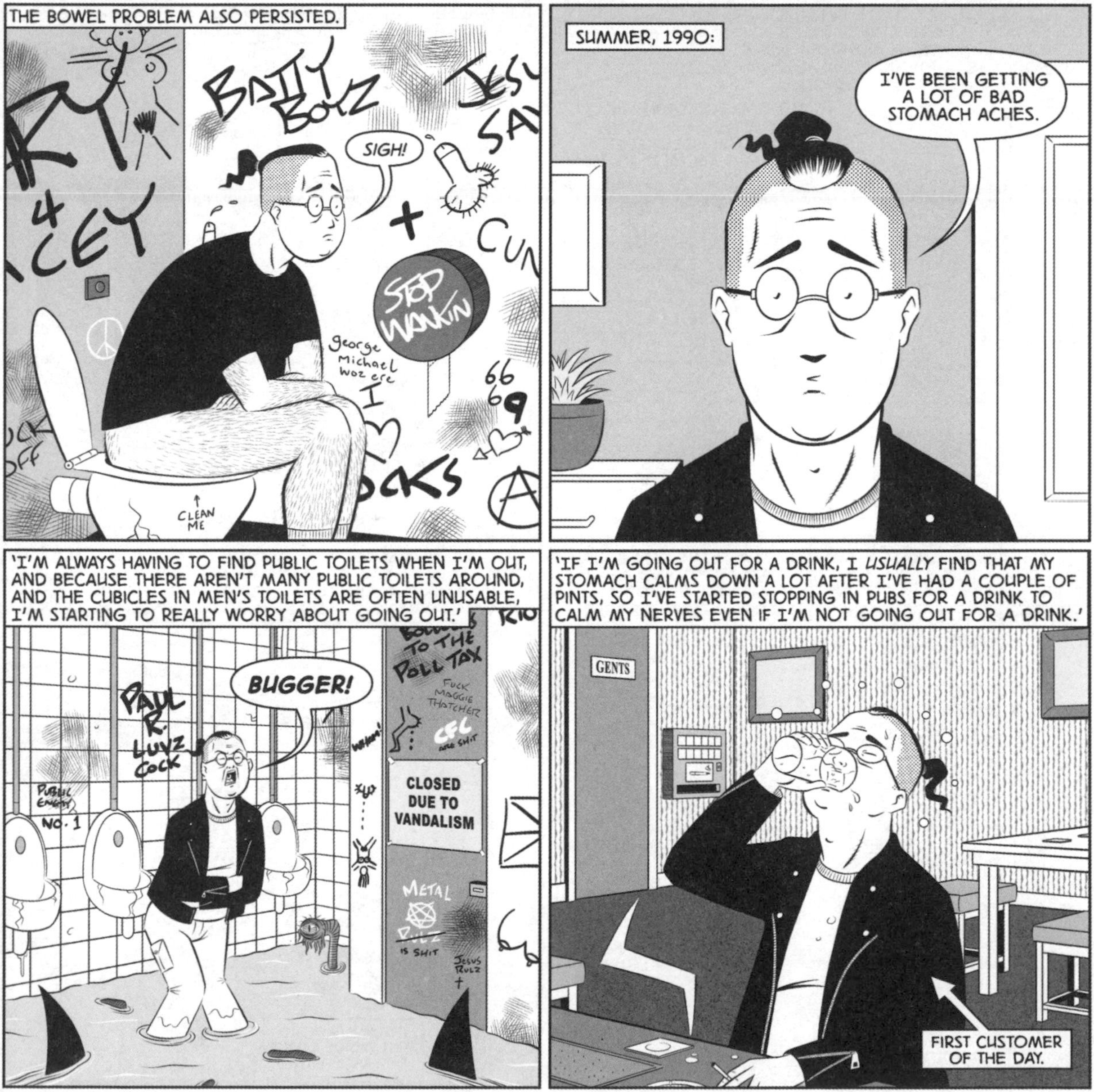
THE BOWEL PROBLEM ALSO PERSISTED.
BATTY BOYZ
SIGH!
STOP WANKIN
george Michael woz ere
CLEAN ME
SUMMER, 1990:
I'VE BEEN GETTING A LOT OF BAD STOMACH ACHES.
'I'M ALWAYS HAVING TO FIND PUBLIC TOILETS WHEN I'M OUT, AND BECAUSE THERE AREN'T MANY PUBLIC TOILETS AROUND, AND THE CUBICLES IN MEN'S TOILETS ARE OFTEN UNUSABLE, I'M STARTING TO REALLY WORRY ABOUT GOING OUT.'
BUGGER!
PAUL R. LUVZ COCK
TO THE POLL TAX
FUCK MAGGIE THATCHER
CLOSED DUE TO VANDALISM
METAL
IS SHIT
JESUS RULZ
'IF I'M GOING OUT FOR A DRINK, I *USUALLY* FIND THAT MY STOMACH CALMS DOWN A LOT AFTER I'VE HAD A COUPLE OF PINTS, SO I'VE STARTED STOPPING IN PUBS FOR A DRINK TO CALM MY NERVES EVEN IF I'M NOT GOING OUT FOR A DRINK.'
GENTS
FIRST CUSTOMER OF THE DAY.

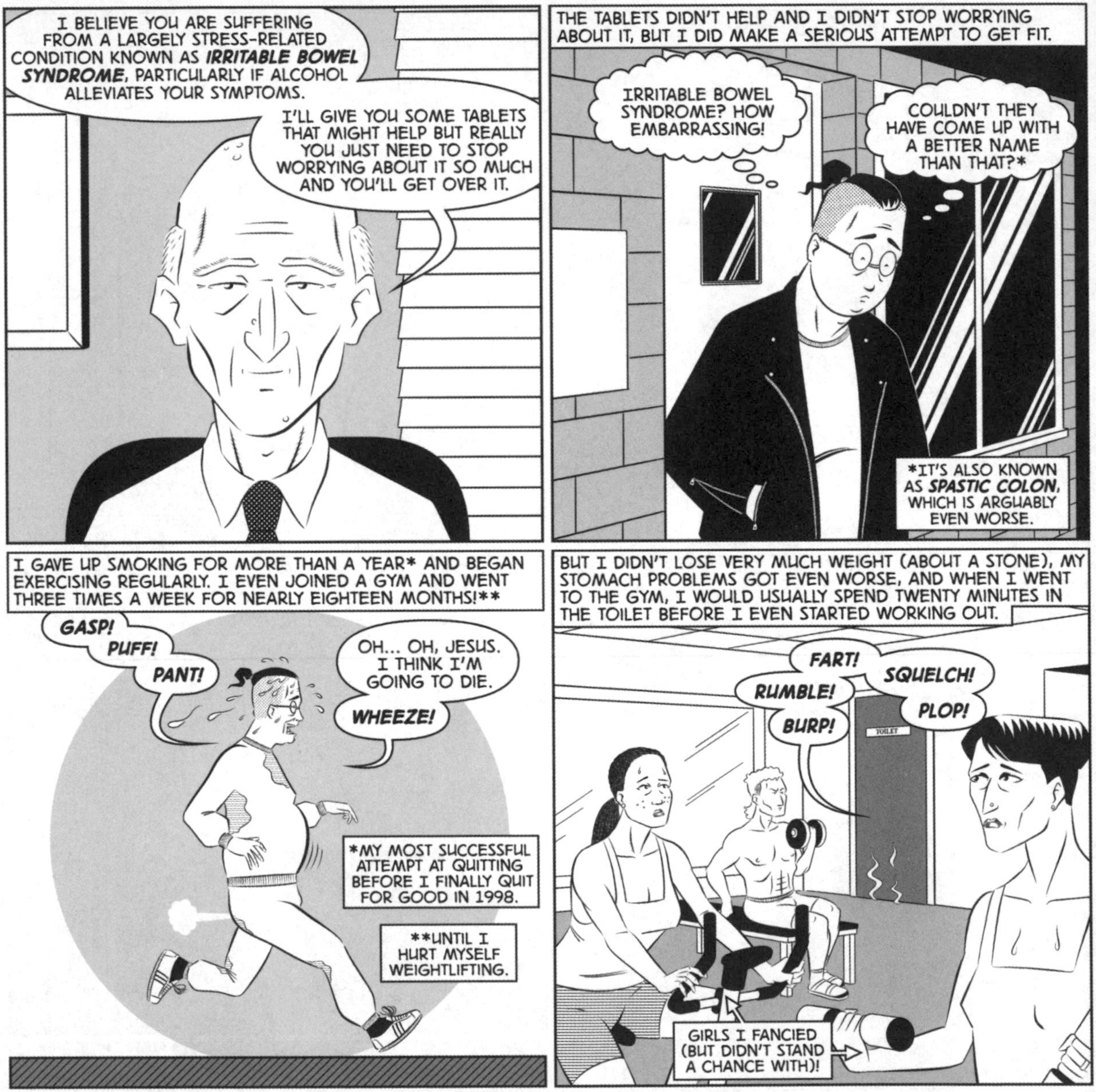
I BELIEVE YOU ARE SUFFERING FROM A LARGELY STRESS-RELATED CONDITION KNOWN AS ***IRRITABLE BOWEL SYNDROME***, PARTICULARLY IF ALCOHOL ALLEVIATES YOUR SYMPTOMS.
I'LL GIVE YOU SOME TABLETS THAT MIGHT HELP BUT REALLY YOU JUST NEED TO STOP WORRYING ABOUT IT SO MUCH AND YOU'LL GET OVER IT.
THE TABLETS DIDN'T HELP AND I DIDN'T STOP WORRYING ABOUT IT, BUT I DID MAKE A SERIOUS ATTEMPT TO GET FIT.
IRRITABLE BOWEL SYNDROME? HOW EMBARRASSING!
COULDN'T THEY HAVE COME UP WITH A BETTER NAME THAN THAT?*
*IT'S ALSO KNOWN AS ***SPASTIC COLON***, WHICH IS ARGUABLY EVEN WORSE.
I GAVE UP SMOKING FOR MORE THAN A YEAR* AND BEGAN EXERCISING REGULARLY. I EVEN JOINED A GYM AND WENT THREE TIMES A WEEK FOR NEARLY EIGHTEEN MONTHS!**
GASP!
PUFF!
PANT!
OH... OH, JESUS. I THINK I'M GOING TO DIE.
WHEEZE!
*MY MOST SUCCESSFUL ATTEMPT AT QUITTING BEFORE I FINALLY QUIT FOR GOOD IN 1998.
**UNTIL I HURT MYSELF WEIGHTLIFTING.
BUT I DIDN'T LOSE VERY MUCH WEIGHT (ABOUT A STONE), MY STOMACH PROBLEMS GOT EVEN WORSE, AND WHEN I WENT TO THE GYM, I WOULD USUALLY SPEND TWENTY MINUTES IN THE TOILET BEFORE I EVEN STARTED WORKING OUT.
FART!
RUMBLE!
BURP!
SQUELCH!
PLOP!
TOILET
GIRLS I FANCIED (BUT DIDN'T STAND A CHANCE WITH)!

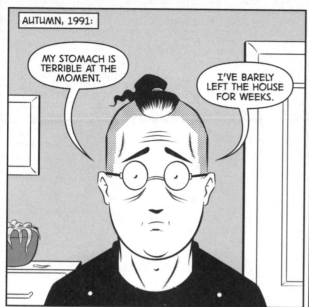

AUTUMN, 1991:

MY STOMACH IS TERRIBLE AT THE MOMENT.

I'VE BARELY LEFT THE HOUSE FOR WEEKS.

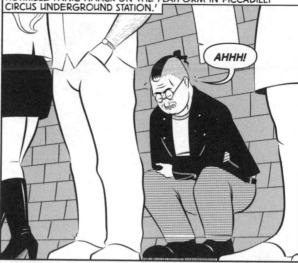

'A FEW WEEKS AGO, I WENT INTO LONDON TO SEE A FILM, STARTED TO GET A STOMACH ACHE ON MY WAY THERE, THEN DOUBLED OVER IN PAIN, NEARLY CRAPPED MYSELF, AND HAD A HORRIBLE PANIC ATTACK ON THE PLATFORM IN PICCADILLY CIRCUS UNDERGROUND STATION.'

AHHH!

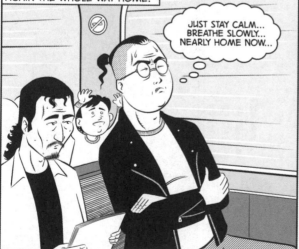

'I SOMEHOW MADE IT TO THE CINEMA, WHERE I WAS MEETING A FRIEND, BUT I SPENT AGES IN THE CINEMA TOILETS BEFORE THE FILM, EVEN LONGER IN THE TOILETS AFTER THE FILM, AND WORRIED ABOUT NEEDING TO GO TO THE TOILET AGAIN THE WHOLE WAY HOME.'

JUST STAY CALM... BREATHE SLOWLY... NEARLY HOME NOW...

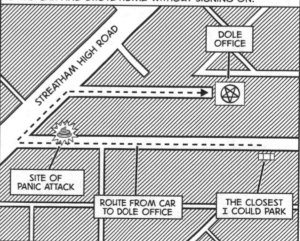

'I'M UNEMPLOYED AT THE MOMENT AND THE ONLY TIME I'VE BEEN OUT SINCE THEN IS WHEN I HAD TO GO AND SIGN ON LAST WEEK. I MANAGED TO DRIVE THERE, BUT AS I WAS WALKING FROM THE CAR TO THE DOLE OFFICE, MY STOMACH GOT REALLY BAD, I HAD A PANIC ATTACK IN THE STREET, RAN BACK TO THE CAR AND DROVE HOME WITHOUT SIGNING ON.'

STREATHAM HIGH ROAD

DOLE OFFICE

SITE OF PANIC ATTACK

ROUTE FROM CAR TO DOLE OFFICE

THE CLOSEST I COULD PARK

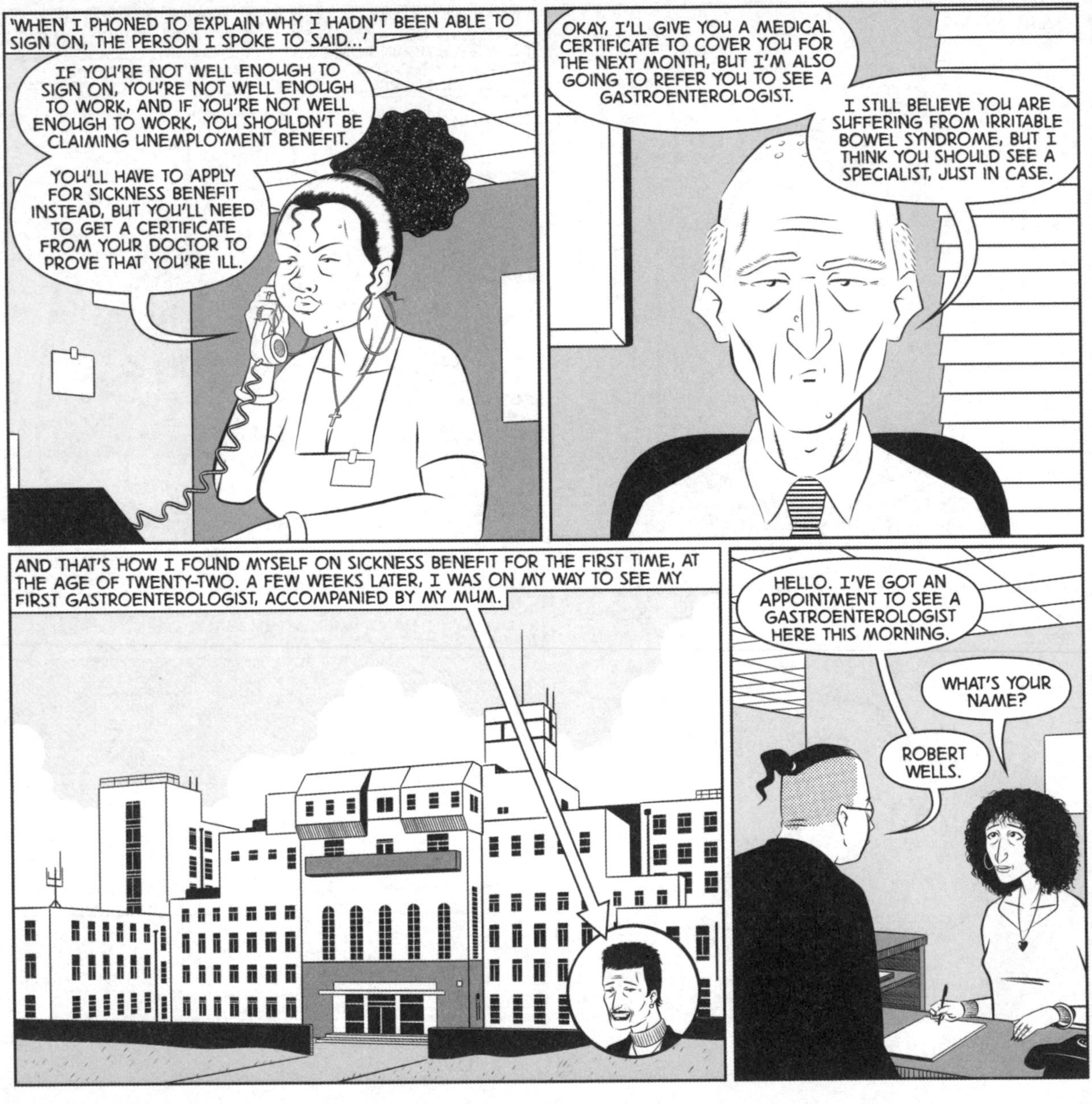

'WHEN I PHONED TO EXPLAIN WHY I HADN'T BEEN ABLE TO SIGN ON, THE PERSON I SPOKE TO SAID...'
IF YOU'RE NOT WELL ENOUGH TO SIGN ON, YOU'RE NOT WELL ENOUGH TO WORK, AND IF YOU'RE NOT WELL ENOUGH TO WORK, YOU SHOULDN'T BE CLAIMING UNEMPLOYMENT BENEFIT.
YOU'LL HAVE TO APPLY FOR SICKNESS BENEFIT INSTEAD, BUT YOU'LL NEED TO GET A CERTIFICATE FROM YOUR DOCTOR TO PROVE THAT YOU'RE ILL.
OKAY, I'LL GIVE YOU A MEDICAL CERTIFICATE TO COVER YOU FOR THE NEXT MONTH, BUT I'M ALSO GOING TO REFER YOU TO SEE A GASTROENTEROLOGIST.
I STILL BELIEVE YOU ARE SUFFERING FROM IRRITABLE BOWEL SYNDROME, BUT I THINK YOU SHOULD SEE A SPECIALIST, JUST IN CASE.
AND THAT'S HOW I FOUND MYSELF ON SICKNESS BENEFIT FOR THE FIRST TIME, AT THE AGE OF TWENTY-TWO. A FEW WEEKS LATER, I WAS ON MY WAY TO SEE MY FIRST GASTROENTEROLOGIST, ACCOMPANIED BY MY MUM.
HELLO. I'VE GOT AN APPOINTMENT TO SEE A GASTROENTEROLOGIST HERE THIS MORNING.
WHAT'S YOUR NAME?
ROBERT WELLS.

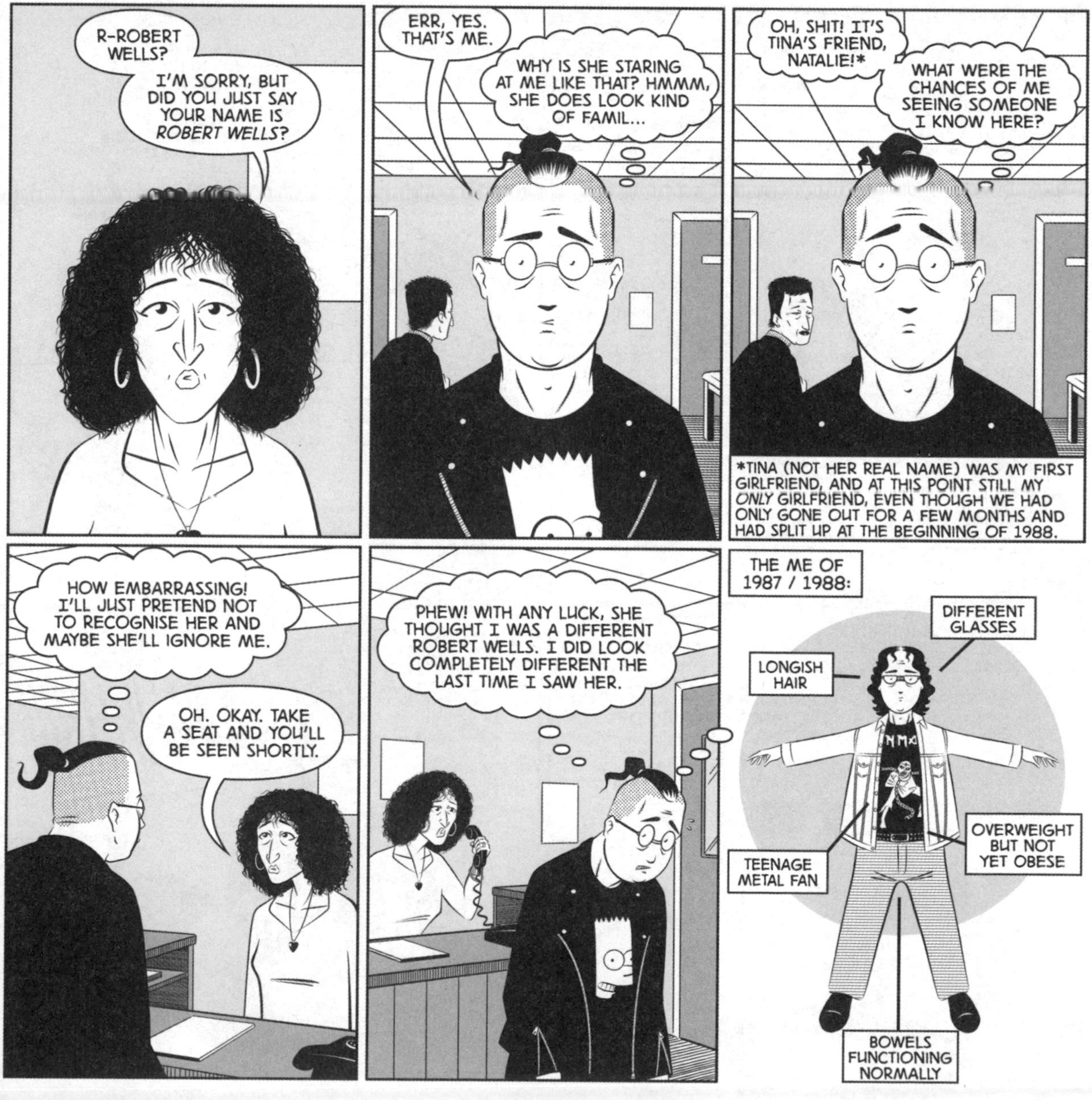
R-ROBERT WELLS?
I'M SORRY, BUT DID YOU JUST SAY YOUR NAME IS *ROBERT WELLS*?
ERR, YES. THAT'S ME.
WHY IS SHE STARING AT ME LIKE THAT? HMMM, SHE DOES LOOK KIND OF FAMIL...
OH, SHIT! IT'S TINA'S FRIEND, NATALIE!*
WHAT WERE THE CHANCES OF ME SEEING SOMEONE I KNOW HERE?
*TINA (NOT HER REAL NAME) WAS MY FIRST GIRLFRIEND, AND AT THIS POINT STILL MY *ONLY* GIRLFRIEND, EVEN THOUGH WE HAD ONLY GONE OUT FOR A FEW MONTHS AND HAD SPLIT UP AT THE BEGINNING OF 1988.
HOW EMBARRASSING! I'LL JUST PRETEND NOT TO RECOGNISE HER AND MAYBE SHE'LL IGNORE ME.
OH. OKAY. TAKE A SEAT AND YOU'LL BE SEEN SHORTLY.
PHEW! WITH ANY LUCK, SHE THOUGHT I WAS A DIFFERENT ROBERT WELLS. I DID LOOK COMPLETELY DIFFERENT THE LAST TIME I SAW HER.
THE ME OF 1987 / 1988:
DIFFERENT GLASSES
LONGISH HAIR
OVERWEIGHT BUT NOT YET OBESE
TEENAGE METAL FAN
BOWELS FUNCTIONING NORMALLY

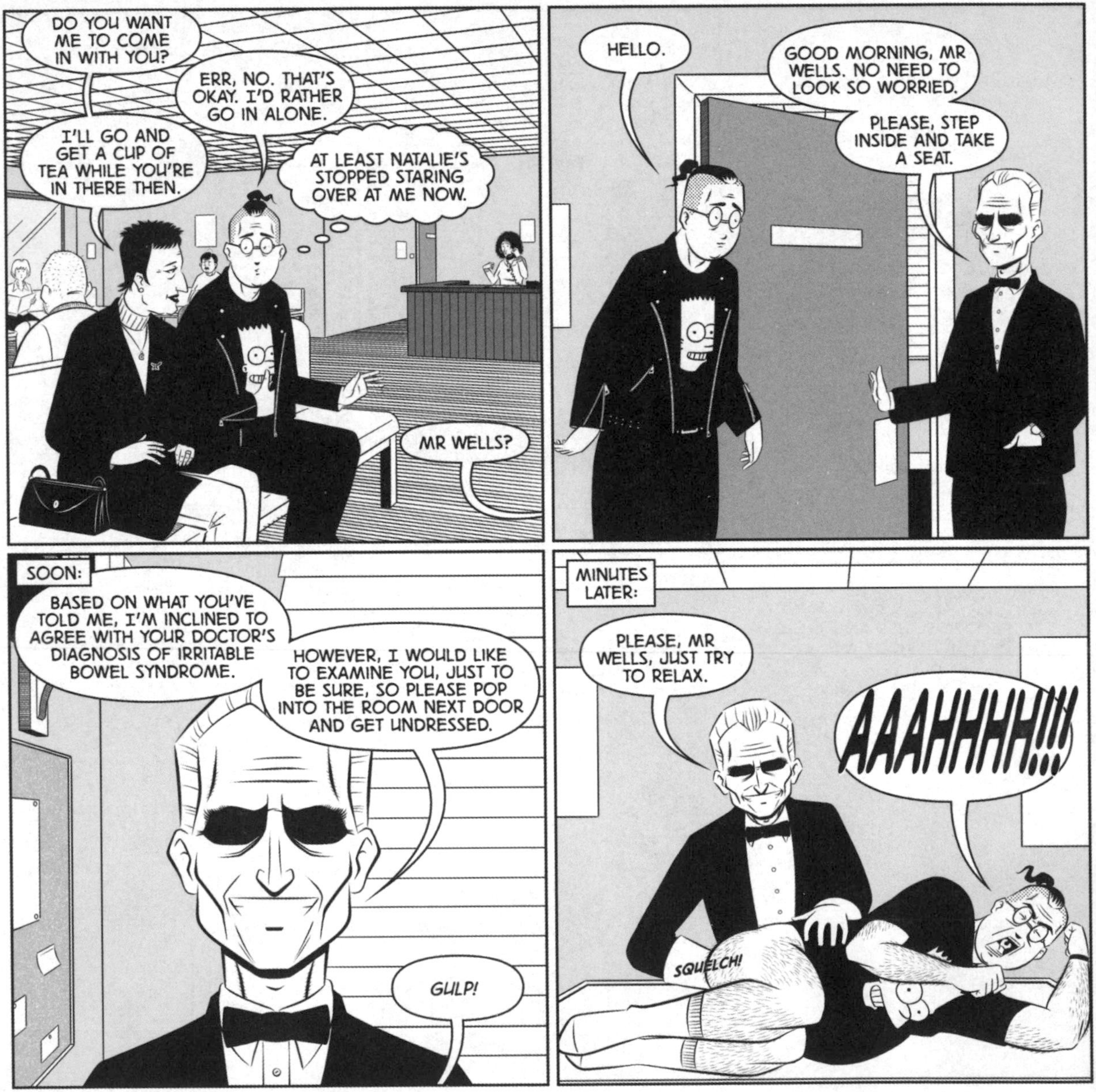

DO YOU WANT ME TO COME IN WITH YOU?
ERR, NO. THAT'S OKAY. I'D RATHER GO IN ALONE.
I'LL GO AND GET A CUP OF TEA WHILE YOU'RE IN THERE THEN.
AT LEAST NATALIE'S STOPPED STARING OVER AT ME NOW.
MR WELLS?
HELLO.
GOOD MORNING, MR WELLS. NO NEED TO LOOK SO WORRIED.
PLEASE, STEP INSIDE AND TAKE A SEAT.
SOON:
BASED ON WHAT YOU'VE TOLD ME, I'M INCLINED TO AGREE WITH YOUR DOCTOR'S DIAGNOSIS OF IRRITABLE BOWEL SYNDROME.
HOWEVER, I WOULD LIKE TO EXAMINE YOU, JUST TO BE SURE, SO PLEASE POP INTO THE ROOM NEXT DOOR AND GET UNDRESSED.
GULP!
MINUTES LATER:
PLEASE, MR WELLS, JUST TRY TO RELAX.
AAAHHHH!!!
SQUELCH!

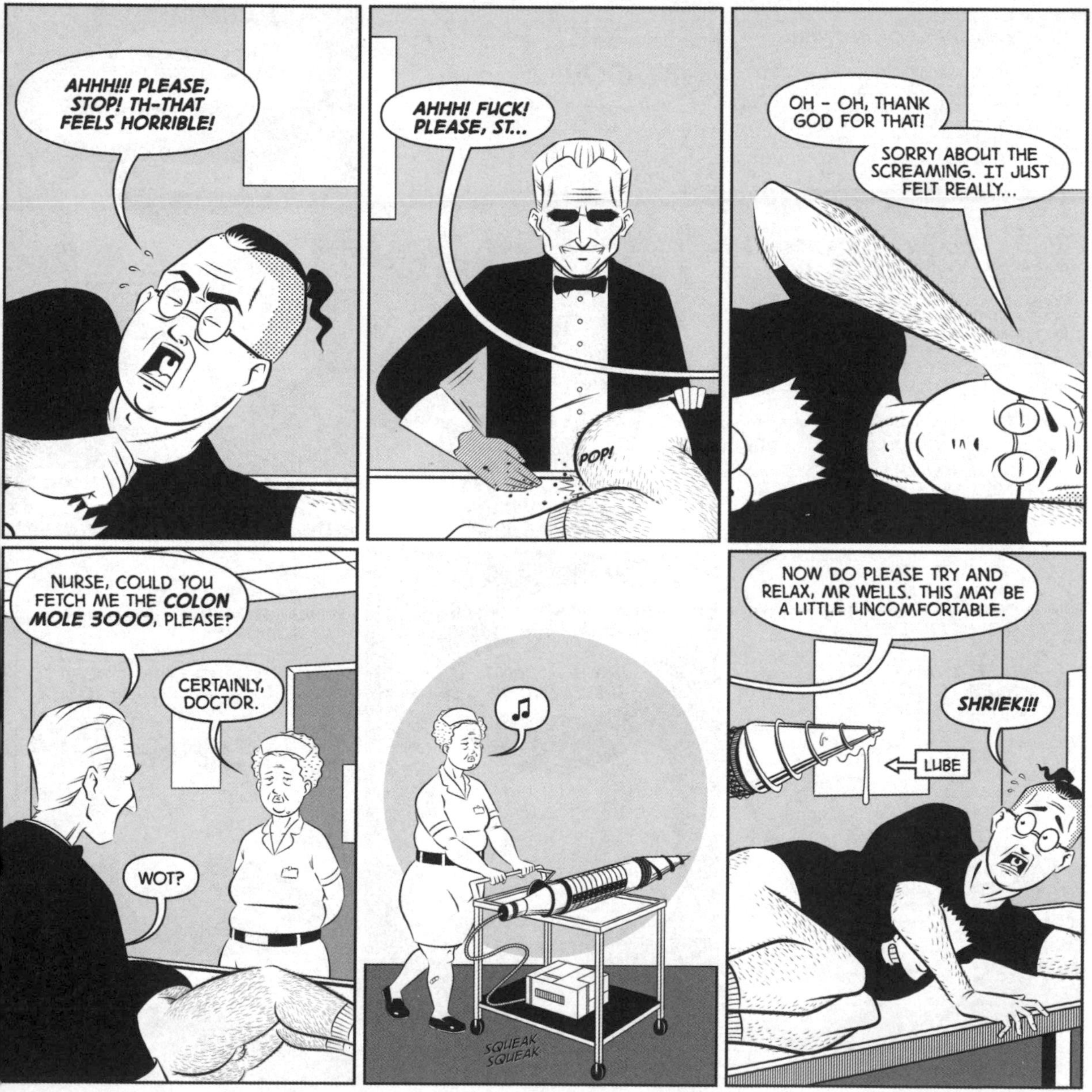
AHHH!!! PLEASE, STOP! TH-THAT FEELS HORRIBLE!
AHHH! FUCK! PLEASE, ST...
POP!
OH - OH, THANK GOD FOR THAT!
SORRY ABOUT THE SCREAMING. IT JUST FELT REALLY...
NURSE, COULD YOU FETCH ME THE COLON MOLE 3000, PLEASE?
CERTAINLY, DOCTOR.
WOT?
♫
SQUEAK SQUEAK
NOW DO PLEASE TRY AND RELAX, MR WELLS. THIS MAY BE A LITTLE UNCOMFORTABLE.
SHRIEK!!!
LUBE

EXAGGERATION NOTICE:

IN CASE IT ISN'T OBVIOUS, I WOULD LIKE TO POINT OUT THAT THIS SCENE HAS BEEN SLIGHTLY EXAGGERATED. IN REALITY, I'M PRETTY SURE THAT THIS DOCTOR DIDN'T STICK HIS ENTIRE HAND UP MY BOTTOM, JUST A FINGER, AND WHILE I DID HAVE A CONTRAPTION OF SOME KIND INSERTED *DEEP* INTO MY BOWELS, I DON'T REMEMBER WHAT IT LOOKED LIKE AND IT CERTAINLY WASN'T CALLED A *COLON MOLE 3000*. I HAVE EXAGGERATED PARTLY FOR COMEDIC EFFECT AND PARTLY TO CONVEY WHAT THIS EXAMINATION FELT LIKE. THIS REALLY WAS THE MOST UNCOMFORTABLE EXAMINATION I HAVE *EVER* EXPERIENCED – LIKE HAVING A COLONOSCOPY CARRIED OUT WITHOUT ANY PREPARATION OR ANAESTHETIC.

HOWEVER, WHILE I HAVE EXAGGERATED THIS SCENE VISUALLY, I ASSURE YOU THAT I HAVE NOT EXAGGERATED MY SCREAMS AT ALL. IN FACT, I PROBABLY SCREAMED AND SWORE *A LOT* MORE THAN THIS.

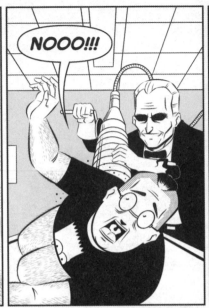

NOOO!!!

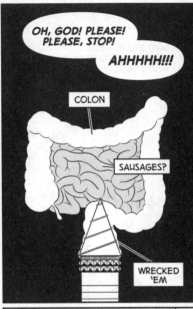

OH, GOD! PLEASE! PLEASE, STOP!

AHHHHH!!!

COLON

SAUSAGES?

WRECKED 'EM

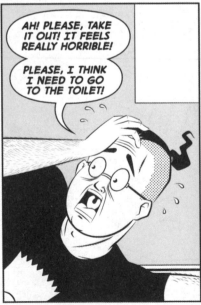

AH! PLEASE, TAKE IT OUT! IT FEELS REALLY HORRIBLE!

PLEASE, I THINK I NEED TO GO TO THE TOILET!

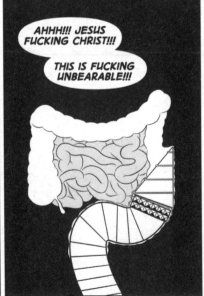

AHHH!!! JESUS FUCKING CHRIST!!!

THIS IS FUCKING UNBEARABLE!!!

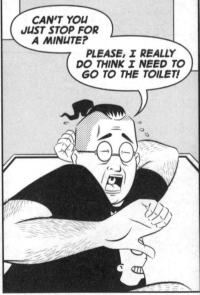

CAN'T YOU JUST STOP FOR A MINUTE?

PLEASE, I REALLY DO THINK I NEED TO GO TO THE TOILET!

AHHH!!! FUCK! IT FEELS LIKE YOU'RE PUSHING ALL THE CRAP BACK UP INSIDE ME!
PLEASE, CAN'T YOU JUST STOP AND LET ME GO TO THE TOILET?
GAHHH!!!
OH, BLOODY HELL! THIS IS AGONY!
HOW MUCH LONGER IS IT GOING TO TAKE?
OH, GOD! I CAN FEEL IT ALL THE WAY UP IN MY CHEST!
PLEASE, TAKE IT OUT! PL...
AAAHHHH!!!
SQUEAK!
AAAAAA

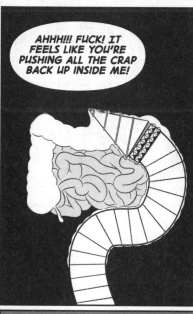

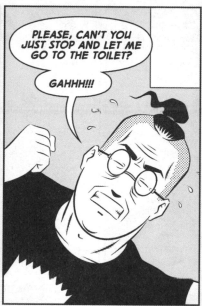

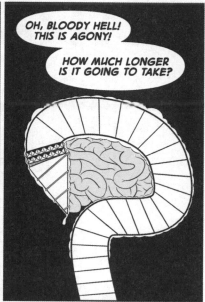

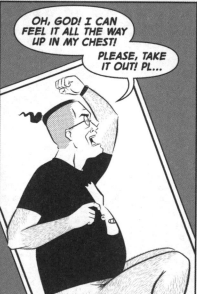

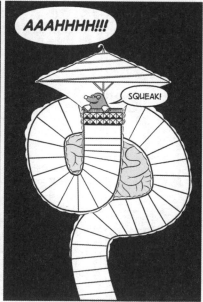

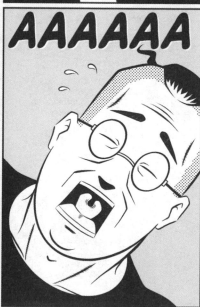

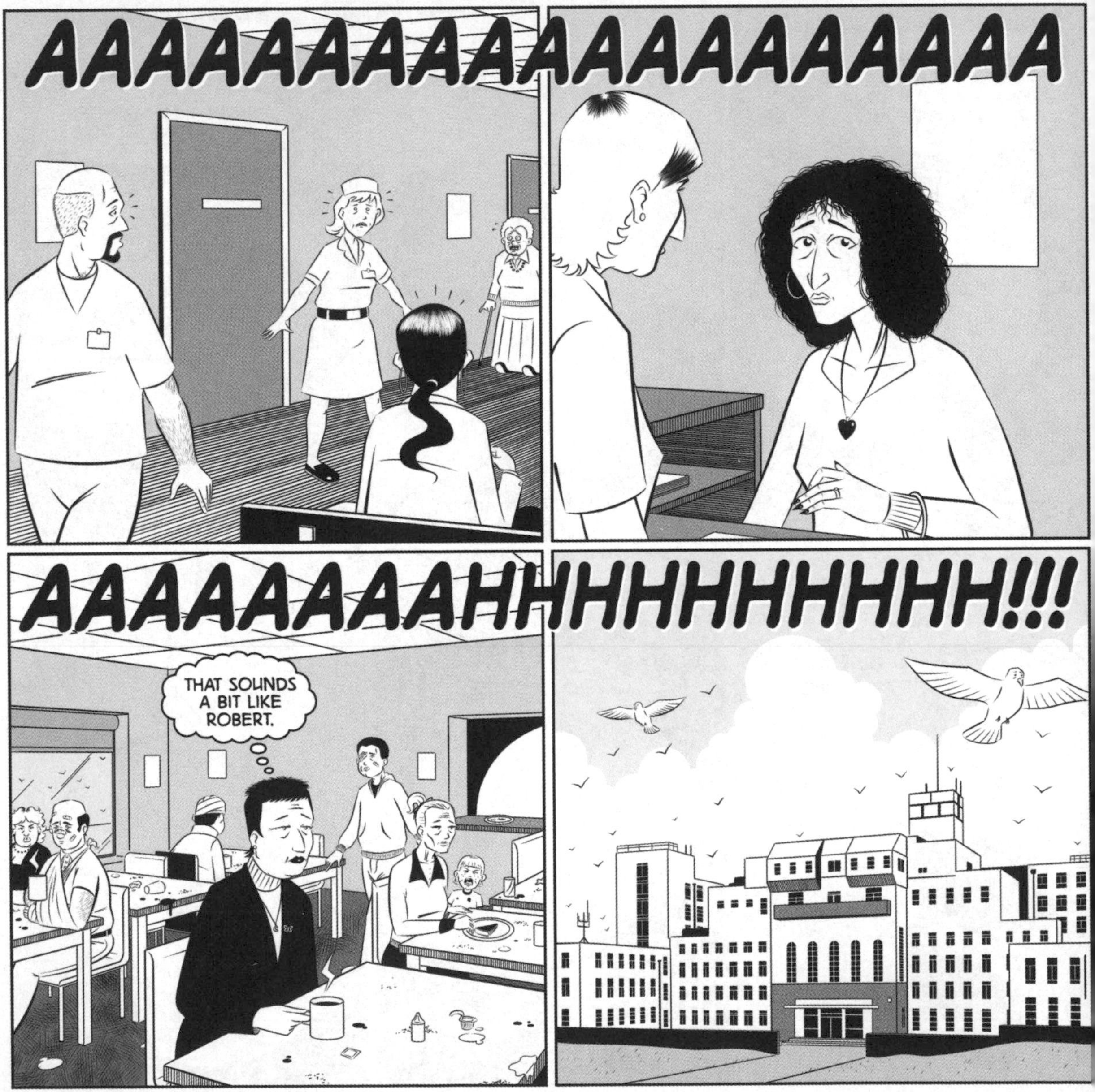
AAAAAAAAAAAAAAAAAAAAAAA
AAAAAAAAAHHHHHHHHHHH!!!
THAT SOUNDS A BIT LIKE ROBERT.

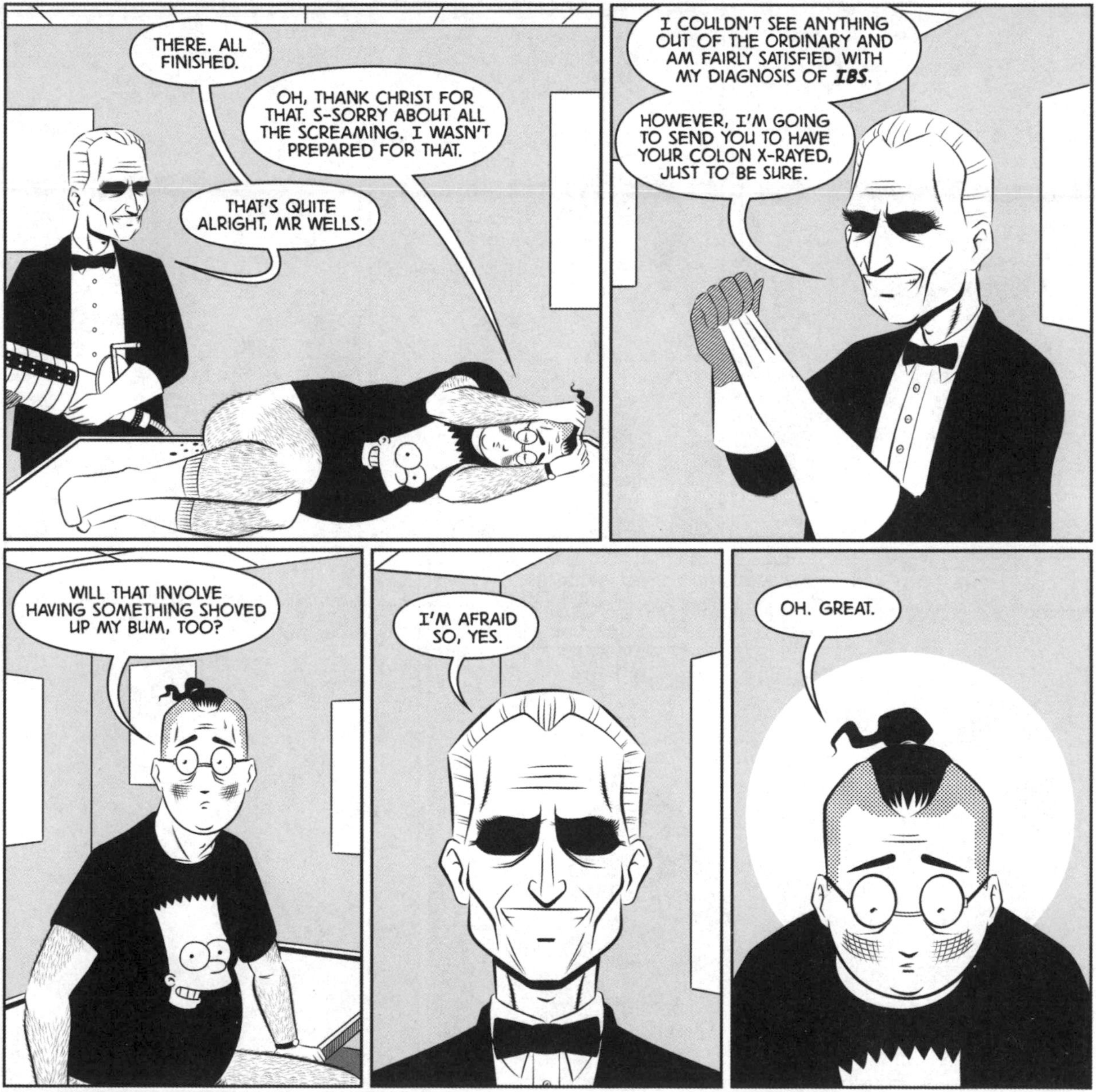
THERE. ALL FINISHED.
OH, THANK CHRIST FOR THAT. S-SORRY ABOUT ALL THE SCREAMING. I WASN'T PREPARED FOR THAT.
THAT'S QUITE ALRIGHT, MR WELLS.
I COULDN'T SEE ANYTHING OUT OF THE ORDINARY AND AM FAIRLY SATISFIED WITH MY DIAGNOSIS OF IBS.
HOWEVER, I'M GOING TO SEND YOU TO HAVE YOUR COLON X-RAYED, JUST TO BE SURE.
WILL THAT INVOLVE HAVING SOMETHING SHOVED UP MY BUM, TOO?
I'M AFRAID SO, YES.
OH. GREAT.

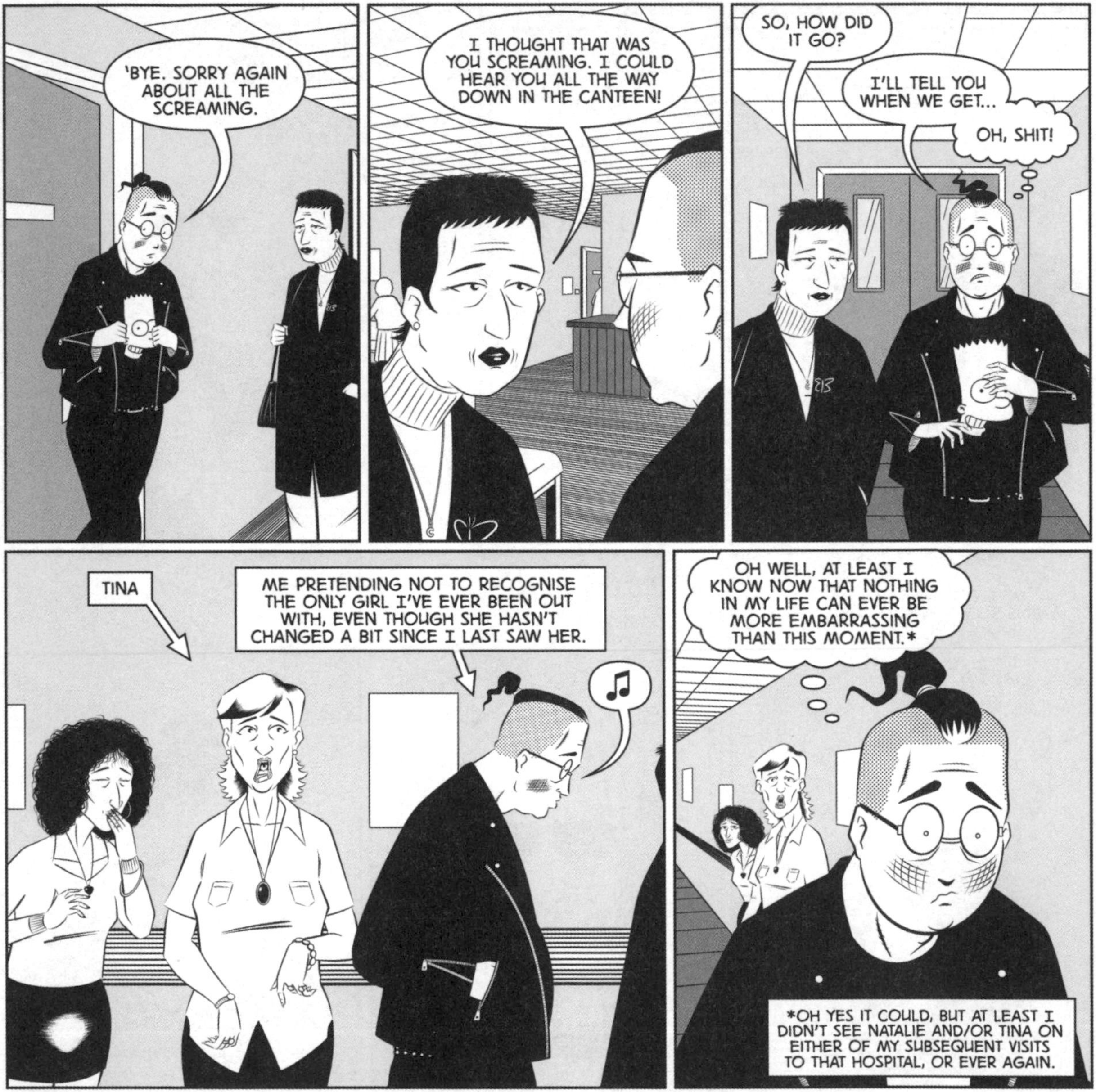
'BYE. SORRY AGAIN ABOUT ALL THE SCREAMING.
I THOUGHT THAT WAS YOU SCREAMING. I COULD HEAR YOU ALL THE WAY DOWN IN THE CANTEEN!
SO, HOW DID IT GO?
I'LL TELL YOU WHEN WE GET...
OH, SHIT!
TINA
ME PRETENDING NOT TO RECOGNISE THE ONLY GIRL I'VE EVER BEEN OUT WITH, EVEN THOUGH SHE HASN'T CHANGED A BIT SINCE I LAST SAW HER.
♫
OH WELL, AT LEAST I KNOW NOW THAT NOTHING IN MY LIFE CAN EVER BE MORE EMBARRASSING THAN THIS MOMENT.*
*OH YES IT COULD, BUT AT LEAST I DIDN'T SEE NATALIE AND/OR TINA ON EITHER OF MY SUBSEQUENT VISITS TO THAT HOSPITAL, OR EVER AGAIN.

A WEEK OR SO LATER, I WAS BACK AT THAT HOSPITAL HAVING MY COLON X-RAYED. HAVING YOUR COLON X-RAYED IS MUCH THE SAME AS HAVING ANY OTHER PART OF YOUR BODY X-RAYED, BUT IN ORDER FOR YOUR COLON TO SHOW UP ON AN X-RAY, YOU FIRST NEED TO HAVE SOMETHING CALLED A *BARIUM ENEMA*.

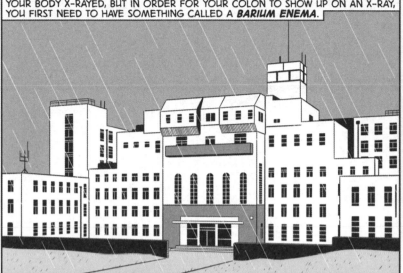

THIS INVOLVES HAVING A TUBE INSERTED INTO YOUR ANUS AND YOUR COLON FILLED WITH A WHITE FLUID CALLED BARIUM.

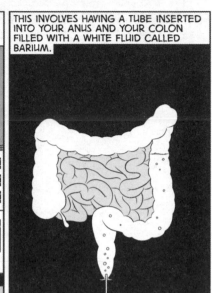

THEN, DURING THE X-RAY, AIR WILL OCCASIONALLY GET PUMPED INTO THE COLON TO INFLATE IT AND HELP MOVE THE BARIUM AROUND.

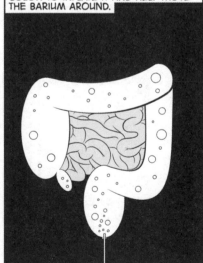

NEEDLESS TO SAY, I WAS DREADING IT. I'D EMPTIED MY BOWELS WITH LAXATIVES BEFORE ARRIVING AT THE HOSPITAL, AS WAS REQUIRED OF ME, BUT I STILL HAD A STOMACH ACHE.

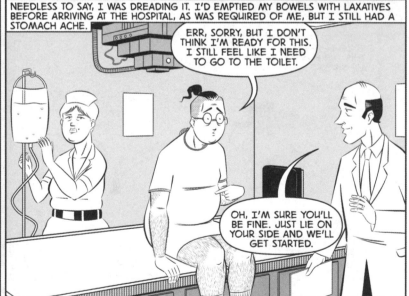

ERR, SORRY, BUT I DON'T THINK I'M READY FOR THIS. I STILL FEEL LIKE I NEED TO GO TO THE TOILET.

OH, I'M SURE YOU'LL BE FINE. JUST LIE ON YOUR SIDE AND WE'LL GET STARTED.

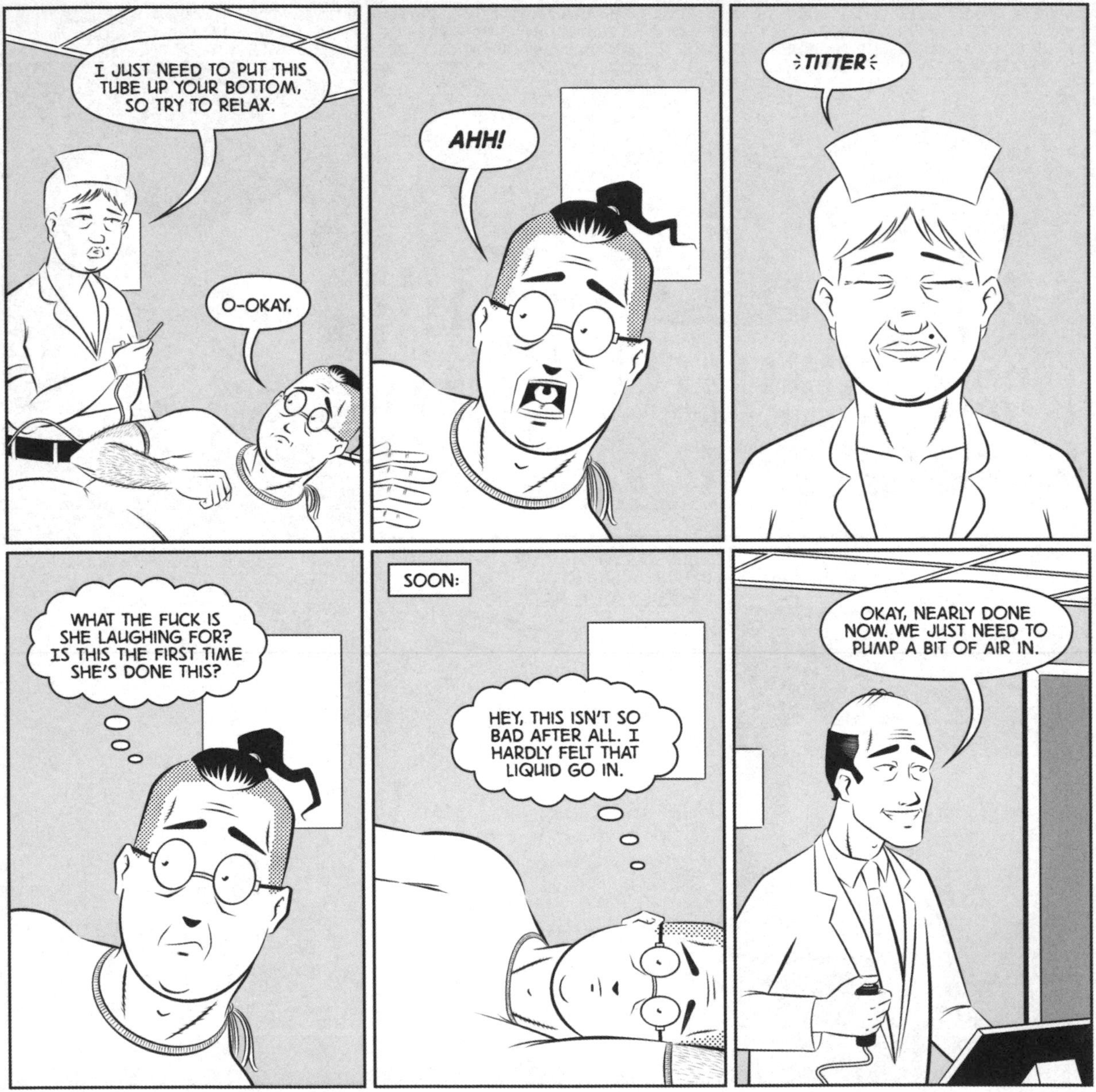
I JUST NEED TO PUT THIS TUBE UP YOUR BOTTOM, SO TRY TO RELAX.
O-OKAY.
AHH!
TITTER
WHAT THE FUCK IS SHE LAUGHING FOR? IS THIS THE FIRST TIME SHE'S DONE THIS?
SOON:
HEY, THIS ISN'T SO BAD AFTER ALL. I HARDLY FELT THAT LIQUID GO IN.
OKAY, NEARLY DONE NOW. WE JUST NEED TO PUMP A BIT OF AIR IN.

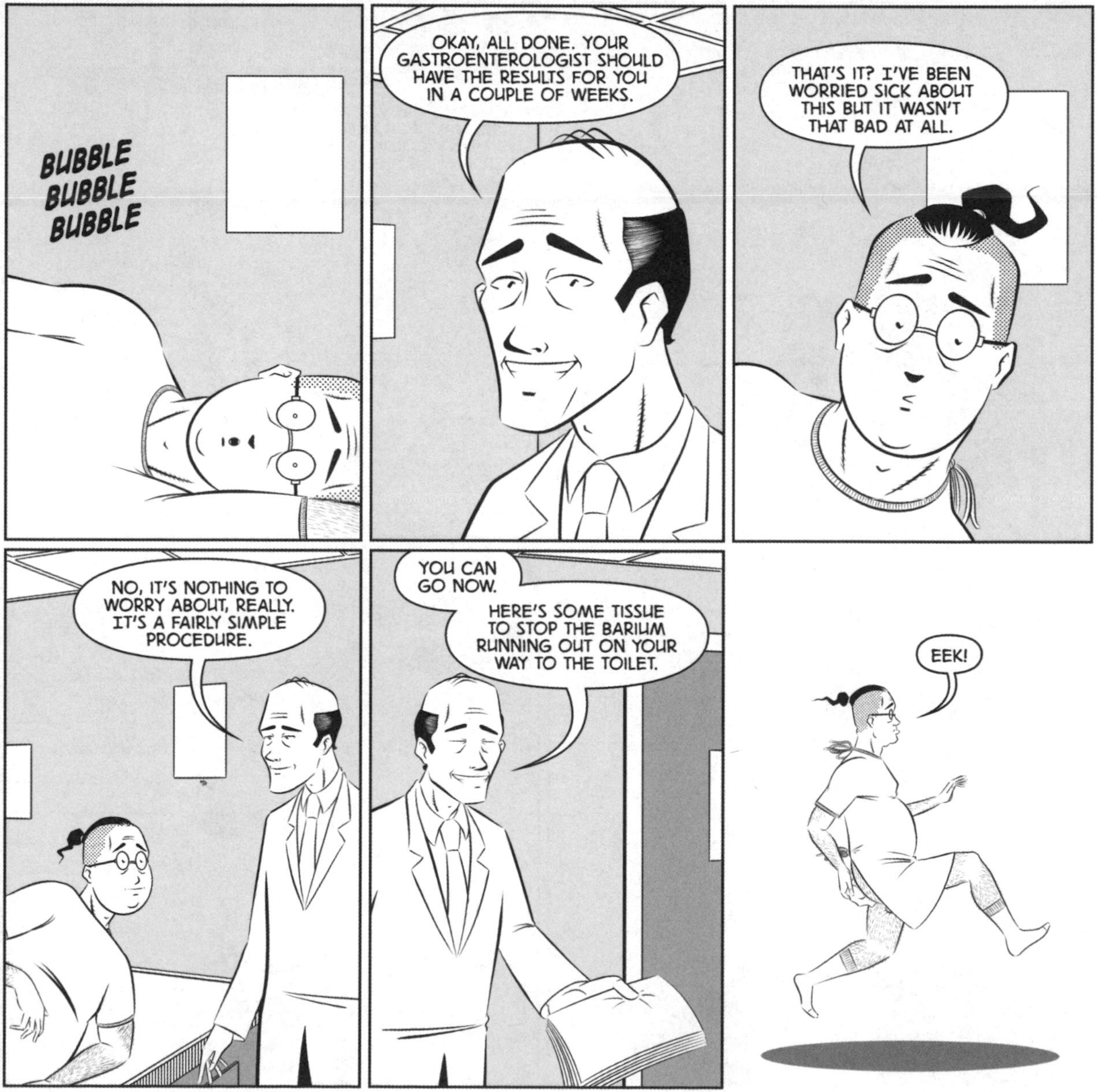
BUBBLE
BUBBLE
BUBBLE
OKAY, ALL DONE. YOUR GASTROENTEROLOGIST SHOULD HAVE THE RESULTS FOR YOU IN A COUPLE OF WEEKS.
THAT'S IT? I'VE BEEN WORRIED SICK ABOUT THIS BUT IT WASN'T THAT BAD AT ALL.
NO, IT'S NOTHING TO WORRY ABOUT, REALLY. IT'S A FAIRLY SIMPLE PROCEDURE.
YOU CAN GO NOW.
HERE'S SOME TISSUE TO STOP THE BARIUM RUNNING OUT ON YOUR WAY TO THE TOILET.
EEK!

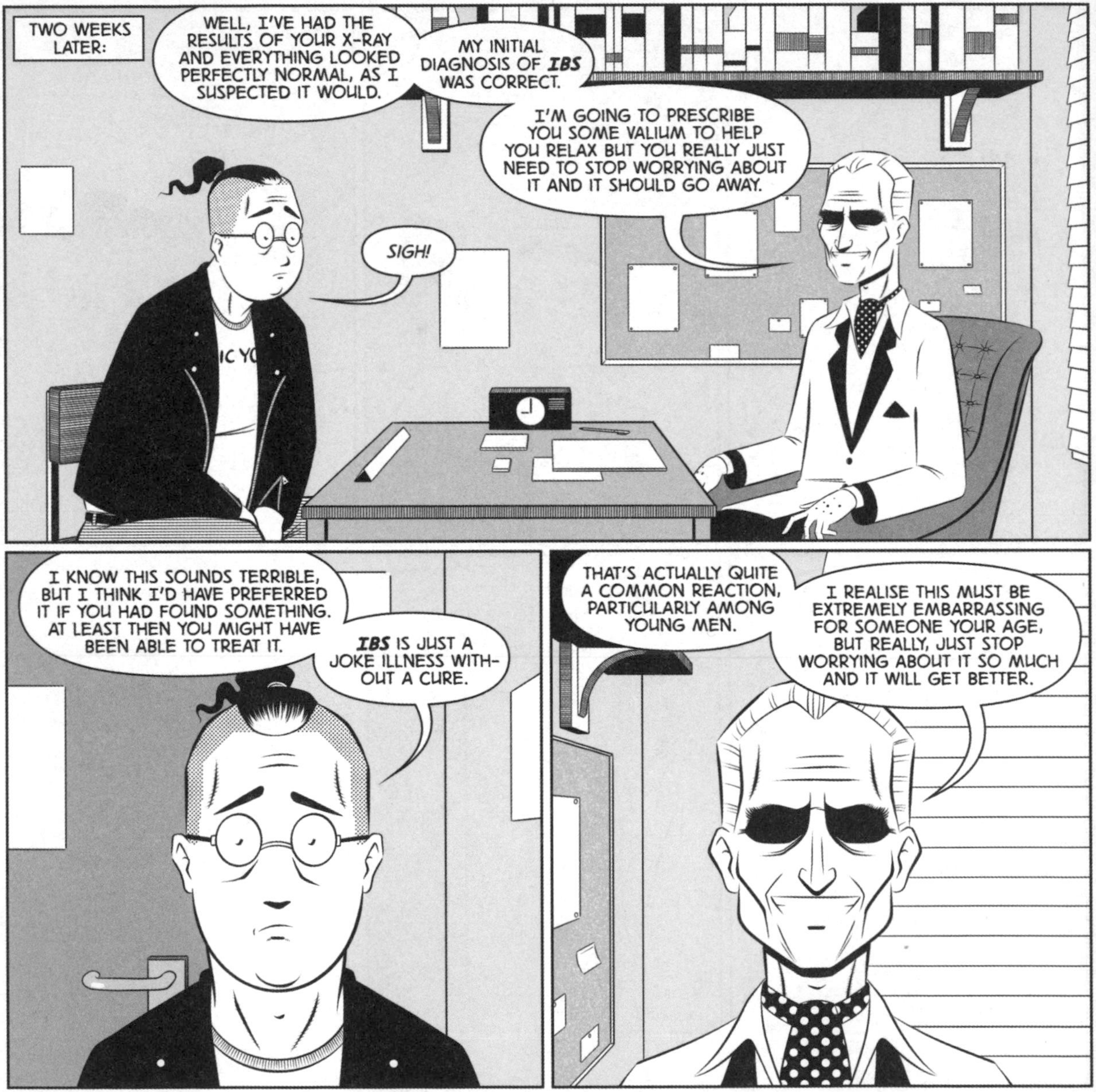
TWO WEEKS LATER:
WELL, I'VE HAD THE RESULTS OF YOUR X-RAY AND EVERYTHING LOOKED PERFECTLY NORMAL, AS I SUSPECTED IT WOULD.
MY INITIAL DIAGNOSIS OF IBS WAS CORRECT.
I'M GOING TO PRESCRIBE YOU SOME VALIUM TO HELP YOU RELAX BUT YOU REALLY JUST NEED TO STOP WORRYING ABOUT IT AND IT SHOULD GO AWAY.
SIGH!
I KNOW THIS SOUNDS TERRIBLE, BUT I THINK I'D HAVE PREFERRED IT IF YOU HAD FOUND SOMETHING. AT LEAST THEN YOU MIGHT HAVE BEEN ABLE TO TREAT IT.
IBS IS JUST A JOKE ILLNESS WITHOUT A CURE.
THAT'S ACTUALLY QUITE A COMMON REACTION, PARTICULARLY AMONG YOUNG MEN.
I REALISE THIS MUST BE EXTREMELY EMBARRASSING FOR SOMEONE YOUR AGE, BUT REALLY, JUST STOP WORRYING ABOUT IT SO MUCH AND IT WILL GET BETTER.

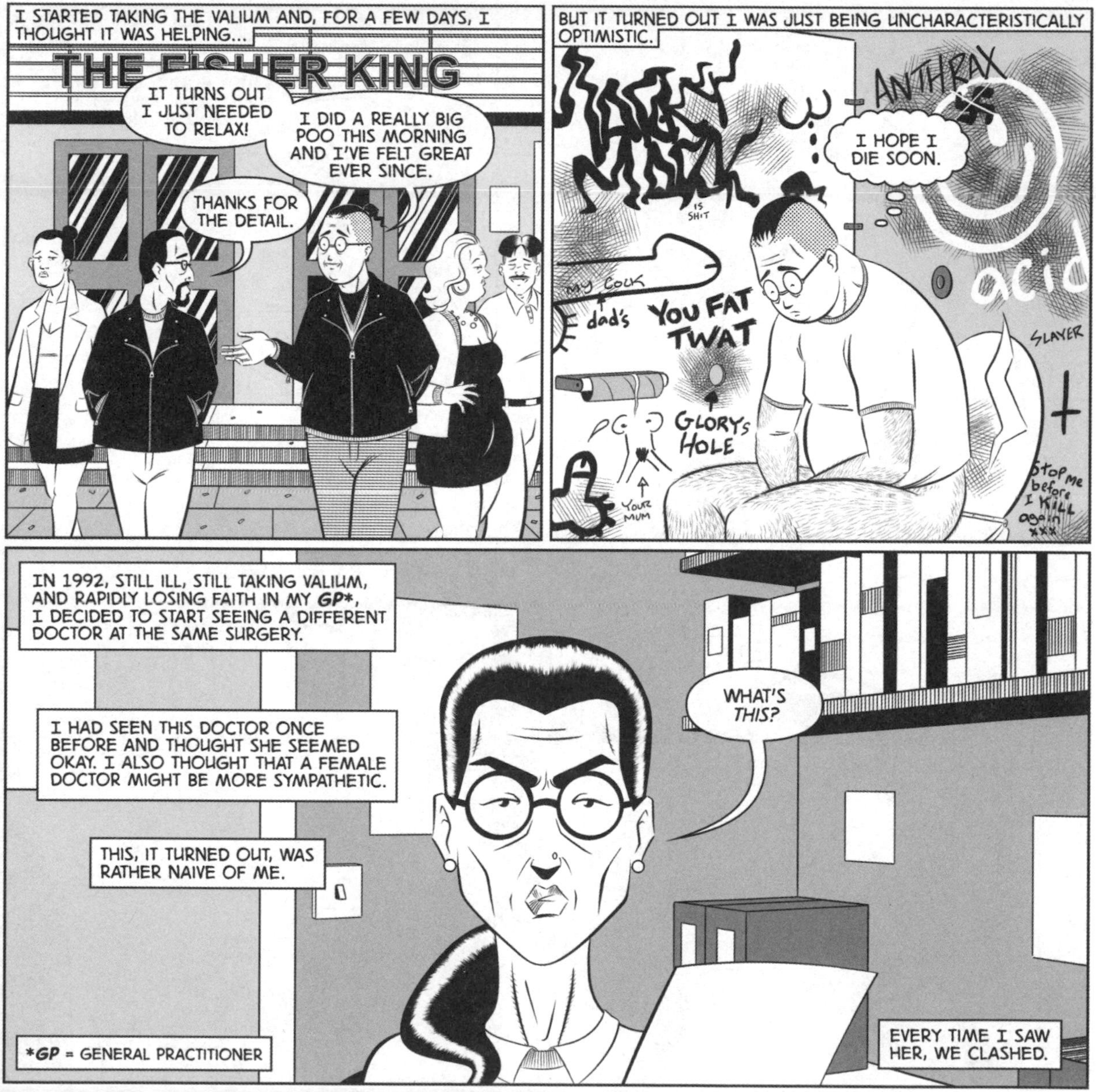
I STARTED TAKING THE VALIUM AND, FOR A FEW DAYS, I THOUGHT IT WAS HELPING...
THE FISHER KING
IT TURNS OUT I JUST NEEDED TO RELAX!
I DID A REALLY BIG POO THIS MORNING AND I'VE FELT GREAT EVER SINCE.
THANKS FOR THE DETAIL.
BUT IT TURNED OUT I WAS JUST BEING UNCHARACTERISTICALLY OPTIMISTIC.
IS SHIT
ANTHRAX
I HOPE I DIE SOON.
MY COCK
dad's
YOU FAT TWAT
acid
SLAYER
GLORY'S HOLE
YOUR MUM
Stop me before I KILL again xxx
IN 1992, STILL ILL, STILL TAKING VALIUM, AND RAPIDLY LOSING FAITH IN MY GP*, I DECIDED TO START SEEING A DIFFERENT DOCTOR AT THE SAME SURGERY.
WHAT'S THIS?
I HAD SEEN THIS DOCTOR ONCE BEFORE AND THOUGHT SHE SEEMED OKAY. I ALSO THOUGHT THAT A FEMALE DOCTOR MIGHT BE MORE SYMPATHETIC.
THIS, IT TURNED OUT, WAS RATHER NAIVE OF ME.
*GP = GENERAL PRACTITIONER
EVERY TIME I SAW HER, WE CLASHED.

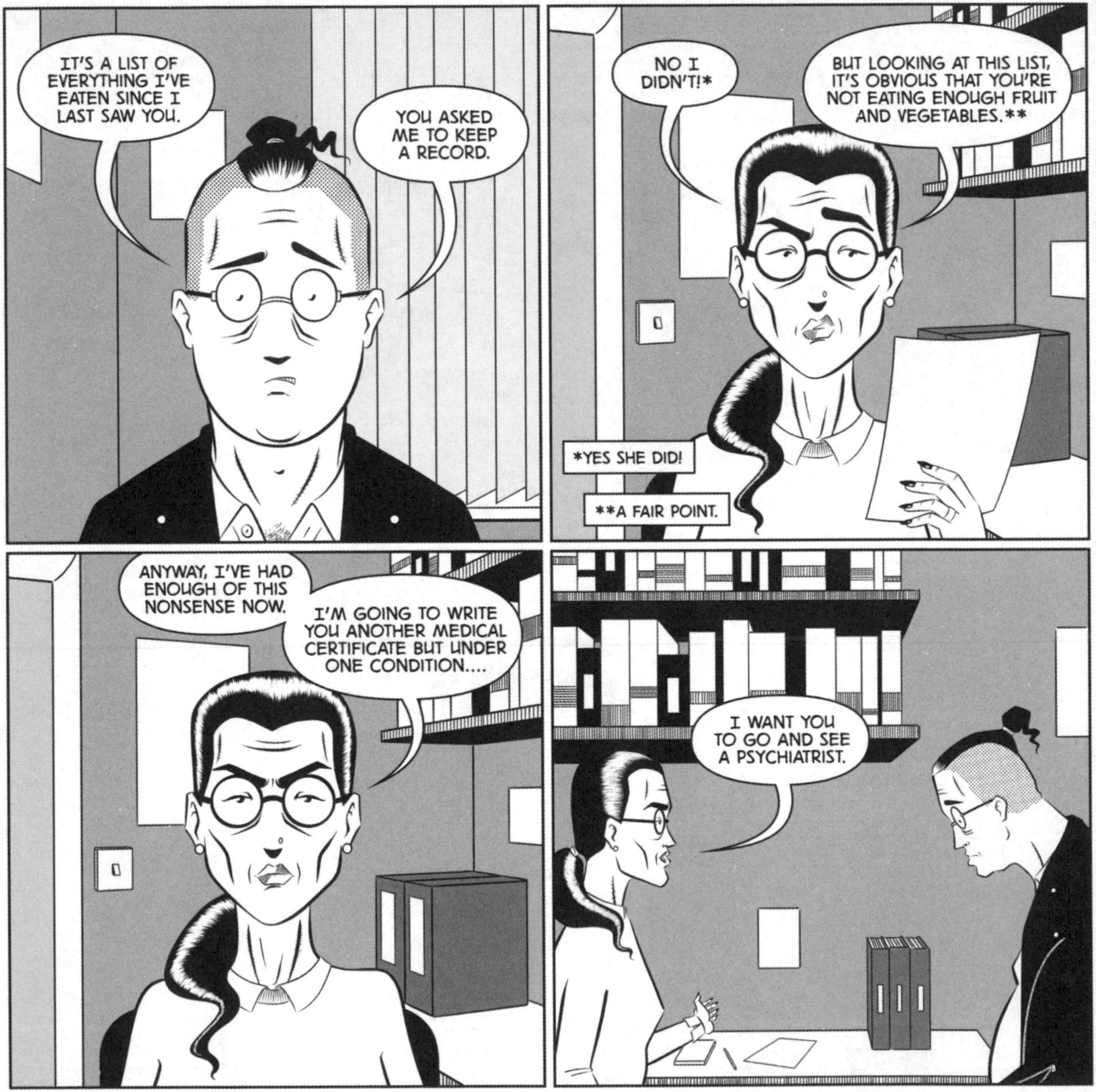
IT'S A LIST OF EVERYTHING I'VE EATEN SINCE I LAST SAW YOU.
YOU ASKED ME TO KEEP A RECORD.
NO I DIDN'T!*
BUT LOOKING AT THIS LIST, IT'S OBVIOUS THAT YOU'RE NOT EATING ENOUGH FRUIT AND VEGETABLES.**
*YES SHE DID!
**A FAIR POINT.
ANYWAY, I'VE HAD ENOUGH OF THIS NONSENSE NOW.
I'M GOING TO WRITE YOU ANOTHER MEDICAL CERTIFICATE BUT UNDER ONE CONDITION....
I WANT YOU TO GO AND SEE A PSYCHIATRIST.

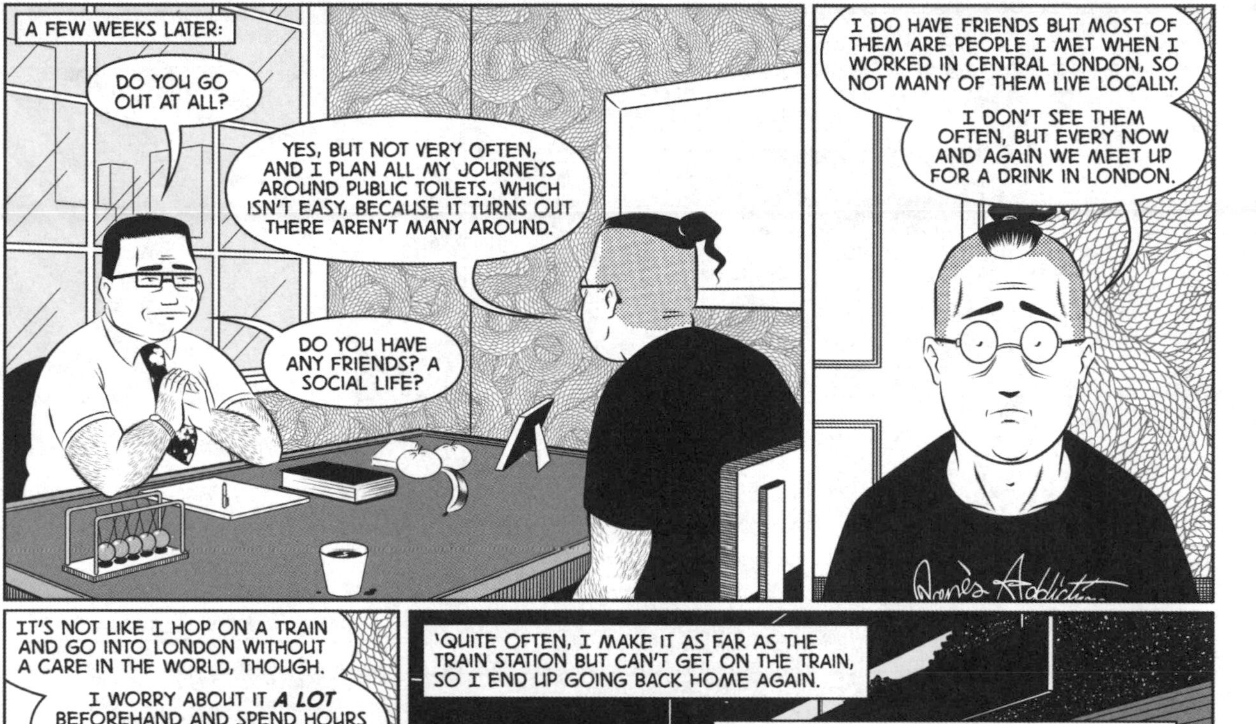

A FEW WEEKS LATER:
DO YOU GO OUT AT ALL?
YES, BUT NOT VERY OFTEN, AND I PLAN ALL MY JOURNEYS AROUND PUBLIC TOILETS, WHICH ISN'T EASY, BECAUSE IT TURNS OUT THERE AREN'T MANY AROUND.
DO YOU HAVE ANY FRIENDS? A SOCIAL LIFE?
I DO HAVE FRIENDS BUT MOST OF THEM ARE PEOPLE I MET WHEN I WORKED IN CENTRAL LONDON, SO NOT MANY OF THEM LIVE LOCALLY.
I DON'T SEE THEM OFTEN, BUT EVERY NOW AND AGAIN WE MEET UP FOR A DRINK IN LONDON.
IT'S NOT LIKE I HOP ON A TRAIN AND GO INTO LONDON WITHOUT A CARE IN THE WORLD, THOUGH.
I WORRY ABOUT IT ***A LOT*** BEFOREHAND AND SPEND HOURS IN THE TOILET BEFORE I LEAVE HOME, IF I MANAGE TO LEAVE HOME AT ALL.
'QUITE OFTEN, I MAKE IT AS FAR AS THE TRAIN STATION BUT CAN'T GET ON THE TRAIN, SO I END UP GOING BACK HOME AGAIN.
'THE TRAIN INTO LONDON IS THE WORST PART OF THE JOURNEY, EVEN THOUGH IT'S ONLY TWENTY MINUTES, BECAUSE I'M TRAPPED AND THERE USUALLY AREN'T ANY TOILETS.'
IT'S NO GOOD, I CAN'T DO IT.

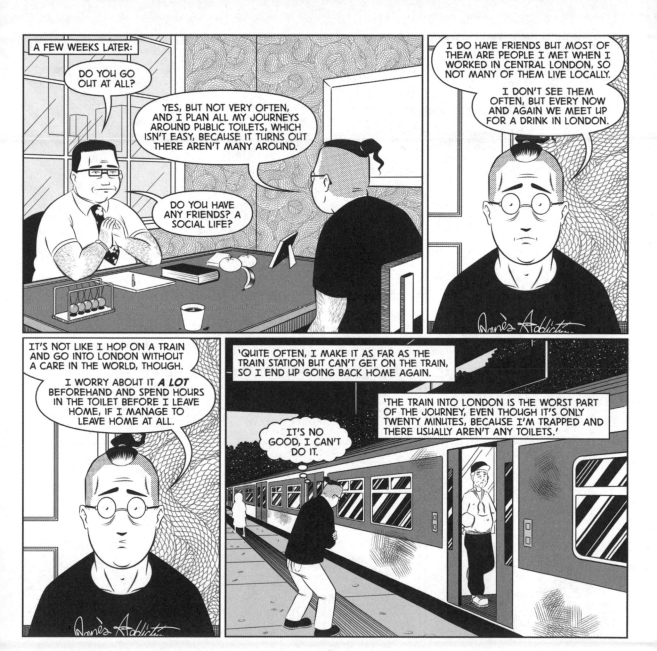

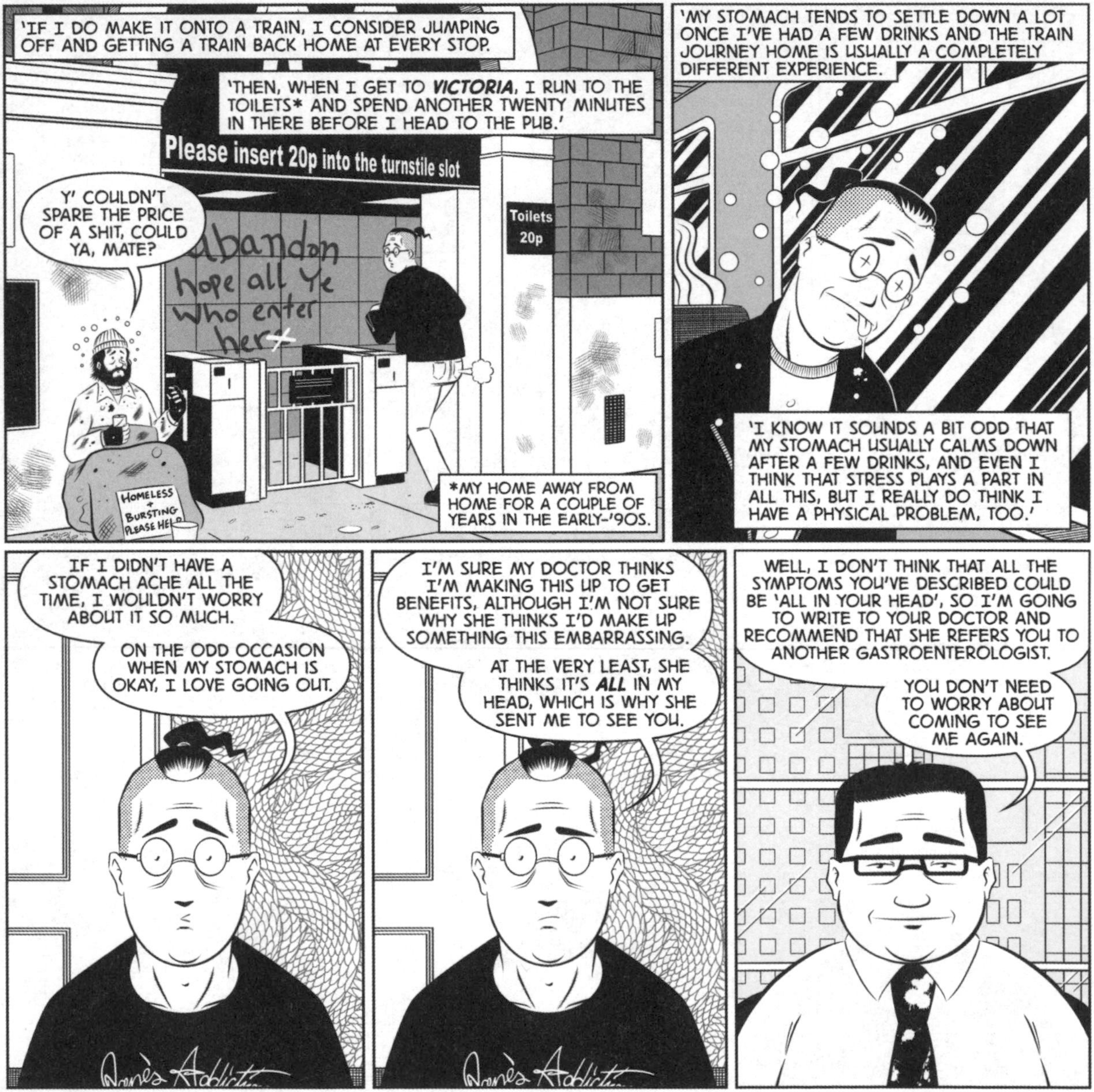
'IF I DO MAKE IT ONTO A TRAIN, I CONSIDER JUMPING OFF AND GETTING A TRAIN BACK HOME AT EVERY STOP.
'THEN, WHEN I GET TO *VICTORIA*, I RUN TO THE TOILETS* AND SPEND ANOTHER TWENTY MINUTES IN THERE BEFORE I HEAD TO THE PUB.'
Please insert 20p into the turnstile slot
Y' COULDN'T SPARE THE PRICE OF A SHIT, COULD YA, MATE?
abandon hope all ye who enter here
Toilets 20p
HOMELESS + BURSTING PLEASE HELP
*MY HOME AWAY FROM HOME FOR A COUPLE OF YEARS IN THE EARLY-'90S.
'MY STOMACH TENDS TO SETTLE DOWN A LOT ONCE I'VE HAD A FEW DRINKS AND THE TRAIN JOURNEY HOME IS USUALLY A COMPLETELY DIFFERENT EXPERIENCE.
'I KNOW IT SOUNDS A BIT ODD THAT MY STOMACH USUALLY CALMS DOWN AFTER A FEW DRINKS, AND EVEN I THINK THAT STRESS PLAYS A PART IN ALL THIS, BUT I REALLY DO THINK I HAVE A PHYSICAL PROBLEM, TOO.'
IF I DIDN'T HAVE A STOMACH ACHE ALL THE TIME, I WOULDN'T WORRY ABOUT IT SO MUCH.
ON THE ODD OCCASION WHEN MY STOMACH IS OKAY, I LOVE GOING OUT.
I'M SURE MY DOCTOR THINKS I'M MAKING THIS UP TO GET BENEFITS, ALTHOUGH I'M NOT SURE WHY SHE THINKS I'D MAKE UP SOMETHING THIS EMBARRASSING.
AT THE VERY LEAST, SHE THINKS IT'S *ALL* IN MY HEAD, WHICH IS WHY SHE SENT ME TO SEE YOU.
WELL, I DON'T THINK THAT ALL THE SYMPTOMS YOU'VE DESCRIBED COULD BE 'ALL IN YOUR HEAD', SO I'M GOING TO WRITE TO YOUR DOCTOR AND RECOMMEND THAT SHE REFERS YOU TO ANOTHER GASTROENTEROLOGIST.
YOU DON'T NEED TO WORRY ABOUT COMING TO SEE ME AGAIN.

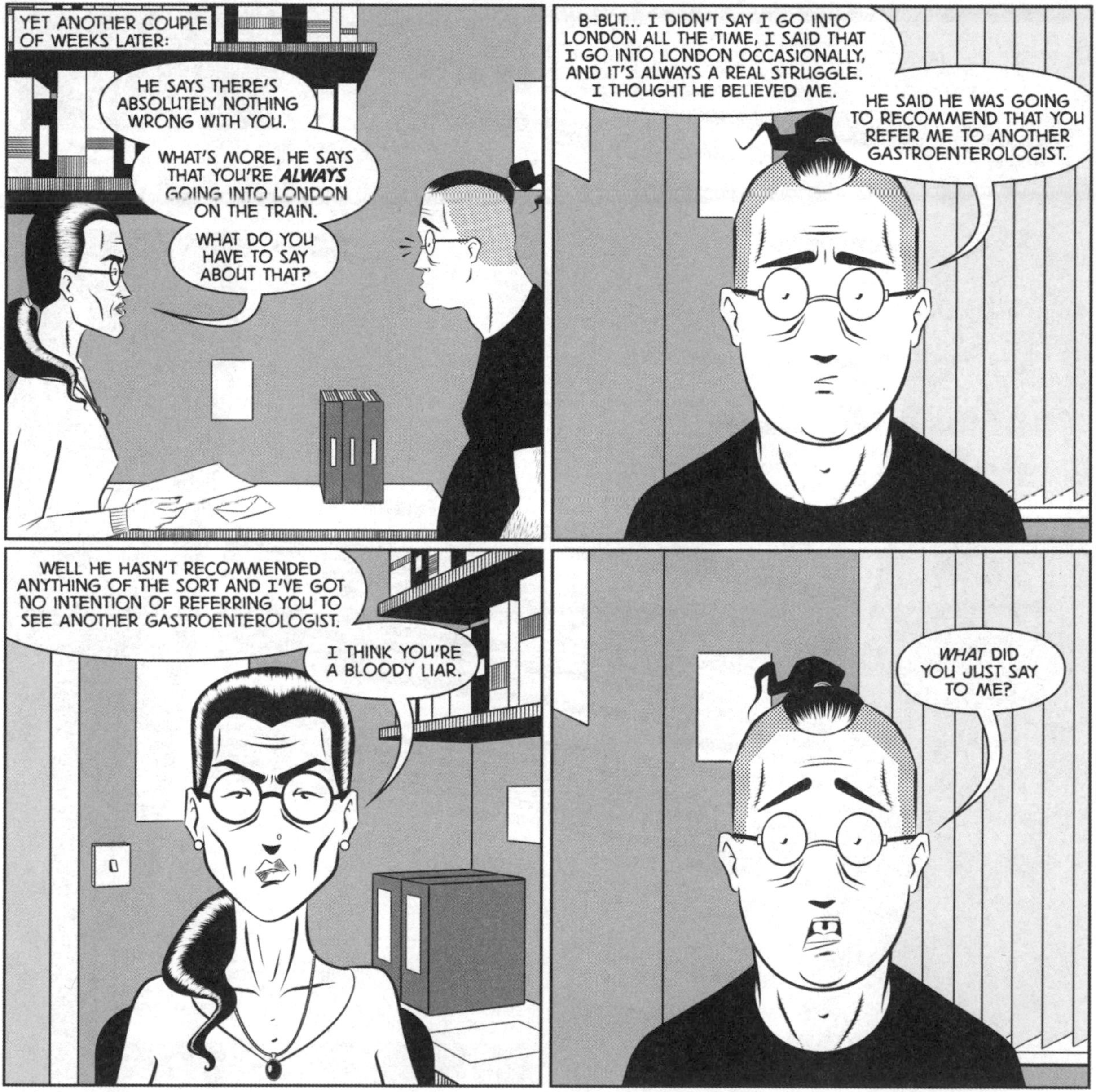
YET ANOTHER COUPLE OF WEEKS LATER:
HE SAYS THERE'S ABSOLUTELY NOTHING WRONG WITH YOU.
WHAT'S MORE, HE SAYS THAT YOU'RE ***ALWAYS*** GOING INTO LONDON ON THE TRAIN.
WHAT DO YOU HAVE TO SAY ABOUT THAT?
B-BUT... I DIDN'T SAY I GO INTO LONDON ALL THE TIME, I SAID THAT I GO INTO LONDON OCCASIONALLY, AND IT'S ALWAYS A REAL STRUGGLE. I THOUGHT HE BELIEVED ME.
HE SAID HE WAS GOING TO RECOMMEND THAT YOU REFER ME TO ANOTHER GASTROENTEROLOGIST.
WELL HE HASN'T RECOMMENDED ANYTHING OF THE SORT AND I'VE GOT NO INTENTION OF REFERRING YOU TO SEE ANOTHER GASTROENTEROLOGIST.
I THINK YOU'RE A BLOODY LIAR.
WHAT DID YOU JUST SAY TO ME?

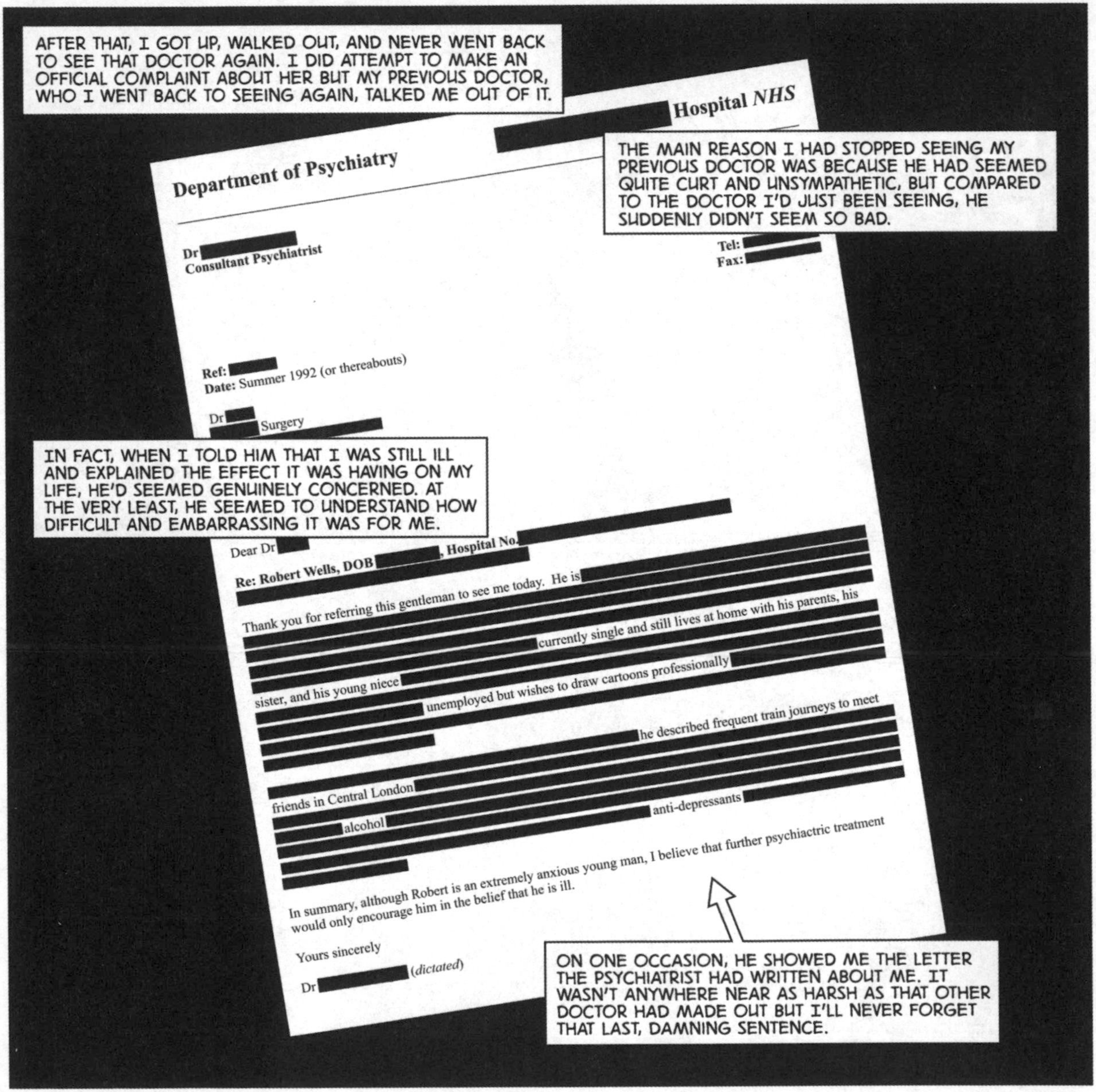

AFTER THAT, I GOT UP, WALKED OUT, AND NEVER WENT BACK TO SEE THAT DOCTOR AGAIN. I DID ATTEMPT TO MAKE AN OFFICIAL COMPLAINT ABOUT HER BUT MY PREVIOUS DOCTOR, WHO I WENT BACK TO SEEING AGAIN, TALKED ME OUT OF IT.
[redacted] Hospital NHS
Department of Psychiatry
THE MAIN REASON I HAD STOPPED SEEING MY PREVIOUS DOCTOR WAS BECAUSE HE HAD SEEMED QUITE CURT AND UNSYMPATHETIC, BUT COMPARED TO THE DOCTOR I'D JUST BEEN SEEING, HE SUDDENLY DIDN'T SEEM SO BAD.
Dr [redacted]
Consultant Psychiatrist
Tel: [redacted]
Fax: [redacted]
Ref: [redacted]
Date: Summer 1992 (or thereabouts)
Dr [redacted]
[redacted] Surgery [redacted]
IN FACT, WHEN I TOLD HIM THAT I WAS STILL ILL AND EXPLAINED THE EFFECT IT WAS HAVING ON MY LIFE, HE'D SEEMED GENUINELY CONCERNED. AT THE VERY LEAST, HE SEEMED TO UNDERSTAND HOW DIFFICULT AND EMBARRASSING IT WAS FOR ME.
[redacted]
Dear Dr [redacted]
Re: Robert Wells, DOB [redacted], Hospital No. [redacted]
Thank you for referring this gentleman to see me today. He is [redacted] currently single and still lives at home with his parents, his [redacted] sister, and his young niece [redacted] unemployed but wishes to draw cartoons professionally [redacted] he described frequent train journeys to meet [redacted] friends in Central London [redacted] alcohol [redacted] anti-depressants [redacted]
In summary, although Robert is an extremely anxious young man, I believe that further psychiactric treatment would only encourage him in the belief that he is ill.
Yours sincerely
Dr [redacted] (dictated)
ON ONE OCCASION, HE SHOWED ME THE LETTER THE PSYCHIATRIST HAD WRITTEN ABOUT ME. IT WASN'T ANYWHERE NEAR AS HARSH AS THAT OTHER DOCTOR HAD MADE OUT BUT I'LL NEVER FORGET THAT LAST, DAMNING SENTENCE.

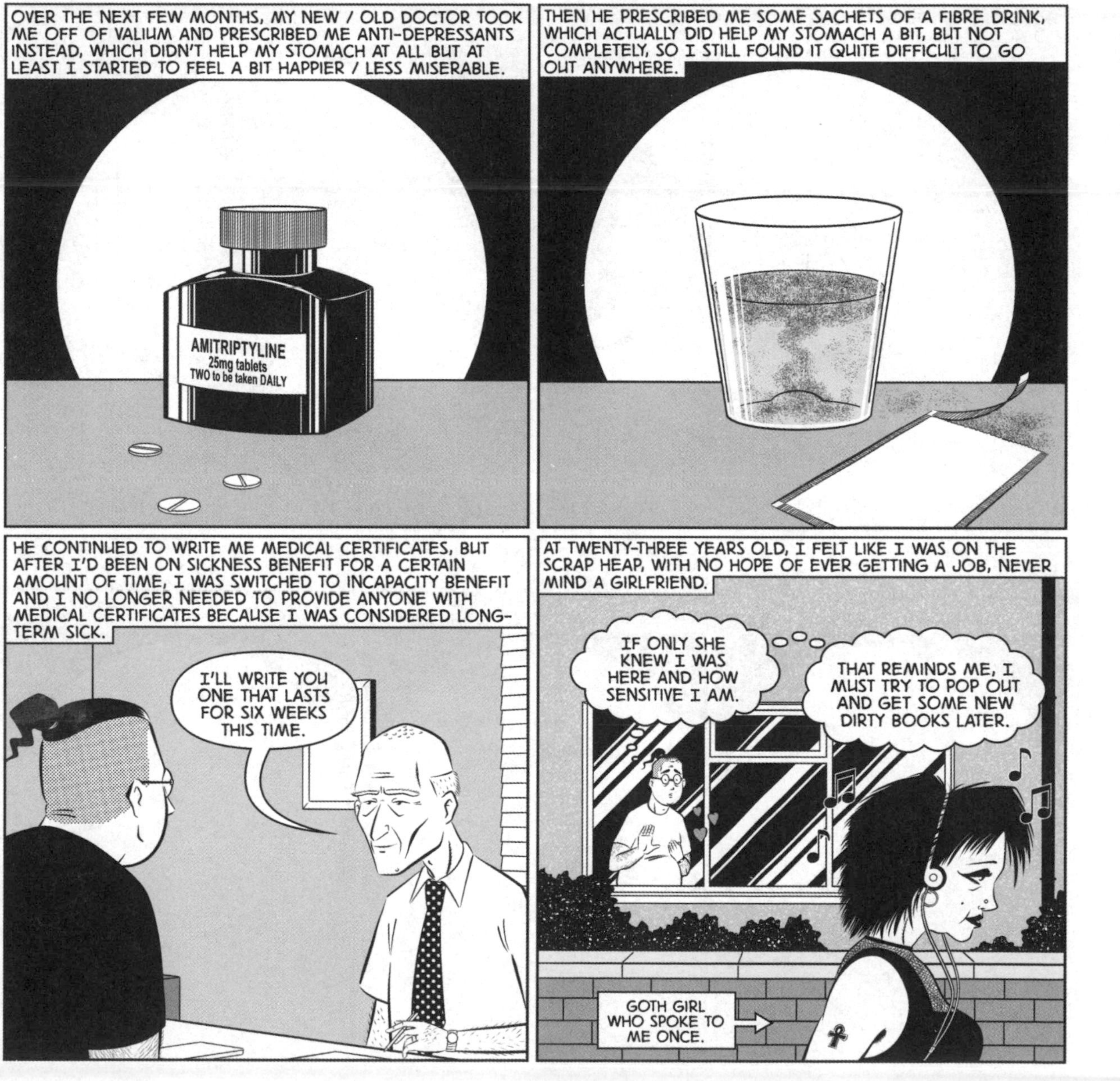
OVER THE NEXT FEW MONTHS, MY NEW / OLD DOCTOR TOOK ME OFF OF VALIUM AND PRESCRIBED ME ANTI-DEPRESSANTS INSTEAD, WHICH DIDN'T HELP MY STOMACH AT ALL BUT AT LEAST I STARTED TO FEEL A BIT HAPPIER / LESS MISERABLE.
AMITRIPTYLINE
25mg tablets
TWO to be taken DAILY
THEN HE PRESCRIBED ME SOME SACHETS OF A FIBRE DRINK, WHICH ACTUALLY DID HELP MY STOMACH A BIT, BUT NOT COMPLETELY, SO I STILL FOUND IT QUITE DIFFICULT TO GO OUT ANYWHERE.
HE CONTINUED TO WRITE ME MEDICAL CERTIFICATES, BUT AFTER I'D BEEN ON SICKNESS BENEFIT FOR A CERTAIN AMOUNT OF TIME, I WAS SWITCHED TO INCAPACITY BENEFIT AND I NO LONGER NEEDED TO PROVIDE ANYONE WITH MEDICAL CERTIFICATES BECAUSE I WAS CONSIDERED LONG-TERM SICK.
I'LL WRITE YOU ONE THAT LASTS FOR SIX WEEKS THIS TIME.
AT TWENTY-THREE YEARS OLD, I FELT LIKE I WAS ON THE SCRAP HEAP, WITH NO HOPE OF EVER GETTING A JOB, NEVER MIND A GIRLFRIEND.
IF ONLY SHE KNEW I WAS HERE AND HOW SENSITIVE I AM.
THAT REMINDS ME, I MUST TRY TO POP OUT AND GET SOME NEW DIRTY BOOKS LATER.
GOTH GIRL WHO SPOKE TO ME ONCE.

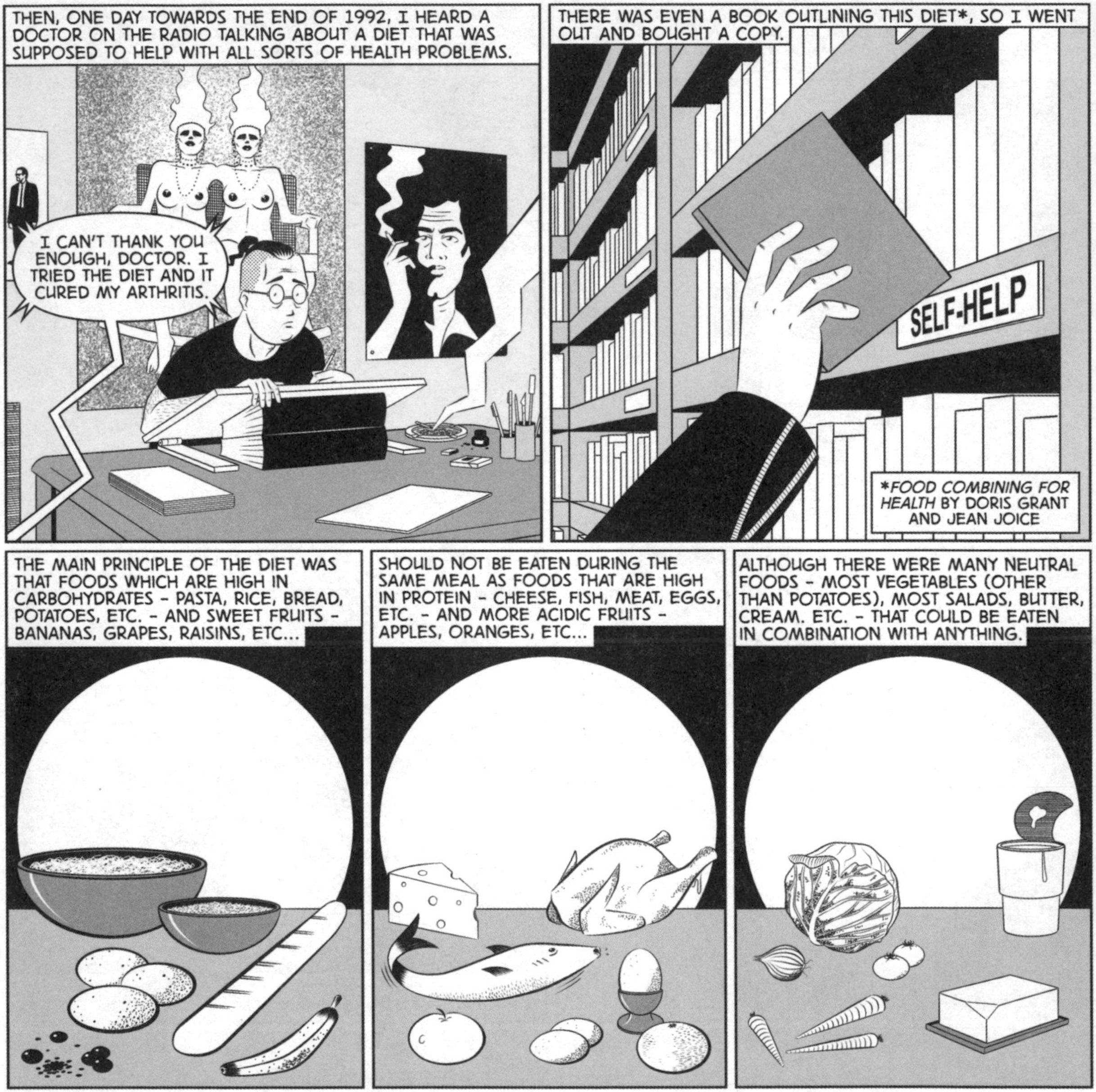
THEN, ONE DAY TOWARDS THE END OF 1992, I HEARD A DOCTOR ON THE RADIO TALKING ABOUT A DIET THAT WAS SUPPOSED TO HELP WITH ALL SORTS OF HEALTH PROBLEMS.
I CAN'T THANK YOU ENOUGH, DOCTOR. I TRIED THE DIET AND IT CURED MY ARTHRITIS.
THERE WAS EVEN A BOOK OUTLINING THIS DIET*, SO I WENT OUT AND BOUGHT A COPY.
SELF-HELP
**FOOD COMBINING FOR HEALTH* BY DORIS GRANT AND JEAN JOICE
THE MAIN PRINCIPLE OF THE DIET WAS THAT FOODS WHICH ARE HIGH IN CARBOHYDRATES - PASTA, RICE, BREAD, POTATOES, ETC. - AND SWEET FRUITS - BANANAS, GRAPES, RAISINS, ETC...
SHOULD NOT BE EATEN DURING THE SAME MEAL AS FOODS THAT ARE HIGH IN PROTEIN - CHEESE, FISH, MEAT, EGGS, ETC. - AND MORE ACIDIC FRUITS - APPLES, ORANGES, ETC...
ALTHOUGH THERE WERE MANY NEUTRAL FOODS - MOST VEGETABLES (OTHER THAN POTATOES), MOST SALADS, BUTTER, CREAM. ETC. - THAT COULD BE EATEN IN COMBINATION WITH ANYTHING.

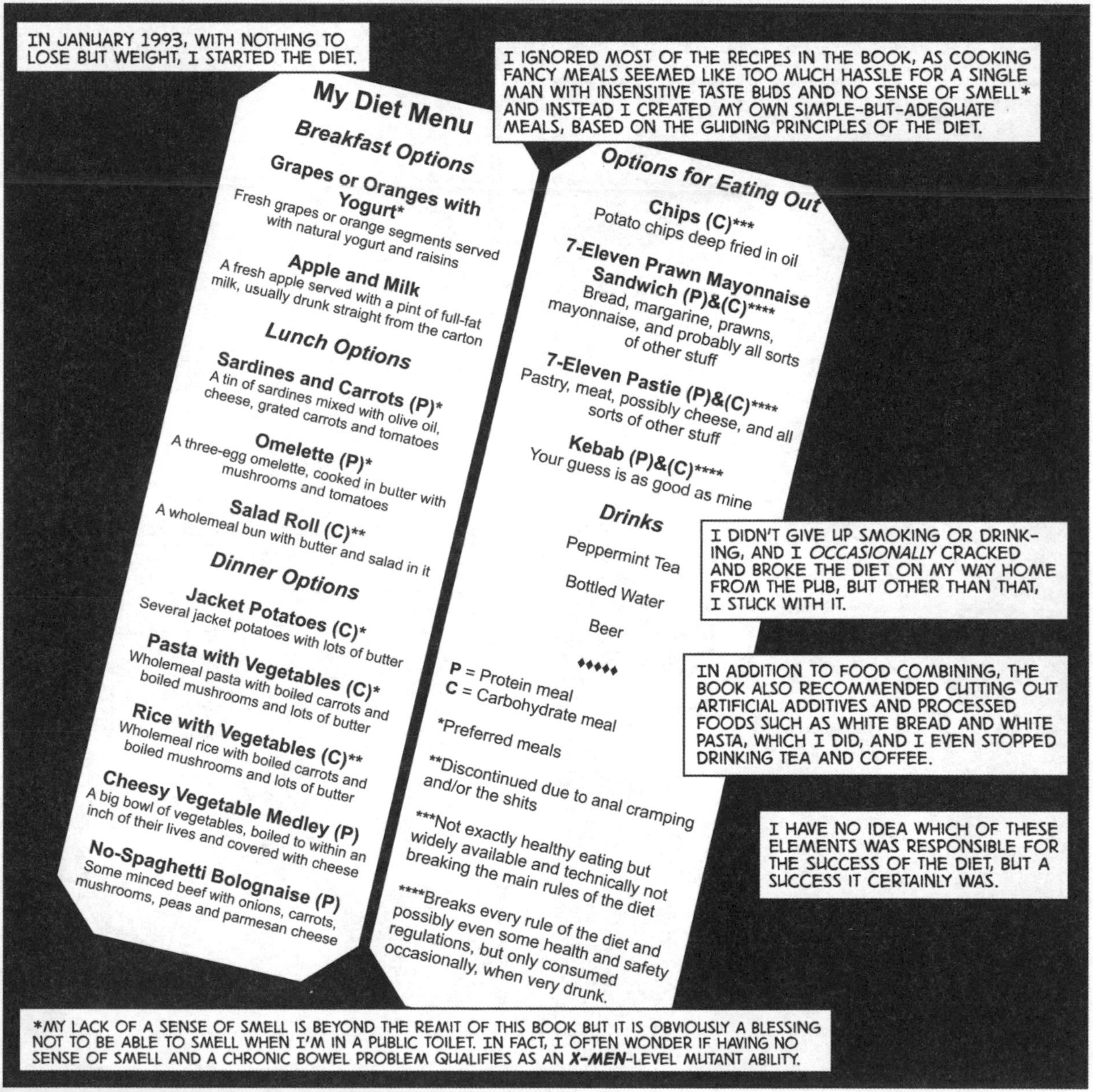
IN JANUARY 1993, WITH NOTHING TO LOSE BUT WEIGHT, I STARTED THE DIET.
I IGNORED MOST OF THE RECIPES IN THE BOOK, AS COOKING FANCY MEALS SEEMED LIKE TOO MUCH HASSLE FOR A SINGLE MAN WITH INSENSITIVE TASTE BUDS AND NO SENSE OF SMELL* AND INSTEAD I CREATED MY OWN SIMPLE-BUT-ADEQUATE MEALS, BASED ON THE GUIDING PRINCIPLES OF THE DIET.
My Diet Menu
Breakfast Options
Grapes or Oranges with Yogurt*
Fresh grapes or orange segments served with natural yogurt and raisins
Apple and Milk
A fresh apple served with a pint of full-fat milk, usually drunk straight from the carton
Lunch Options
Sardines and Carrots (P)*
A tin of sardines mixed with olive oil, cheese, grated carrots and tomatoes
Omelette (P)*
A three-egg omelette, cooked in butter with mushrooms and tomatoes
Salad Roll (C)**
A wholemeal bun with butter and salad in it
Dinner Options
Jacket Potatoes (C)*
Several jacket potatoes with lots of butter
Pasta with Vegetables (C)*
Wholemeal pasta with boiled carrots and boiled mushrooms and lots of butter
Rice with Vegetables (C)**
Wholemeal rice with boiled carrots and boiled mushrooms and lots of butter
Cheesy Vegetable Medley (P)
A big bowl of vegetables, boiled to within an inch of their lives and covered with cheese
No-Spaghetti Bolognaise (P)
Some minced beef with onions, carrots, mushrooms, peas and parmesan cheese
Options for Eating Out
Chips (C)***
Potato chips deep fried in oil
7-Eleven Prawn Mayonnaise Sandwich (P)&(C)****
Bread, margarine, prawns, mayonnaise, and probably all sorts of other stuff
7-Eleven Pastie (P)&(C)****
Pastry, meat, possibly cheese, and all sorts of other stuff
Kebab (P)&(C)****
Your guess is as good as mine
Drinks
Peppermint Tea
Bottled Water
Beer
♦♦♦♦♦
P = Protein meal
C = Carbohydrate meal
*Preferred meals
**Discontinued due to anal cramping and/or the shits
***Not exactly healthy eating but widely available and technically not breaking the main rules of the diet
****Breaks every rule of the diet and possibly even some health and safety regulations, but only consumed occasionally, when very drunk.
I DIDN'T GIVE UP SMOKING OR DRINKING, AND I *OCCASIONALLY* CRACKED AND BROKE THE DIET ON MY WAY HOME FROM THE PUB, BUT OTHER THAN THAT, I STUCK WITH IT.
IN ADDITION TO FOOD COMBINING, THE BOOK ALSO RECOMMENDED CUTTING OUT ARTIFICIAL ADDITIVES AND PROCESSED FOODS SUCH AS WHITE BREAD AND WHITE PASTA, WHICH I DID, AND I EVEN STOPPED DRINKING TEA AND COFFEE.
I HAVE NO IDEA WHICH OF THESE ELEMENTS WAS RESPONSIBLE FOR THE SUCCESS OF THE DIET, BUT A SUCCESS IT CERTAINLY WAS.
*MY LACK OF A SENSE OF SMELL IS BEYOND THE REMIT OF THIS BOOK BUT IT IS OBVIOUSLY A BLESSING NOT TO BE ABLE TO SMELL WHEN I'M IN A PUBLIC TOILET. IN FACT, I OFTEN WONDER IF HAVING NO SENSE OF SMELL AND A CHRONIC BOWEL PROBLEM QUALIFIES AS AN ***X-MEN***-LEVEL MUTANT ABILITY.

WITHIN DAYS, MY STOMACH SYMPTOMS STARTED TO IMPROVE. AND AS AN ADDED BONUS, IN JUST A FEW MONTHS, I LOST ALL OF MY EXCESS WEIGHT, FALLING FROM SEVENTEEN-AND-A-HALF STONE TO TWELVE-AND-A-HALF STONE - THE IDEAL WEIGHT FOR MY HEIGHT.

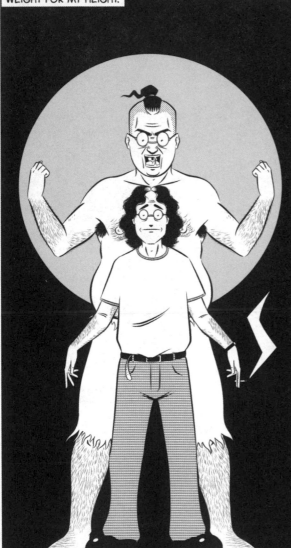

MY STOMACH WAS NEVER 100% BETTER - IT WAS STILL A BIT DODGY IN THE MORNINGS AND I WOULDN'T EVEN THINK ABOUT LEAVING THE HOUSE UNTIL I'D HAD A BOWEL MOVE-MENT* - BUT IT GOT SO MUCH BETTER THAT I STARTED TO TELL PEOPLE THAT...

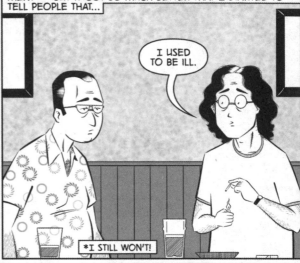

I USED TO BE ILL.

*I STILL WON'T!

I STOPPED TAKING THE FIBRE DRINK, STOPPED TAKING ANTI-DEPRESSANTS AND I STOPPED CLAIMING INCAPACITY BENEFIT.

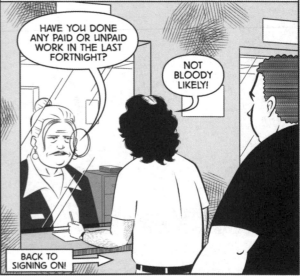

HAVE YOU DONE ANY PAID OR UNPAID WORK IN THE LAST FORTNIGHT?

NOT BLOODY LIKELY!

BACK TO SIGNING ON!

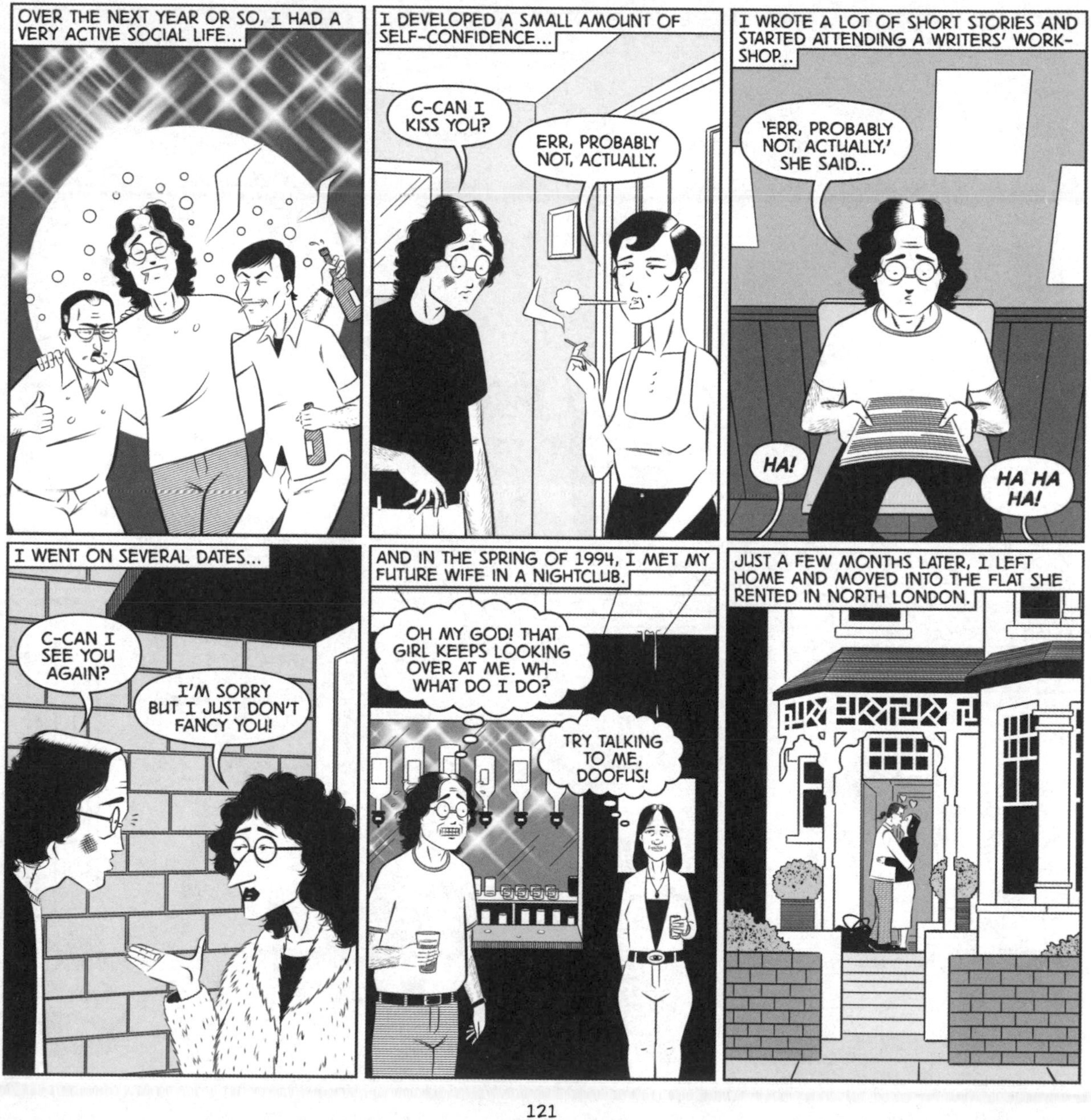
OVER THE NEXT YEAR OR SO, I HAD A VERY ACTIVE SOCIAL LIFE...
I DEVELOPED A SMALL AMOUNT OF SELF-CONFIDENCE...
C-CAN I KISS YOU?
ERR, PROBABLY NOT, ACTUALLY.
I WROTE A LOT OF SHORT STORIES AND STARTED ATTENDING A WRITERS' WORK-SHOP...
'ERR, PROBABLY NOT, ACTUALLY,' SHE SAID...
HA!
HA HA HA!
I WENT ON SEVERAL DATES...
C-CAN I SEE YOU AGAIN?
I'M SORRY BUT I JUST DON'T FANCY YOU!
AND IN THE SPRING OF 1994, I MET MY FUTURE WIFE IN A NIGHTCLUB.
OH MY GOD! THAT GIRL KEEPS LOOKING OVER AT ME. WH-WHAT DO I DO?
TRY TALKING TO ME, DOOFUS!
JUST A FEW MONTHS LATER, I LEFT HOME AND MOVED INTO THE FLAT SHE RENTED IN NORTH LONDON.

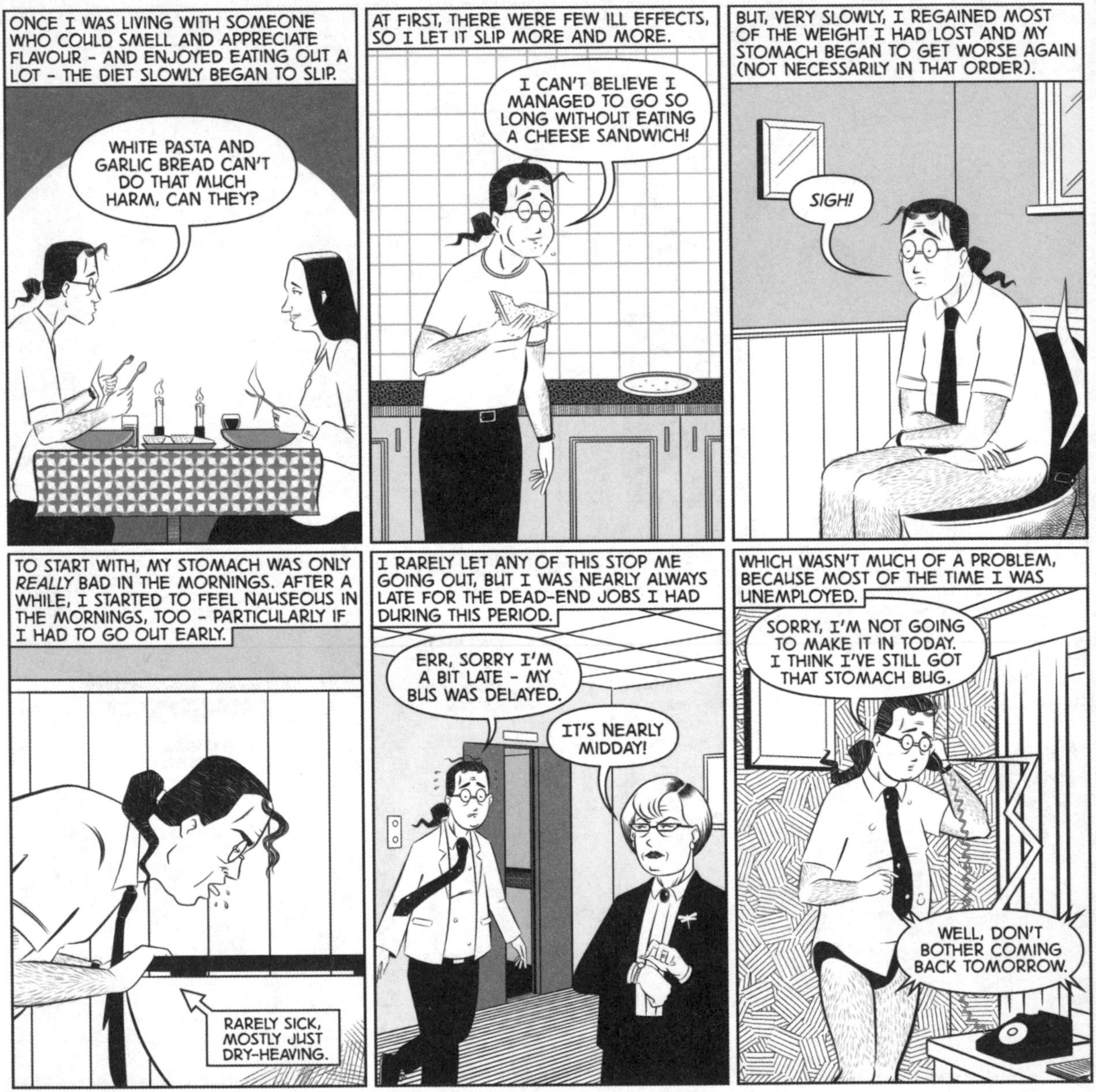
ONCE I WAS LIVING WITH SOMEONE WHO COULD SMELL AND APPRECIATE FLAVOUR - AND ENJOYED EATING OUT A LOT - THE DIET SLOWLY BEGAN TO SLIP.
WHITE PASTA AND GARLIC BREAD CAN'T DO THAT MUCH HARM, CAN THEY?
AT FIRST, THERE WERE FEW ILL EFFECTS, SO I LET IT SLIP MORE AND MORE.
I CAN'T BELIEVE I MANAGED TO GO SO LONG WITHOUT EATING A CHEESE SANDWICH!
BUT, VERY SLOWLY, I REGAINED MOST OF THE WEIGHT I HAD LOST AND MY STOMACH BEGAN TO GET WORSE AGAIN (NOT NECESSARILY IN THAT ORDER).
SIGH!
TO START WITH, MY STOMACH WAS ONLY *REALLY* BAD IN THE MORNINGS. AFTER A WHILE, I STARTED TO FEEL NAUSEOUS IN THE MORNINGS, TOO - PARTICULARLY IF I HAD TO GO OUT EARLY.
RARELY SICK, MOSTLY JUST DRY-HEAVING.
I RARELY LET ANY OF THIS STOP ME GOING OUT, BUT I WAS NEARLY ALWAYS LATE FOR THE DEAD-END JOBS I HAD DURING THIS PERIOD.
ERR, SORRY I'M A BIT LATE - MY BUS WAS DELAYED.
IT'S NEARLY MIDDAY!
WHICH WASN'T MUCH OF A PROBLEM, BECAUSE MOST OF THE TIME I WAS UNEMPLOYED.
SORRY, I'M NOT GOING TO MAKE IT IN TODAY. I THINK I'VE STILL GOT THAT STOMACH BUG.
WELL, DON'T BOTHER COMING BACK TOMORROW.

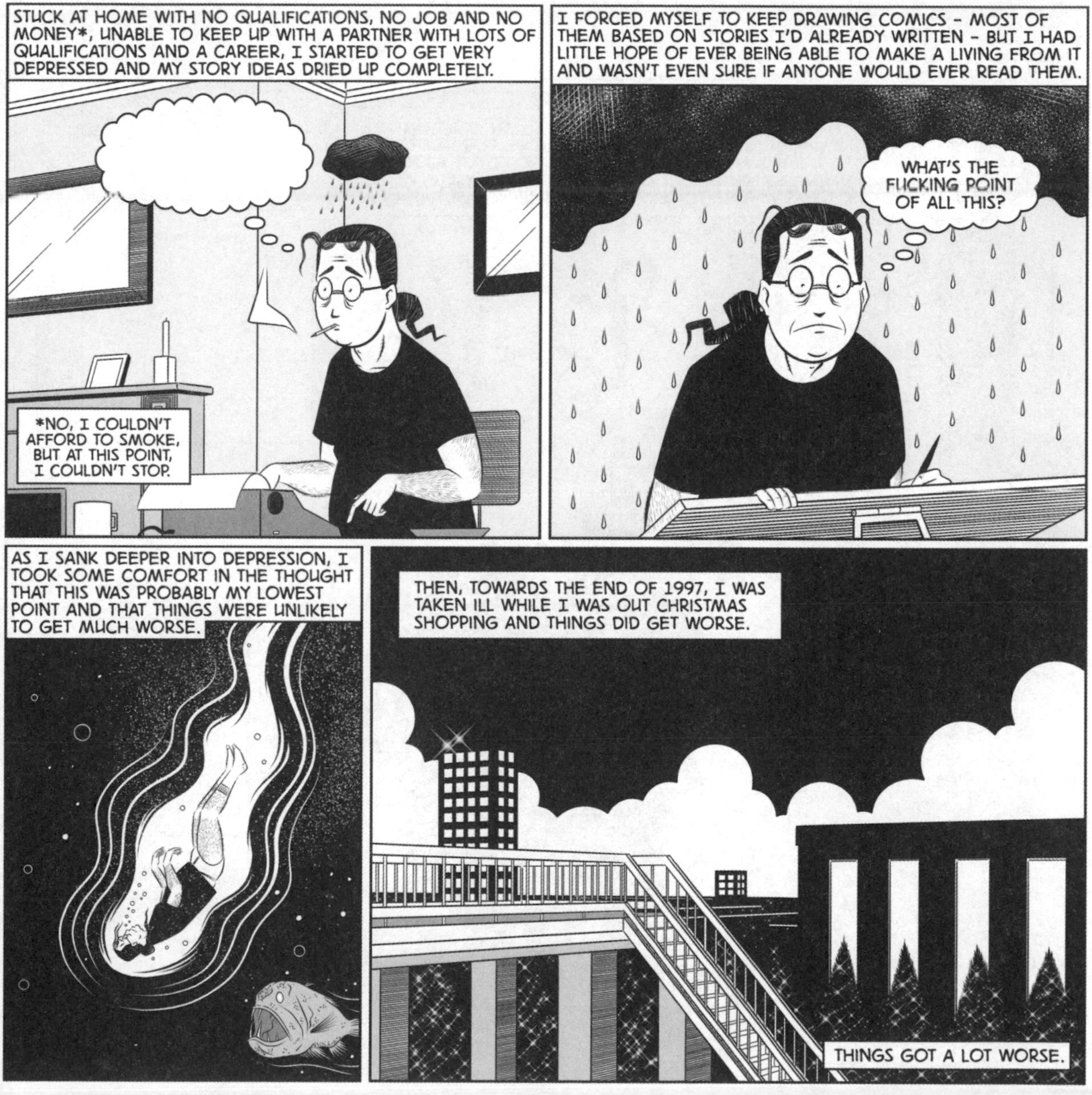
STUCK AT HOME WITH NO QUALIFICATIONS, NO JOB AND NO MONEY*, UNABLE TO KEEP UP WITH A PARTNER WITH LOTS OF QUALIFICATIONS AND A CAREER, I STARTED TO GET VERY DEPRESSED AND MY STORY IDEAS DRIED UP COMPLETELY.
*NO, I COULDN'T AFFORD TO SMOKE, BUT AT THIS POINT, I COULDN'T STOP.
I FORCED MYSELF TO KEEP DRAWING COMICS - MOST OF THEM BASED ON STORIES I'D ALREADY WRITTEN - BUT I HAD LITTLE HOPE OF EVER BEING ABLE TO MAKE A LIVING FROM IT AND WASN'T EVEN SURE IF ANYONE WOULD EVER READ THEM.
WHAT'S THE FUCKING POINT OF ALL THIS?
AS I SANK DEEPER INTO DEPRESSION, I TOOK SOME COMFORT IN THE THOUGHT THAT THIS WAS PROBABLY MY LOWEST POINT AND THAT THINGS WERE UNLIKELY TO GET MUCH WORSE.
THEN, TOWARDS THE END OF 1997, I WAS TAKEN ILL WHILE I WAS OUT CHRISTMAS SHOPPING AND THINGS DID GET WORSE.
THINGS GOT A LOT WORSE.

7. DOCTORS & NURSES (& CARROTS)

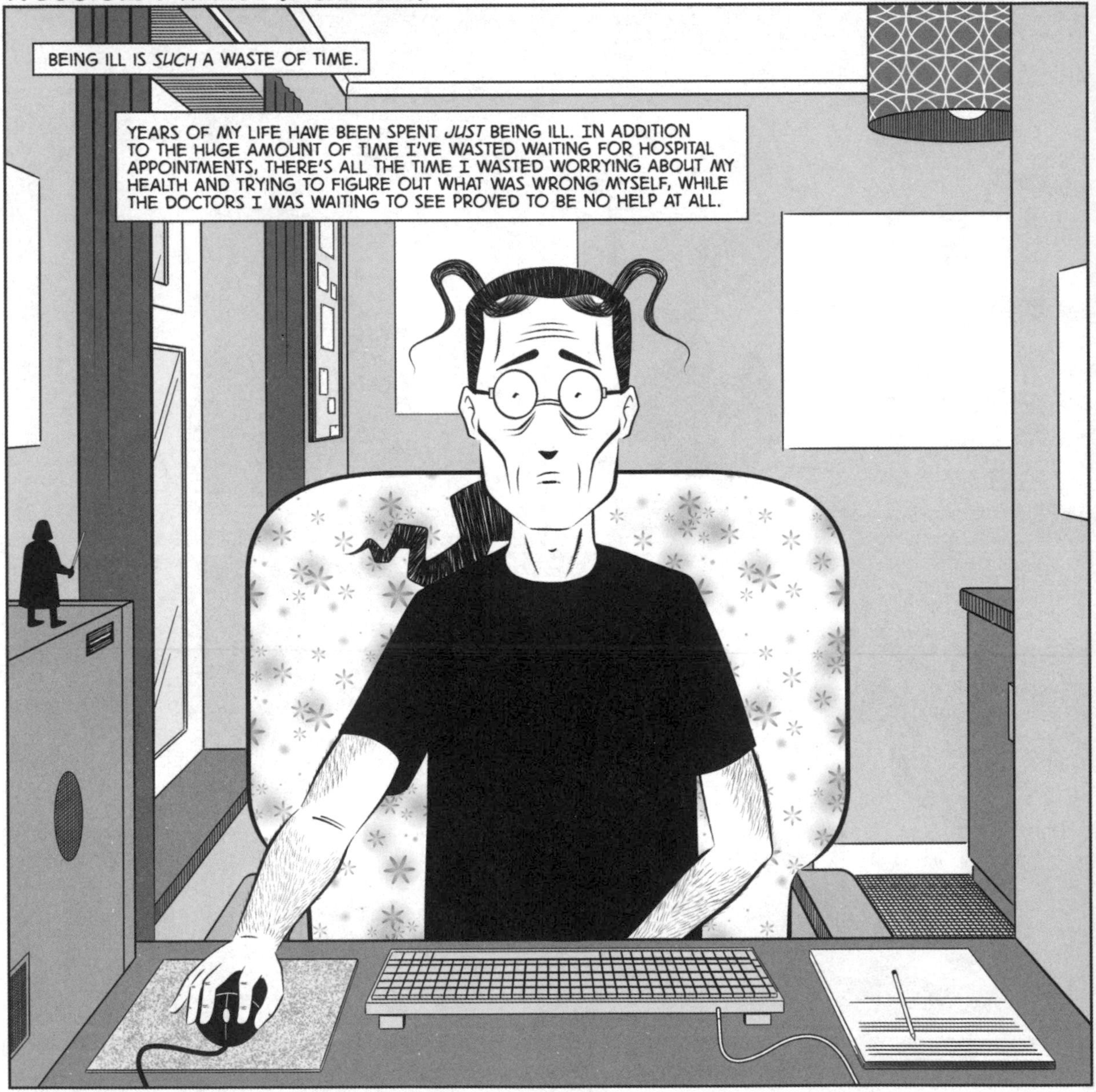
BEING ILL IS *SUCH* A WASTE OF TIME.
YEARS OF MY LIFE HAVE BEEN SPENT *JUST* BEING ILL. IN ADDITION TO THE HUGE AMOUNT OF TIME I'VE WASTED WAITING FOR HOSPITAL APPOINTMENTS, THERE'S ALL THE TIME I WASTED WORRYING ABOUT MY HEALTH AND TRYING TO FIGURE OUT WHAT WAS WRONG MYSELF, WHILE THE DOCTORS I WAS WAITING TO SEE PROVED TO BE NO HELP AT ALL.

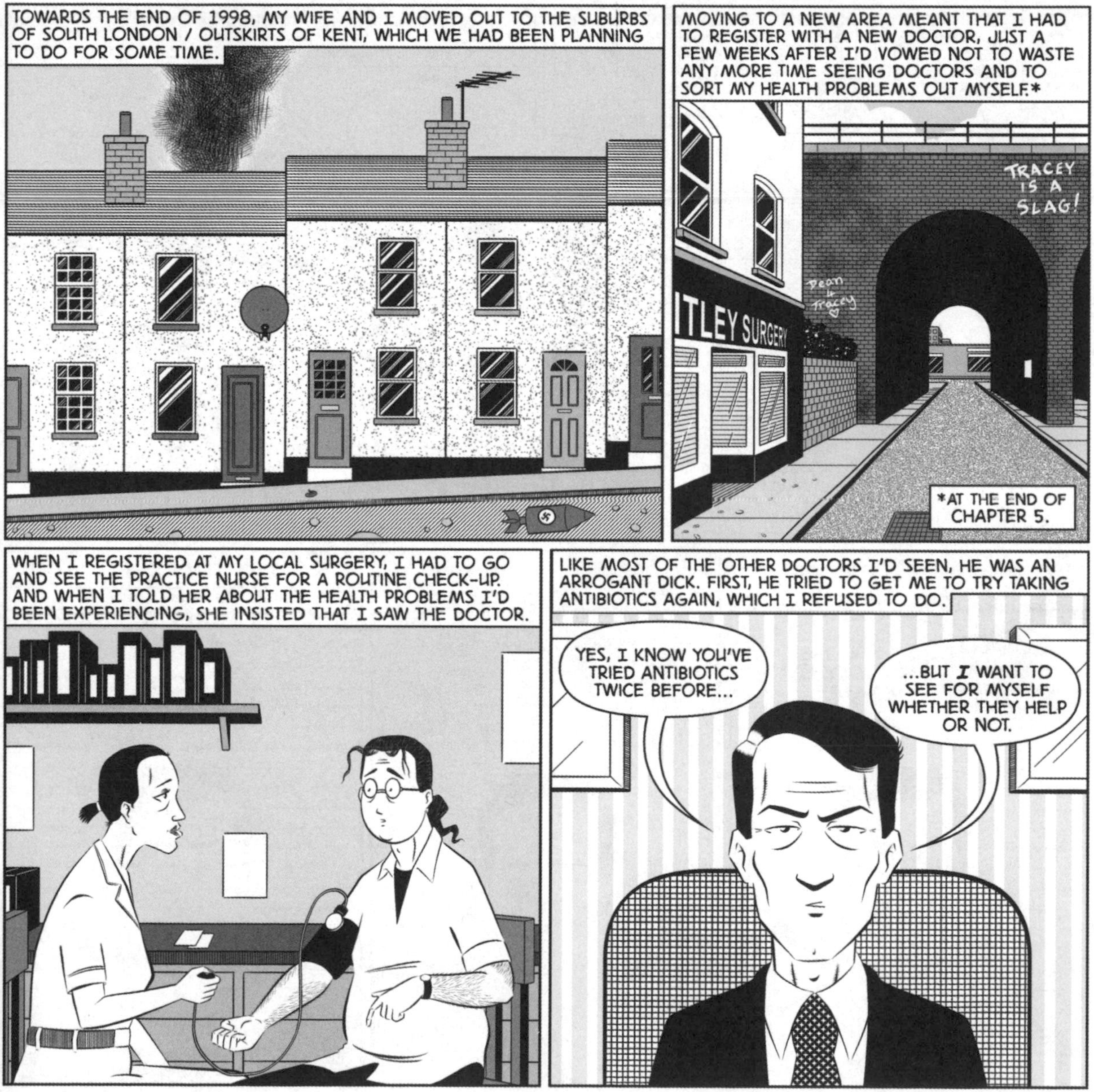
TOWARDS THE END OF 1998, MY WIFE AND I MOVED OUT TO THE SUBURBS OF SOUTH LONDON / OUTSKIRTS OF KENT, WHICH WE HAD BEEN PLANNING TO DO FOR SOME TIME.
MOVING TO A NEW AREA MEANT THAT I HAD TO REGISTER WITH A NEW DOCTOR, JUST A FEW WEEKS AFTER I'D VOWED NOT TO WASTE ANY MORE TIME SEEING DOCTORS AND TO SORT MY HEALTH PROBLEMS OUT MYSELF.*
TRACEY IS A SLAG!
TLEY SURGERY
*AT THE END OF CHAPTER 5.
WHEN I REGISTERED AT MY LOCAL SURGERY, I HAD TO GO AND SEE THE PRACTICE NURSE FOR A ROUTINE CHECK-UP. AND WHEN I TOLD HER ABOUT THE HEALTH PROBLEMS I'D BEEN EXPERIENCING, SHE INSISTED THAT I SAW THE DOCTOR.
LIKE MOST OF THE OTHER DOCTORS I'D SEEN, HE WAS AN ARROGANT DICK. FIRST, HE TRIED TO GET ME TO TRY TAKING ANTIBIOTICS AGAIN, WHICH I REFUSED TO DO.
YES, I KNOW YOU'VE TRIED ANTIBIOTICS TWICE BEFORE...
...BUT *I* WANT TO SEE FOR MYSELF WHETHER THEY HELP OR NOT.

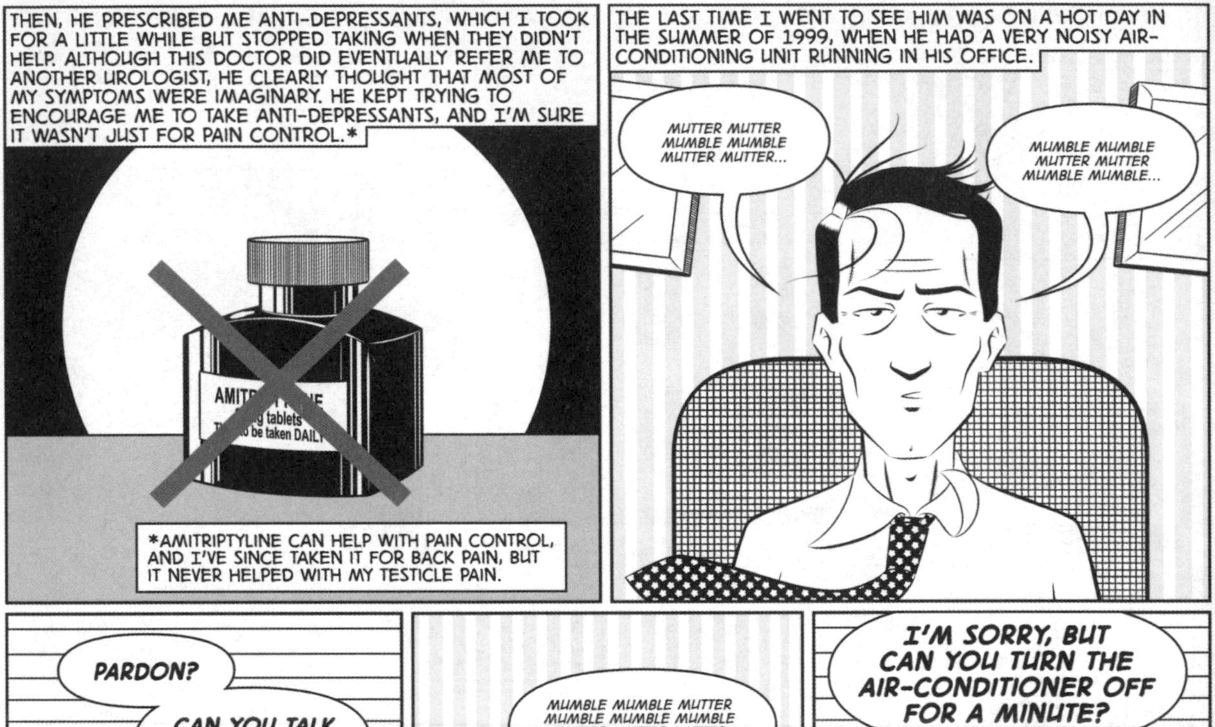

THEN, HE PRESCRIBED ME ANTI-DEPRESSANTS, WHICH I TOOK FOR A LITTLE WHILE BUT STOPPED TAKING WHEN THEY DIDN'T HELP. ALTHOUGH THIS DOCTOR DID EVENTUALLY REFER ME TO ANOTHER UROLOGIST, HE CLEARLY THOUGHT THAT MOST OF MY SYMPTOMS WERE IMAGINARY. HE KEPT TRYING TO ENCOURAGE ME TO TAKE ANTI-DEPRESSANTS, AND I'M SURE IT WASN'T JUST FOR PAIN CONTROL.*

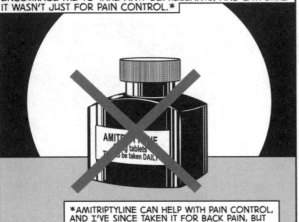

AMITRIPTYLINE
...ng tablets
T...to be taken DAILY

*AMITRIPTYLINE CAN HELP WITH PAIN CONTROL, AND I'VE SINCE TAKEN IT FOR BACK PAIN, BUT IT NEVER HELPED WITH MY TESTICLE PAIN.

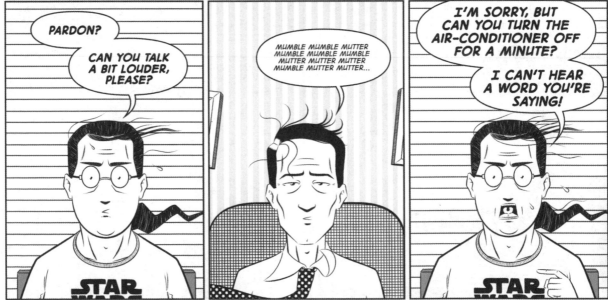

THE LAST TIME I WENT TO SEE HIM WAS ON A HOT DAY IN THE SUMMER OF 1999, WHEN HE HAD A VERY NOISY AIR-CONDITIONING UNIT RUNNING IN HIS OFFICE.

MUTTER MUTTER MUMBLE MUMBLE MUTTER MUTTER...

MUMBLE MUMBLE MUTTER MUTTER MUMBLE MUMBLE...

PARDON?

CAN YOU TALK A BIT LOUDER, PLEASE?

MUMBLE MUMBLE MUTTER MUMBLE MUMBLE MUMBLE MUTTER MUTTER MUTTER MUMBLE MUTTER MUTTER...

I'M SORRY, BUT CAN YOU TURN THE AIR-CONDITIONER OFF FOR A MINUTE?

I CAN'T HEAR A WORD YOU'RE SAYING!

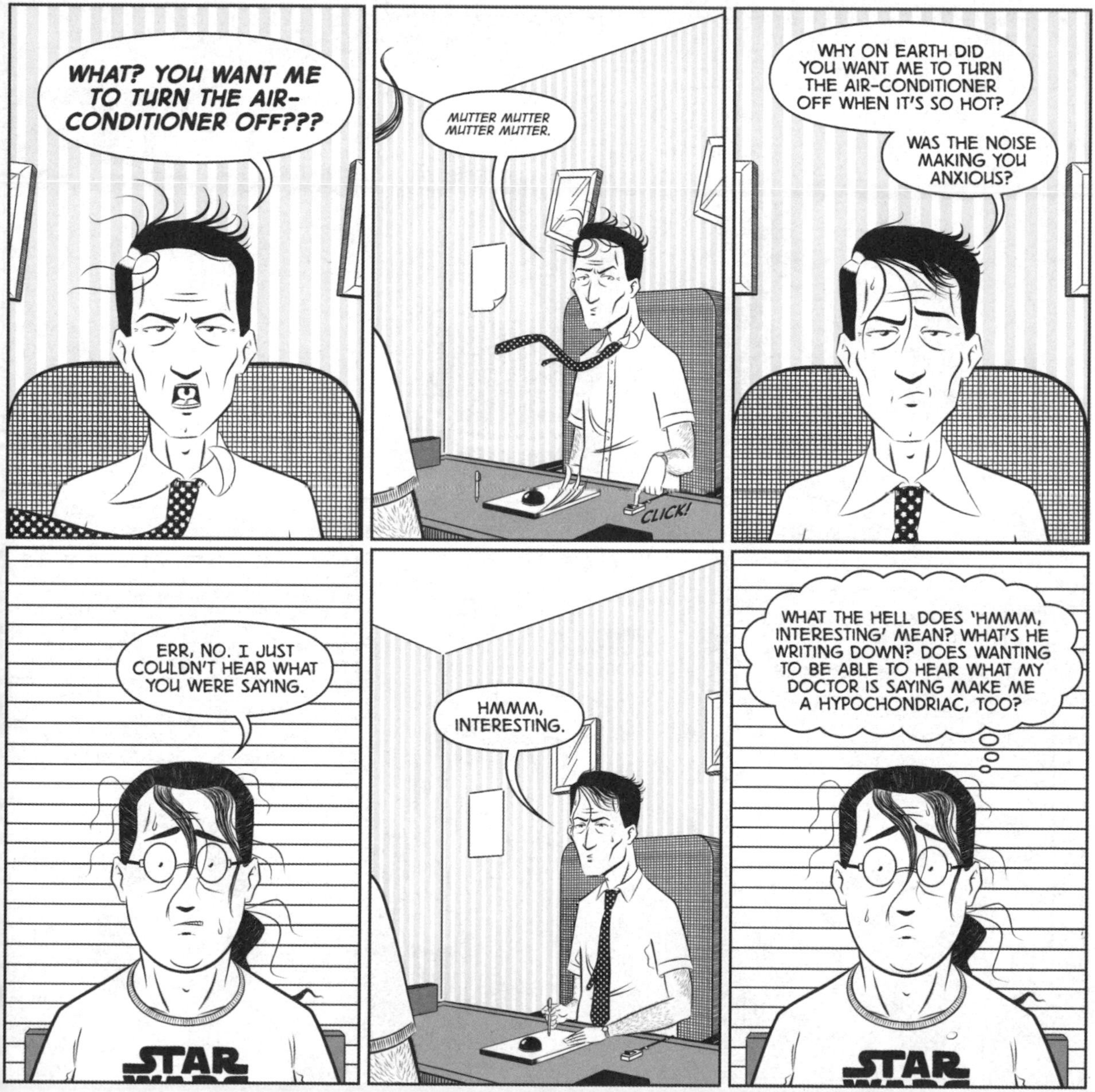
WHAT? YOU WANT ME TO TURN THE AIR-CONDITIONER OFF???
MUTTER MUTTER MUTTER MUTTER.
CLICK!
WHY ON EARTH DID YOU WANT ME TO TURN THE AIR-CONDITIONER OFF WHEN IT'S SO HOT?
WAS THE NOISE MAKING YOU ANXIOUS?
ERR, NO. I JUST COULDN'T HEAR WHAT YOU WERE SAYING.
STAR
HMMM, INTERESTING.
WHAT THE HELL DOES 'HMMM, INTERESTING' MEAN? WHAT'S HE WRITING DOWN? DOES WANTING TO BE ABLE TO HEAR WHAT MY DOCTOR IS SAYING MAKE ME A HYPOCHONDRIAC, TOO?
STAR

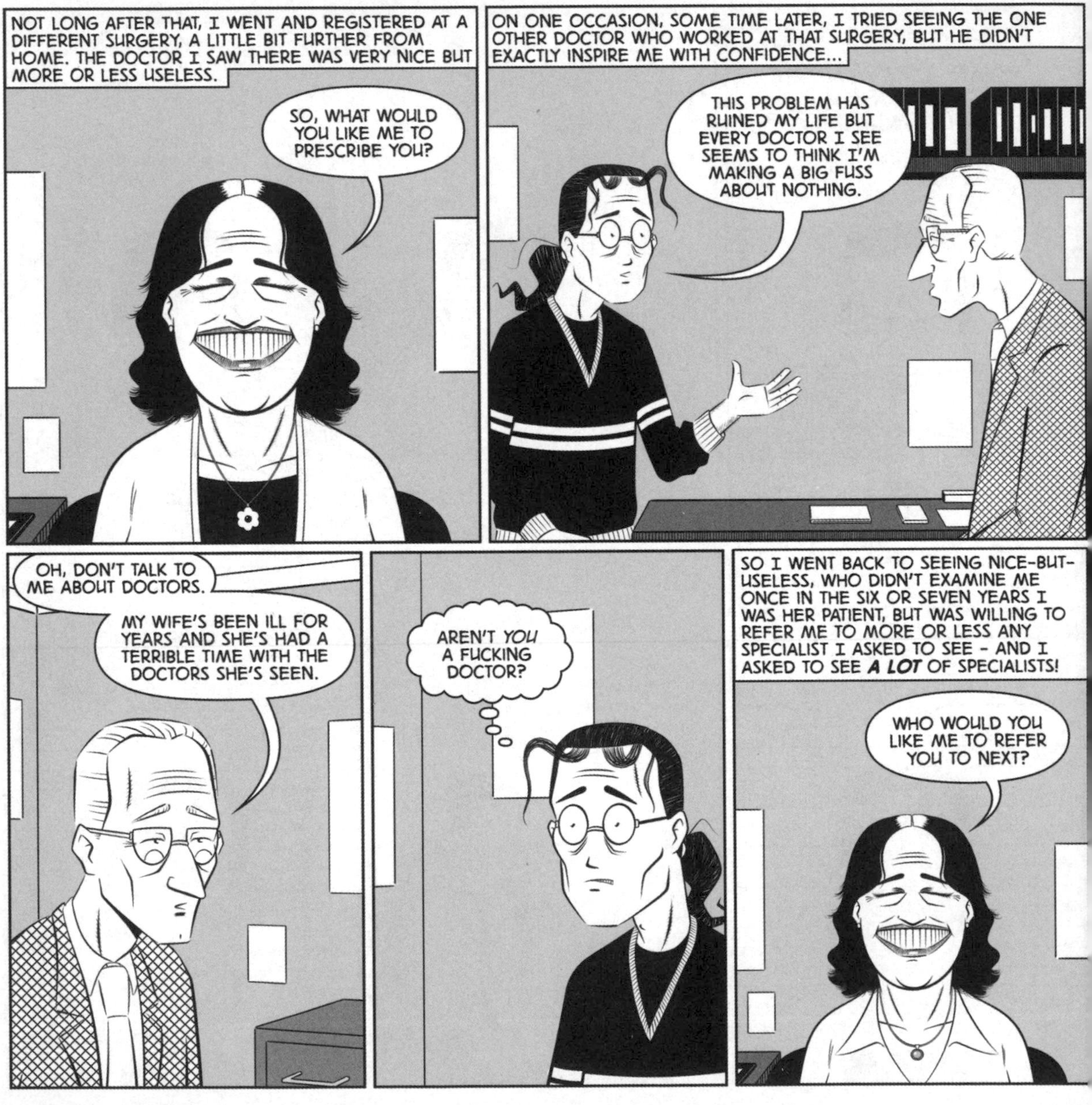

NOT LONG AFTER THAT, I WENT AND REGISTERED AT A DIFFERENT SURGERY, A LITTLE BIT FURTHER FROM HOME. THE DOCTOR I SAW THERE WAS VERY NICE BUT MORE OR LESS USELESS.
SO, WHAT WOULD YOU LIKE ME TO PRESCRIBE YOU?
ON ONE OCCASION, SOME TIME LATER, I TRIED SEEING THE ONE OTHER DOCTOR WHO WORKED AT THAT SURGERY, BUT HE DIDN'T EXACTLY INSPIRE ME WITH CONFIDENCE...
THIS PROBLEM HAS RUINED MY LIFE BUT EVERY DOCTOR I SEE SEEMS TO THINK I'M MAKING A BIG FUSS ABOUT NOTHING.
OH, DON'T TALK TO ME ABOUT DOCTORS.
MY WIFE'S BEEN ILL FOR YEARS AND SHE'S HAD A TERRIBLE TIME WITH THE DOCTORS SHE'S SEEN.
AREN'T *YOU* A FUCKING DOCTOR?
SO I WENT BACK TO SEEING NICE-BUT-USELESS, WHO DIDN'T EXAMINE ME ONCE IN THE SIX OR SEVEN YEARS I WAS HER PATIENT, BUT WAS WILLING TO REFER ME TO MORE OR LESS ANY SPECIALIST I ASKED TO SEE - AND I ASKED TO SEE ***A LOT*** OF SPECIALISTS!
WHO WOULD YOU LIKE ME TO REFER YOU TO NEXT?

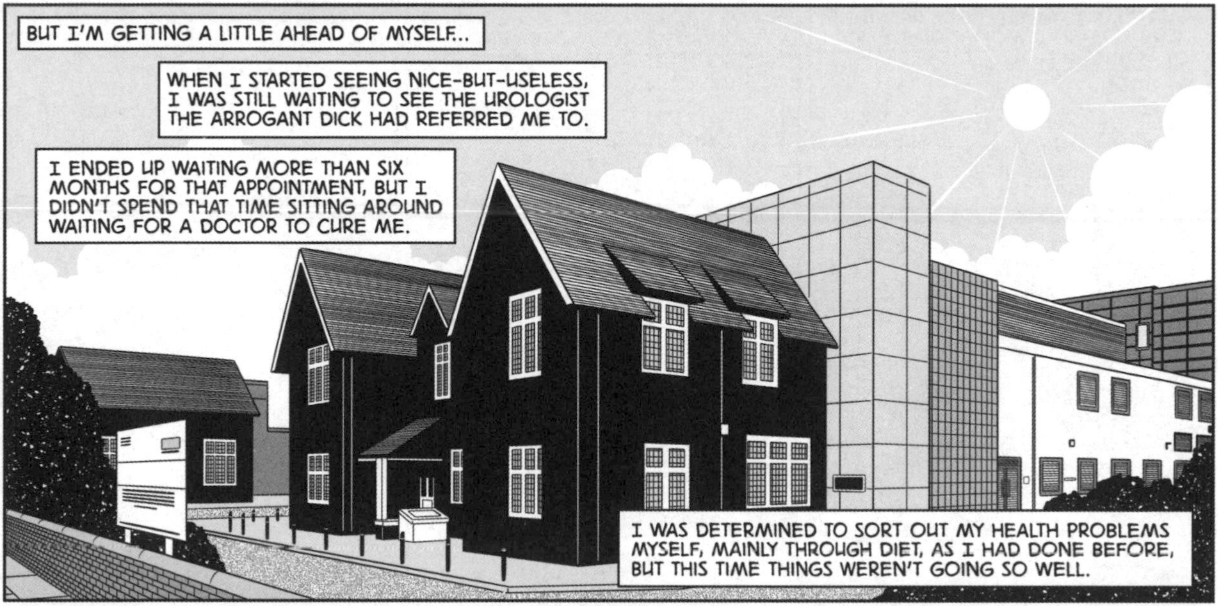
BUT I'M GETTING A LITTLE AHEAD OF MYSELF...
WHEN I STARTED SEEING NICE-BUT-USELESS, I WAS STILL WAITING TO SEE THE UROLOGIST THE ARROGANT DICK HAD REFERRED ME TO.
I ENDED UP WAITING MORE THAN SIX MONTHS FOR THAT APPOINTMENT, BUT I DIDN'T SPEND THAT TIME SITTING AROUND WAITING FOR A DOCTOR TO CURE ME.
I WAS DETERMINED TO SORT OUT MY HEALTH PROBLEMS MYSELF, MAINLY THROUGH DIET, AS I HAD DONE BEFORE, BUT THIS TIME THINGS WEREN'T GOING SO WELL.

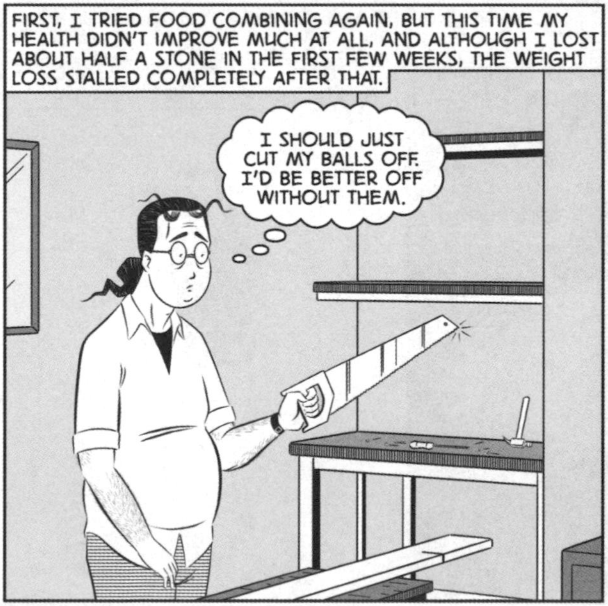
FIRST, I TRIED FOOD COMBINING AGAIN, BUT THIS TIME MY HEALTH DIDN'T IMPROVE MUCH AT ALL, AND ALTHOUGH I LOST ABOUT HALF A STONE IN THE FIRST FEW WEEKS, THE WEIGHT LOSS STALLED COMPLETELY AFTER THAT.
I SHOULD JUST CUT MY BALLS OFF. I'D BE BETTER OFF WITHOUT THEM.

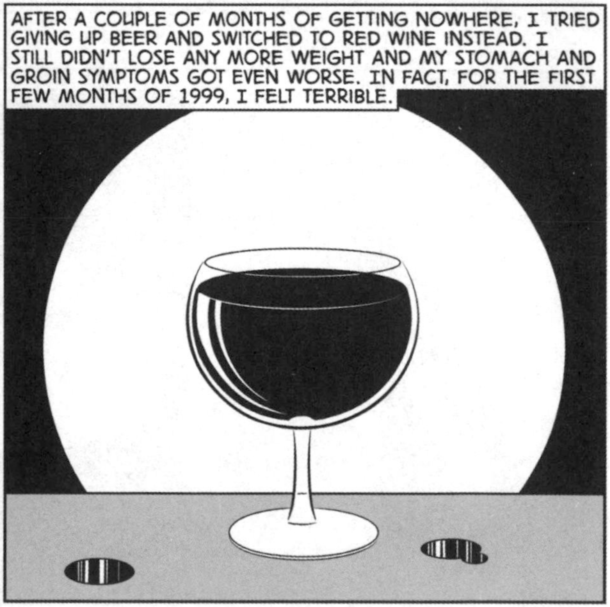
AFTER A COUPLE OF MONTHS OF GETTING NOWHERE, I TRIED GIVING UP BEER AND SWITCHED TO RED WINE INSTEAD. I STILL DIDN'T LOSE ANY MORE WEIGHT AND MY STOMACH AND GROIN SYMPTOMS GOT EVEN WORSE. IN FACT, FOR THE FIRST FEW MONTHS OF 1999, I FELT TERRIBLE.

MOST DAYS, I WOULD WAKE UP WITH MY GROIN FEELING UNCOMFORTABLE, BUT NOT UNBEARABLY SO.

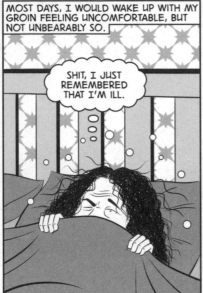

SHIT, I JUST REMEMBERED THAT I'M ILL.

THINGS WOULD TIGHTEN UP A BIT AFTER MY MORNING BOWEL MOVEMENT...

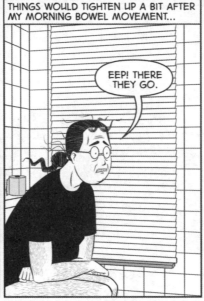

EEP! THERE THEY GO.

BUT WOULD USUALLY EASE OFF AGAIN IN A HOT BATH.

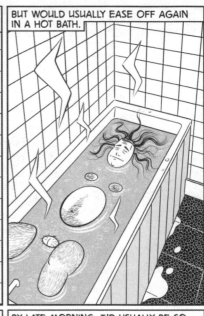

THEN, AS THE MORNING WENT ON, THE TIGHTNESS IN MY GROIN WOULD GET WORSE AND WORSE.

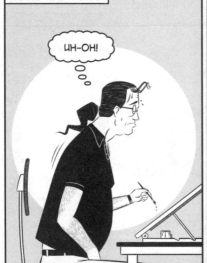

UH-OH!

I'D GET THAT HORRIBLE, SICKLY ACHE ON THE RIGHT SIDE OF MY GROIN AND THE BACK OF MY LEFT TESTICLE WOULD START TO THROB WITH PAIN.

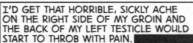

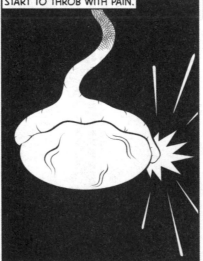

BY LATE MORNING, I'D USUALLY BE SO UNCOMFORTABLE THAT I'D BE UNABLE TO REMAIN SEATED, SO I'D PACE AROUND THE HOUSE, DREADING WHAT MIGHT HAPPEN IF THINGS GOT EVEN WORSE.

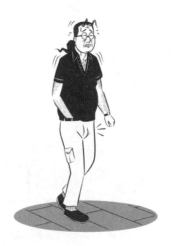

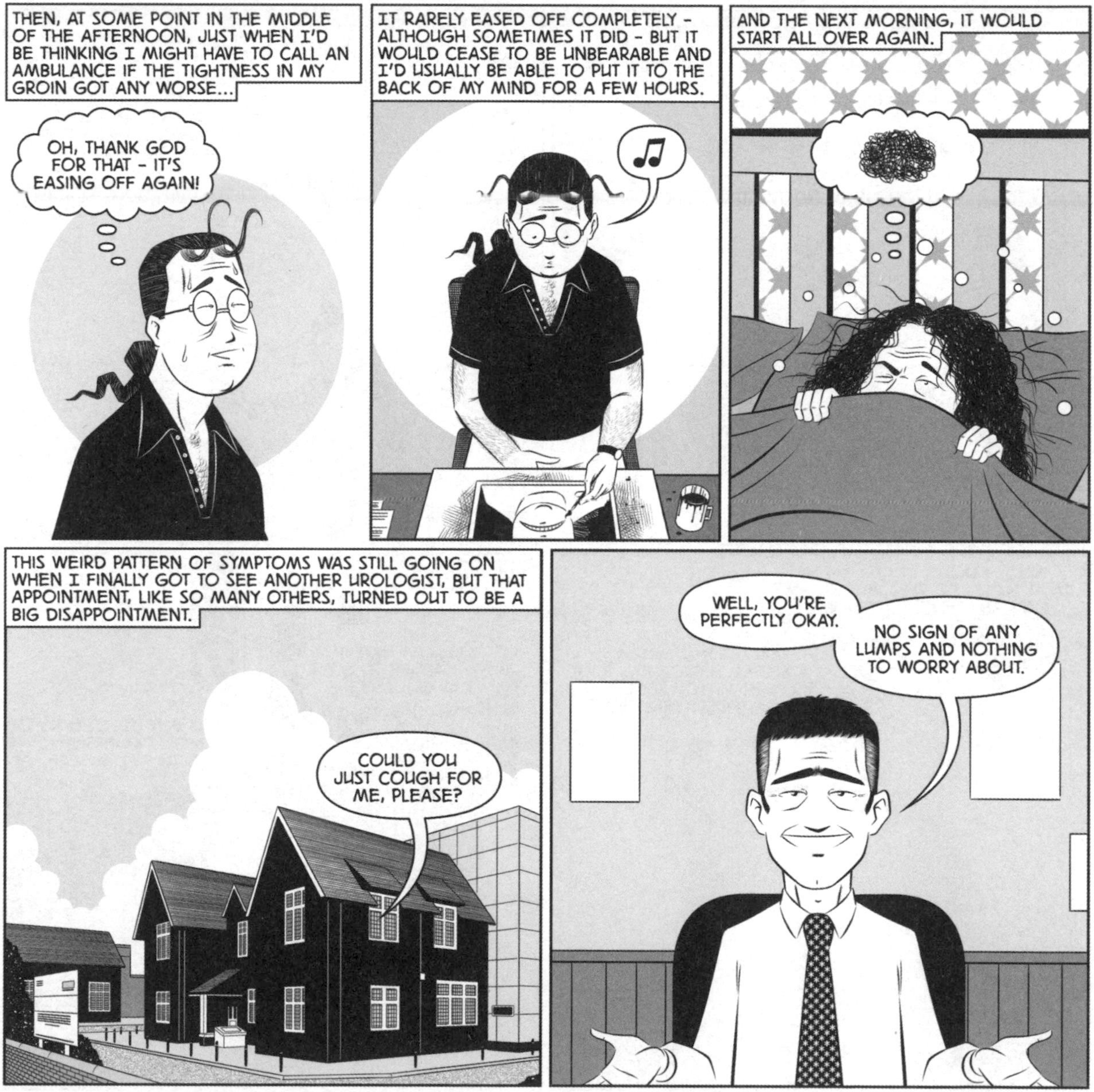
THEN, AT SOME POINT IN THE MIDDLE OF THE AFTERNOON, JUST WHEN I'D BE THINKING I MIGHT HAVE TO CALL AN AMBULANCE IF THE TIGHTNESS IN MY GROIN GOT ANY WORSE...
OH, THANK GOD FOR THAT - IT'S EASING OFF AGAIN!
IT RARELY EASED OFF COMPLETELY - ALTHOUGH SOMETIMES IT DID - BUT IT WOULD CEASE TO BE UNBEARABLE AND I'D USUALLY BE ABLE TO PUT IT TO THE BACK OF MY MIND FOR A FEW HOURS.
AND THE NEXT MORNING, IT WOULD START ALL OVER AGAIN.
THIS WEIRD PATTERN OF SYMPTOMS WAS STILL GOING ON WHEN I FINALLY GOT TO SEE ANOTHER UROLOGIST, BUT THAT APPOINTMENT, LIKE SO MANY OTHERS, TURNED OUT TO BE A BIG DISAPPOINTMENT.
COULD YOU JUST COUGH FOR ME, PLEASE?
WELL, YOU'RE PERFECTLY OKAY.
NO SIGN OF ANY LUMPS AND NOTHING TO WORRY ABOUT.

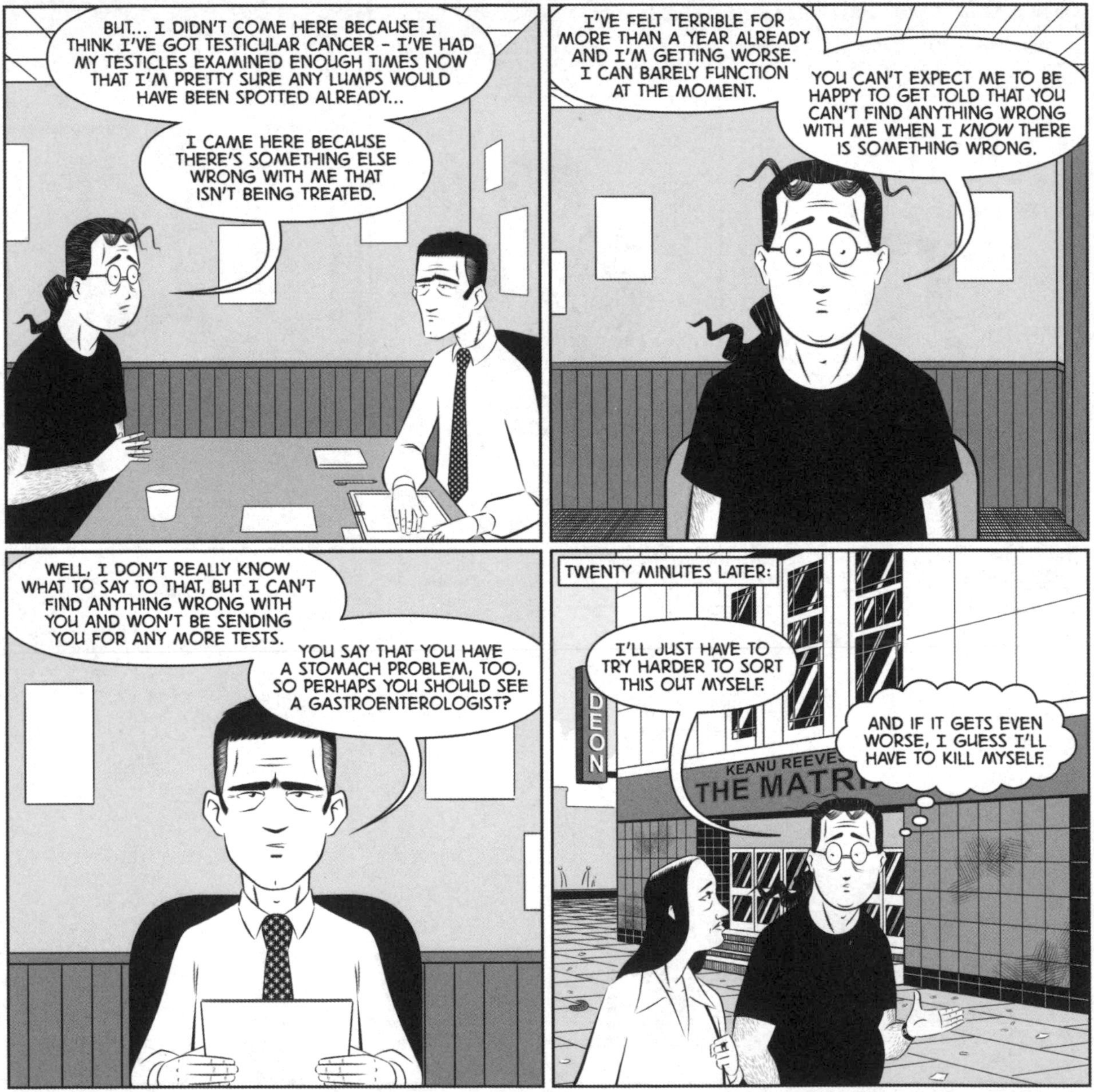
BUT... I DIDN'T COME HERE BECAUSE I THINK I'VE GOT TESTICULAR CANCER - I'VE HAD MY TESTICLES EXAMINED ENOUGH TIMES NOW THAT I'M PRETTY SURE ANY LUMPS WOULD HAVE BEEN SPOTTED ALREADY...
I CAME HERE BECAUSE THERE'S SOMETHING ELSE WRONG WITH ME THAT ISN'T BEING TREATED.
I'VE FELT TERRIBLE FOR MORE THAN A YEAR ALREADY AND I'M GETTING WORSE. I CAN BARELY FUNCTION AT THE MOMENT.
YOU CAN'T EXPECT ME TO BE HAPPY TO GET TOLD THAT YOU CAN'T FIND ANYTHING WRONG WITH ME WHEN I *KNOW* THERE IS SOMETHING WRONG.
WELL, I DON'T REALLY KNOW WHAT TO SAY TO THAT, BUT I CAN'T FIND ANYTHING WRONG WITH YOU AND WON'T BE SENDING YOU FOR ANY MORE TESTS.
YOU SAY THAT YOU HAVE A STOMACH PROBLEM, TOO, SO PERHAPS YOU SHOULD SEE A GASTROENTEROLOGIST?
TWENTY MINUTES LATER:
DEON
KEANU REEVES
THE MATRI
I'LL JUST HAVE TO TRY HARDER TO SORT THIS OUT MYSELF.
AND IF IT GETS EVEN WORSE, I GUESS I'LL HAVE TO KILL MYSELF.

IN THE SPRING OF 1999, I STOPPED DRINKING RED WINE AND WENT BACK TO BEER, AFTER NOTICING THAT I USUALLY FELT WORSE AT THE BEGINNING OF THE WEEK AFTER DRINKING WINE (INDOORS) AT THE WEEKEND.

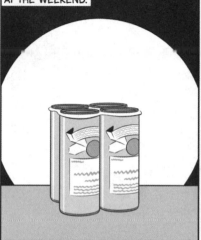

SOME OF MY SYMPTOMS IMPROVED IMMEDIATELY: THE PAIN AT THE BACK OF MY LEFT TESTICLE DISAPPEARED, AND THAT THING WHERE MY GROIN WOULD GET SLOWLY MORE UNCOMFORTABLE THROUGHOUT THE MORNING, BEFORE SUDDENLY EASING OFF AGAIN IN THE AFTERNOON, ALSO STOPPED.

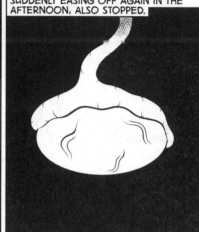

UNFORTUNATELY, ALTHOUGH I WOULD OFTEN HAVE ONE OR TWO DAYS A WEEK WHEN I WASN'T *TOO* BAD, MY GROIN STILL FELT HORRIBLY UNCOMFORTABLE MOST OF THE TIME.

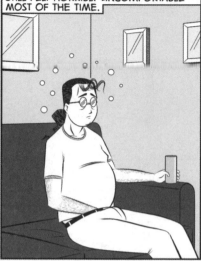

I STARTED TO HAVE TROUBLE FINDING COMFORTABLE NEW UNDERWEAR, AND I'D USUALLY END UP BUYING MULTIPLE PAIRS OF PANTS THAT WERE TOO UNCOMFORTABLE TO WEAR BEFORE I FOUND SOME THAT WERE OKAY.

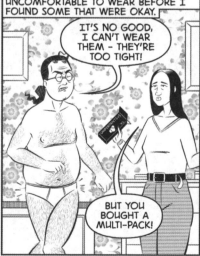

IT'S NO GOOD, I CAN'T WEAR THEM - THEY'RE TOO TIGHT!

BUT YOU BOUGHT A MULTI-PACK!

WHEN I DID FIND A PAIR THAT WERE REASONABLY COMFORTABLE, I'D WEAR THEM UNTIL THEY WERE FALLING APART (WASHING THEM AFTER EVERY WEAR, OF COURSE).

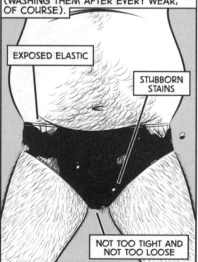

EXPOSED ELASTIC

STUBBORN STAINS

NOT TOO TIGHT AND NOT TOO LOOSE

MEANWHILE, ALL THE UNCOMFORTABLE PAIRS, WHICH WERE NON-RETURNABLE BY THE TIME I'D TRIED THEM ON, WOULD GET PUT IN A BULGING BIN-LINER FULL OF BARELY-WORN PANTS, IN THE HOPE THAT ONE DAY I'D BE ABLE TO WEAR SOME OF THEM.

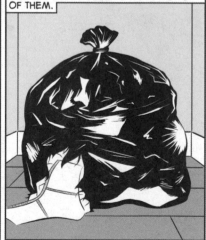

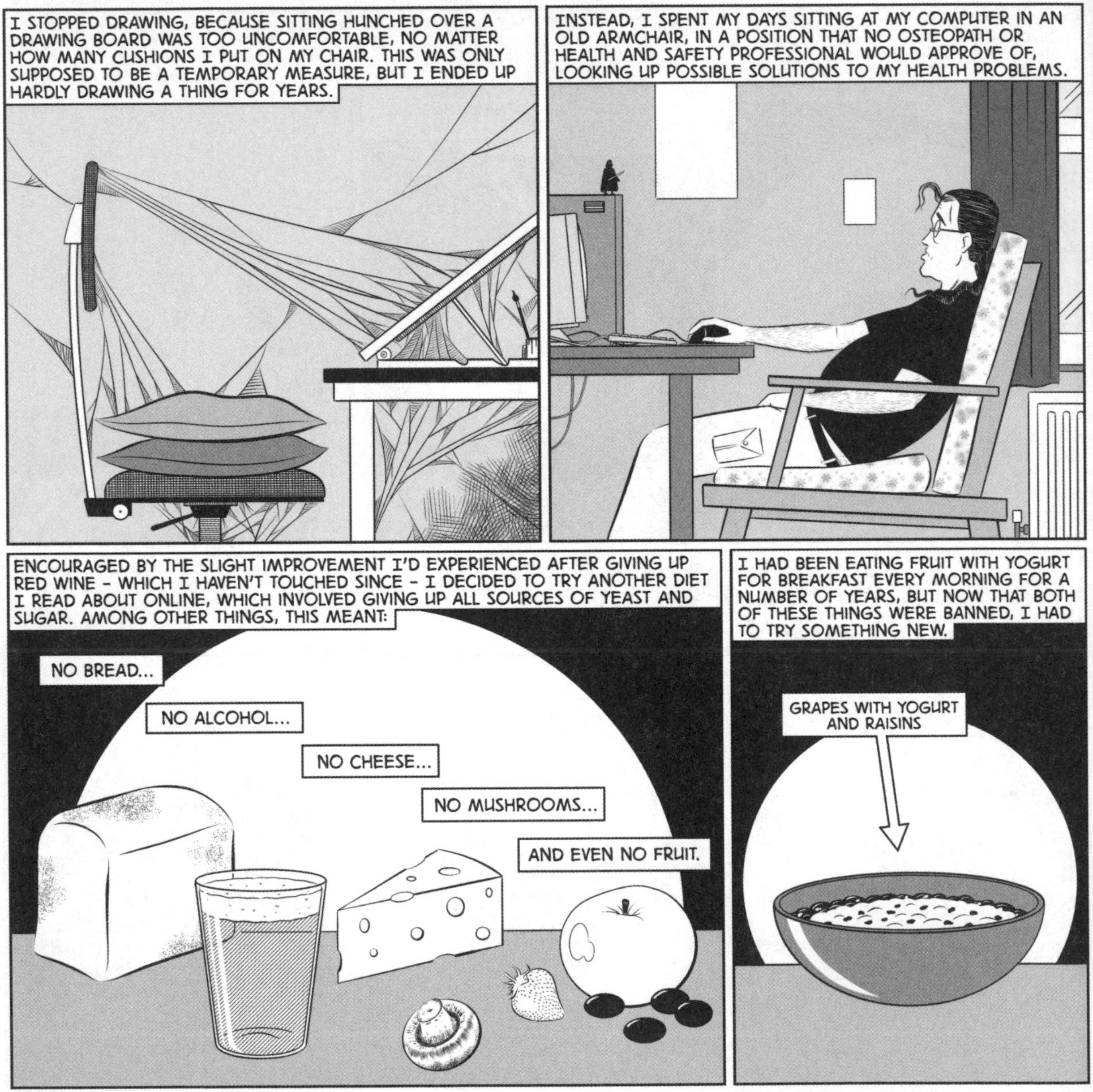
I STOPPED DRAWING, BECAUSE SITTING HUNCHED OVER A DRAWING BOARD WAS TOO UNCOMFORTABLE, NO MATTER HOW MANY CUSHIONS I PUT ON MY CHAIR. THIS WAS ONLY SUPPOSED TO BE A TEMPORARY MEASURE, BUT I ENDED UP HARDLY DRAWING A THING FOR YEARS.
INSTEAD, I SPENT MY DAYS SITTING AT MY COMPUTER IN AN OLD ARMCHAIR, IN A POSITION THAT NO OSTEOPATH OR HEALTH AND SAFETY PROFESSIONAL WOULD APPROVE OF, LOOKING UP POSSIBLE SOLUTIONS TO MY HEALTH PROBLEMS.
ENCOURAGED BY THE SLIGHT IMPROVEMENT I'D EXPERIENCED AFTER GIVING UP RED WINE - WHICH I HAVEN'T TOUCHED SINCE - I DECIDED TO TRY ANOTHER DIET I READ ABOUT ONLINE, WHICH INVOLVED GIVING UP ALL SOURCES OF YEAST AND SUGAR. AMONG OTHER THINGS, THIS MEANT:
NO BREAD...
NO ALCOHOL...
NO CHEESE...
NO MUSHROOMS...
AND EVEN NO FRUIT.
I HAD BEEN EATING FRUIT WITH YOGURT FOR BREAKFAST EVERY MORNING FOR A NUMBER OF YEARS, BUT NOW THAT BOTH OF THESE THINGS WERE BANNED, I HAD TO TRY SOMETHING NEW.
GRAPES WITH YOGURT AND RAISINS

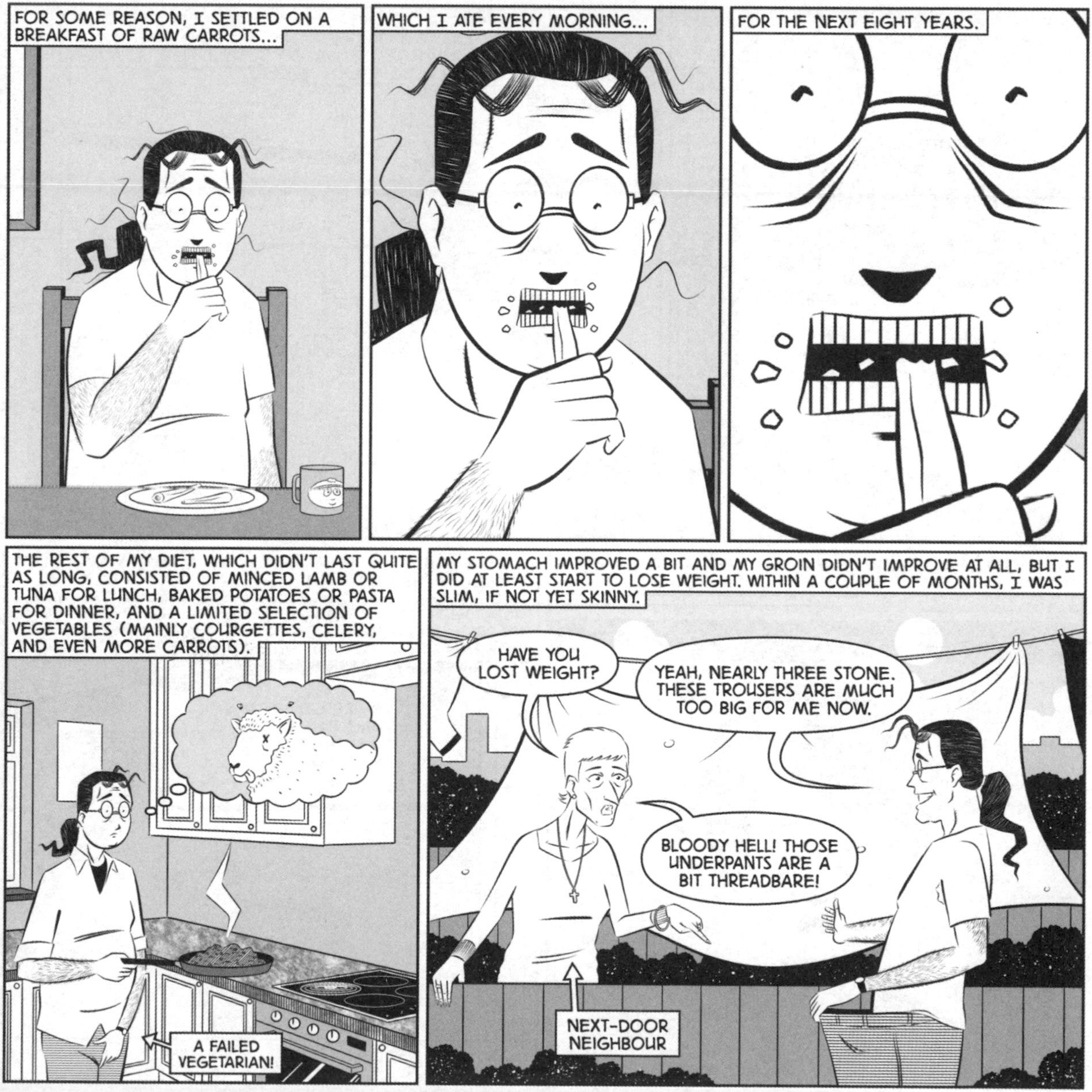
FOR SOME REASON, I SETTLED ON A BREAKFAST OF RAW CARROTS...
WHICH I ATE EVERY MORNING...
FOR THE NEXT EIGHT YEARS.
THE REST OF MY DIET, WHICH DIDN'T LAST QUITE AS LONG, CONSISTED OF MINCED LAMB OR TUNA FOR LUNCH, BAKED POTATOES OR PASTA FOR DINNER, AND A LIMITED SELECTION OF VEGETABLES (MAINLY COURGETTES, CELERY, AND EVEN MORE CARROTS).
A FAILED VEGETARIAN!
MY STOMACH IMPROVED A BIT AND MY GROIN DIDN'T IMPROVE AT ALL, BUT I DID AT LEAST START TO LOSE WEIGHT. WITHIN A COUPLE OF MONTHS, I WAS SLIM, IF NOT YET SKINNY.
HAVE YOU LOST WEIGHT?
YEAH, NEARLY THREE STONE. THESE TROUSERS ARE MUCH TOO BIG FOR ME NOW.
BLOODY HELL! THOSE UNDERPANTS ARE A BIT THREADBARE!
NEXT-DOOR NEIGHBOUR

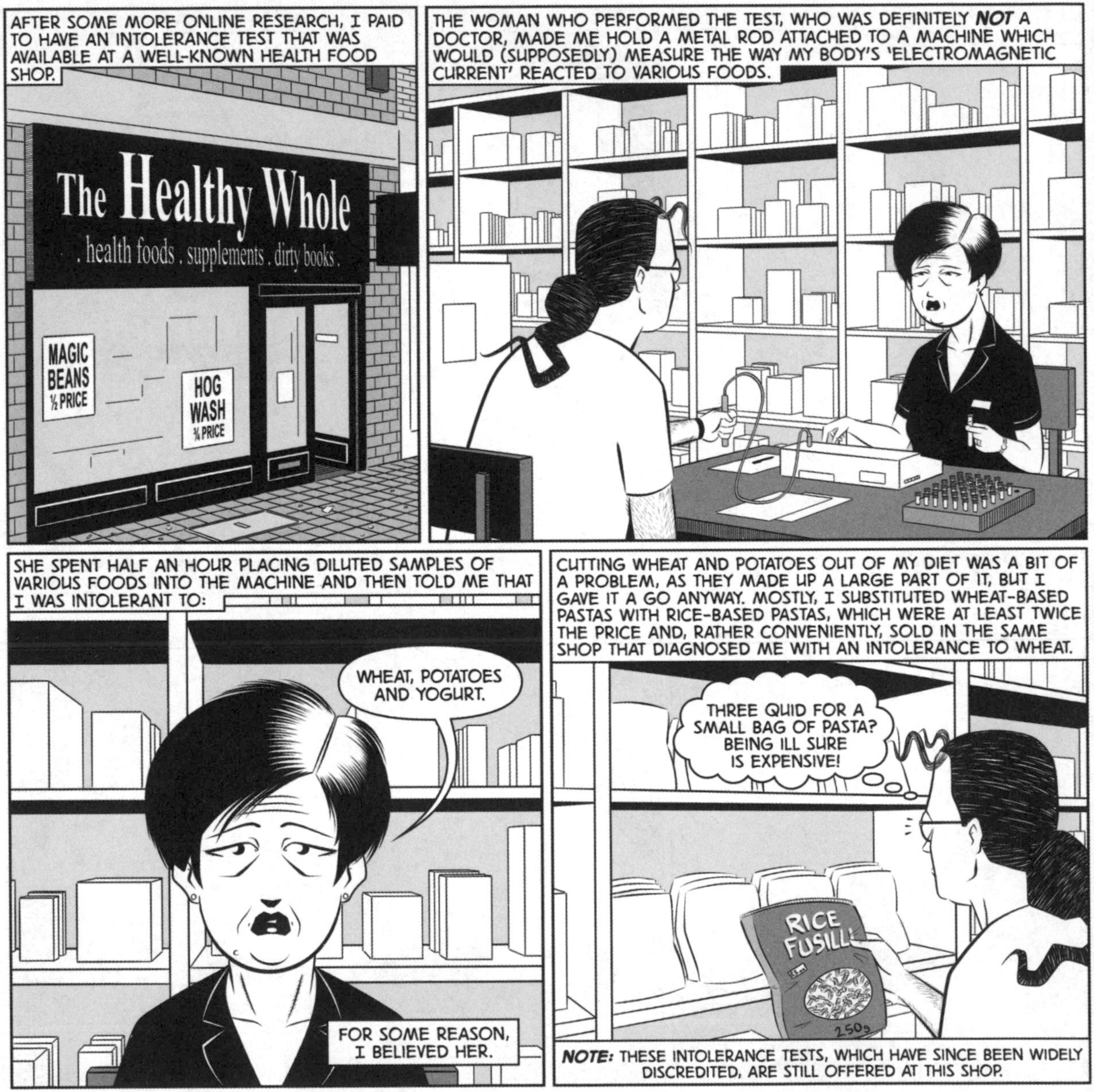
AFTER SOME MORE ONLINE RESEARCH, I PAID TO HAVE AN INTOLERANCE TEST THAT WAS AVAILABLE AT A WELL-KNOWN HEALTH FOOD SHOP.
The Healthy Whole
. health foods . supplements . dirty books .
MAGIC BEANS ½ PRICE
HOG WASH ¾ PRICE
THE WOMAN WHO PERFORMED THE TEST, WHO WAS DEFINITELY ***NOT*** A DOCTOR, MADE ME HOLD A METAL ROD ATTACHED TO A MACHINE WHICH WOULD (SUPPOSEDLY) MEASURE THE WAY MY BODY'S 'ELECTROMAGNETIC CURRENT' REACTED TO VARIOUS FOODS.
SHE SPENT HALF AN HOUR PLACING DILUTED SAMPLES OF VARIOUS FOODS INTO THE MACHINE AND THEN TOLD ME THAT I WAS INTOLERANT TO:
WHEAT, POTATOES AND YOGURT.
FOR SOME REASON, I BELIEVED HER.
CUTTING WHEAT AND POTATOES OUT OF MY DIET WAS A BIT OF A PROBLEM, AS THEY MADE UP A LARGE PART OF IT, BUT I GAVE IT A GO ANYWAY. MOSTLY, I SUBSTITUTED WHEAT-BASED PASTAS WITH RICE-BASED PASTAS, WHICH WERE AT LEAST TWICE THE PRICE AND, RATHER CONVENIENTLY, SOLD IN THE SAME SHOP THAT DIAGNOSED ME WITH AN INTOLERANCE TO WHEAT.
THREE QUID FOR A SMALL BAG OF PASTA? BEING ILL SURE IS EXPENSIVE!
RICE FUSILL
250g
NOTE: THESE INTOLERANCE TESTS, WHICH HAVE SINCE BEEN WIDELY DISCREDITED, ARE STILL OFFERED AT THIS SHOP.

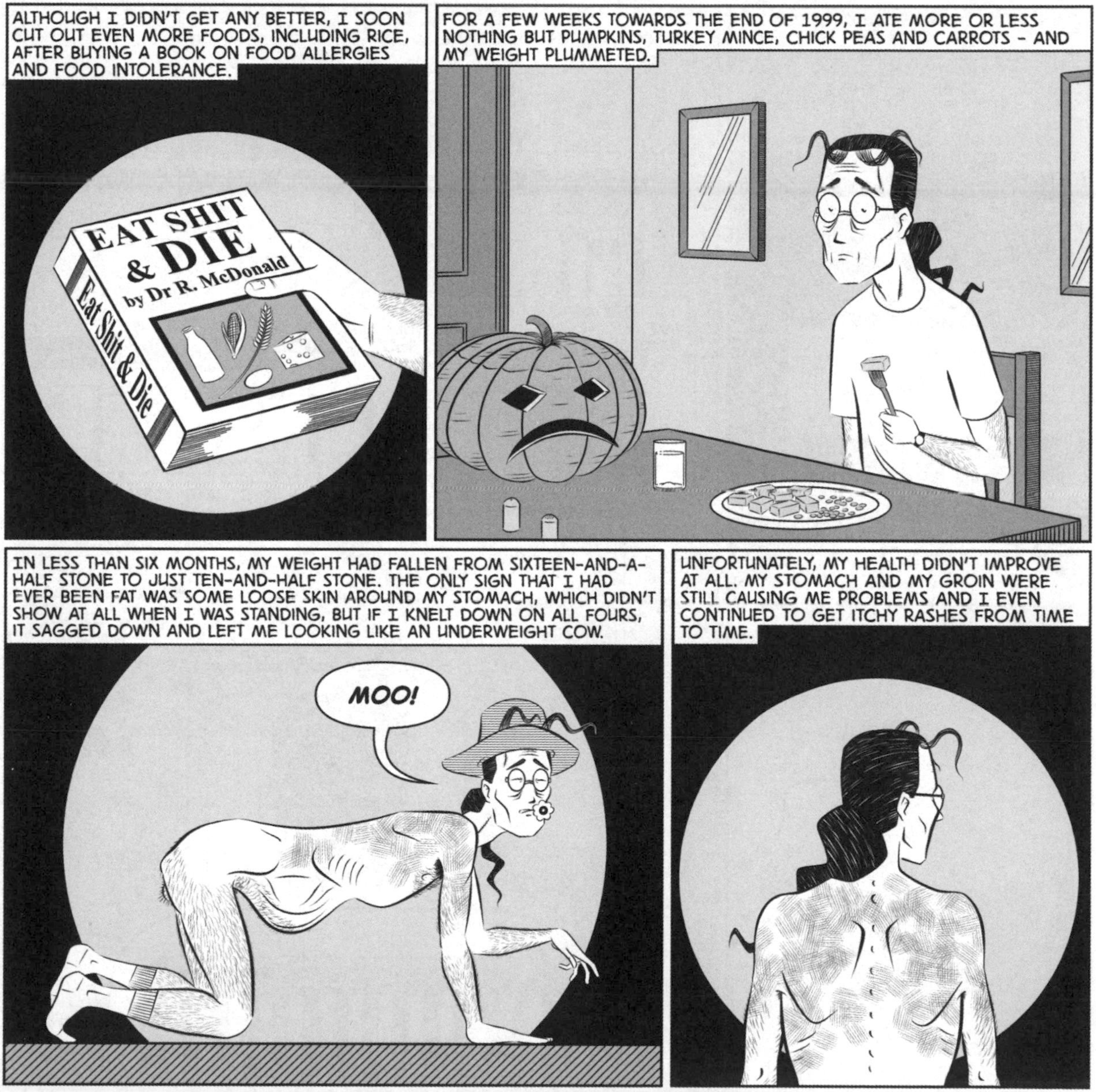
ALTHOUGH I DIDN'T GET ANY BETTER, I SOON CUT OUT EVEN MORE FOODS, INCLUDING RICE, AFTER BUYING A BOOK ON FOOD ALLERGIES AND FOOD INTOLERANCE.
EAT SHIT & DIE
by Dr R. McDonald
Eat Shit & Die
FOR A FEW WEEKS TOWARDS THE END OF 1999, I ATE MORE OR LESS NOTHING BUT PUMPKINS, TURKEY MINCE, CHICK PEAS AND CARROTS – AND MY WEIGHT PLUMMETED.
IN LESS THAN SIX MONTHS, MY WEIGHT HAD FALLEN FROM SIXTEEN-AND-A-HALF STONE TO JUST TEN-AND-HALF STONE. THE ONLY SIGN THAT I HAD EVER BEEN FAT WAS SOME LOOSE SKIN AROUND MY STOMACH, WHICH DIDN'T SHOW AT ALL WHEN I WAS STANDING, BUT IF I KNELT DOWN ON ALL FOURS, IT SAGGED DOWN AND LEFT ME LOOKING LIKE AN UNDERWEIGHT COW.
MOO!
UNFORTUNATELY, MY HEALTH DIDN'T IMPROVE AT ALL. MY STOMACH AND MY GROIN WERE STILL CAUSING ME PROBLEMS AND I EVEN CONTINUED TO GET ITCHY RASHES FROM TIME TO TIME.

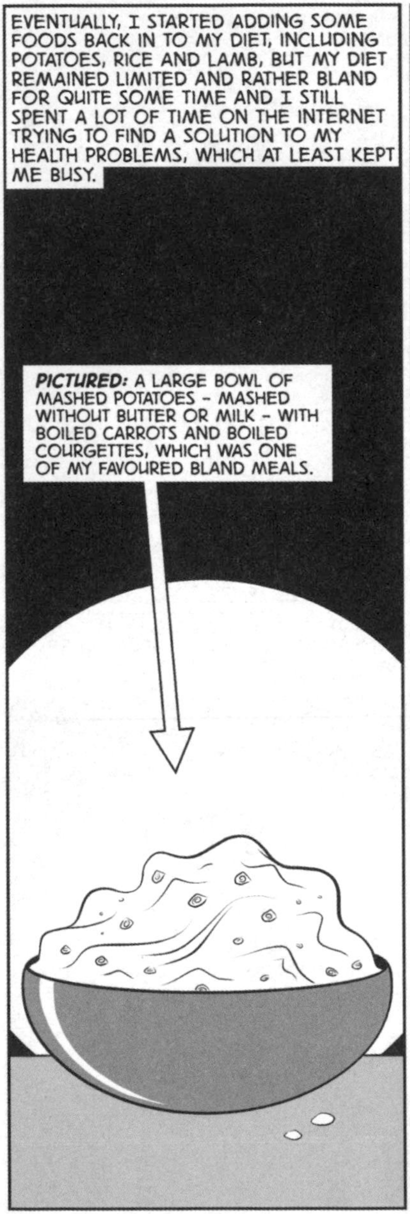
EVENTUALLY, I STARTED ADDING SOME FOODS BACK IN TO MY DIET, INCLUDING POTATOES, RICE AND LAMB, BUT MY DIET REMAINED LIMITED AND RATHER BLAND FOR QUITE SOME TIME AND I STILL SPENT A LOT OF TIME ON THE INTERNET TRYING TO FIND A SOLUTION TO MY HEALTH PROBLEMS, WHICH AT LEAST KEPT ME BUSY.
PICTURED: A LARGE BOWL OF MASHED POTATOES - MASHED WITHOUT BUTTER OR MILK - WITH BOILED CARROTS AND BOILED COURGETTES, WHICH WAS ONE OF MY FAVOURED BLAND MEALS.

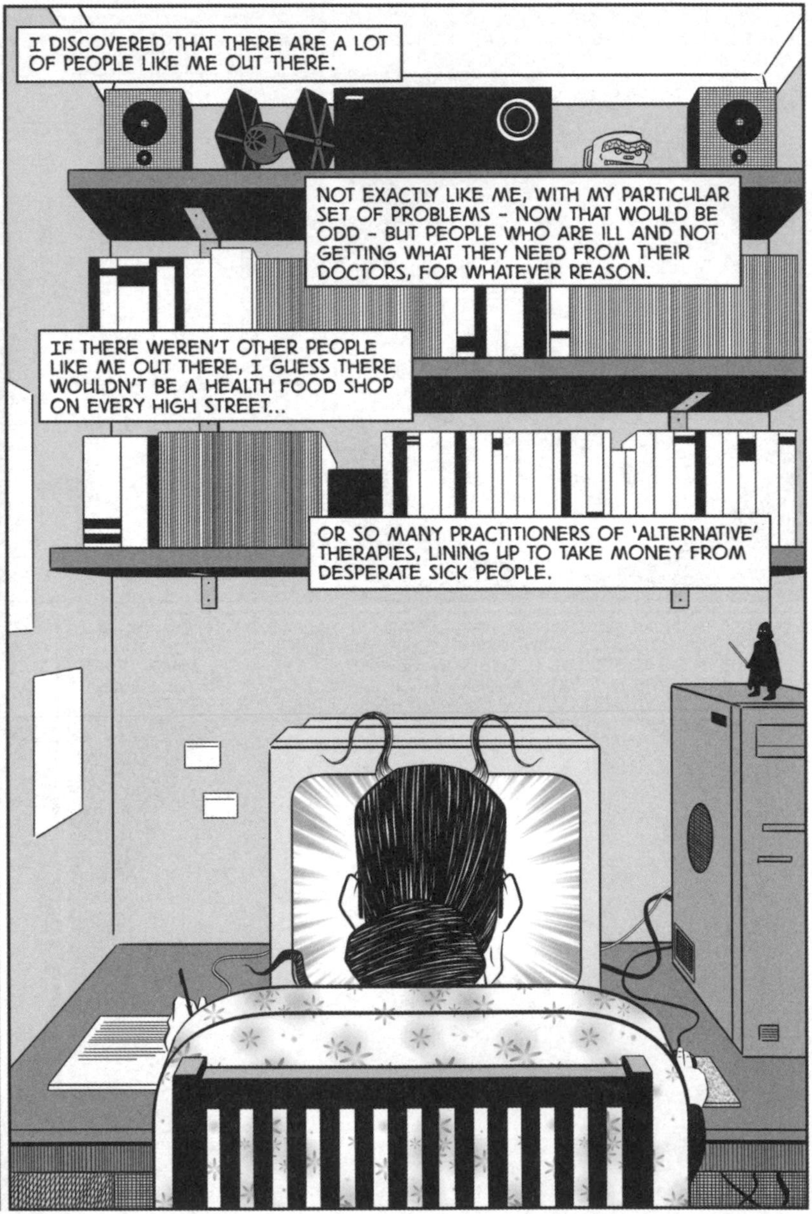
I DISCOVERED THAT THERE ARE A LOT OF PEOPLE LIKE ME OUT THERE.
NOT EXACTLY LIKE ME, WITH MY PARTICULAR SET OF PROBLEMS - NOW THAT WOULD BE ODD - BUT PEOPLE WHO ARE ILL AND NOT GETTING WHAT THEY NEED FROM THEIR DOCTORS, FOR WHATEVER REASON.
IF THERE WEREN'T OTHER PEOPLE LIKE ME OUT THERE, I GUESS THERE WOULDN'T BE A HEALTH FOOD SHOP ON EVERY HIGH STREET...
OR SO MANY PRACTITIONERS OF 'ALTERNATIVE' THERAPIES, LINING UP TO TAKE MONEY FROM DESPERATE SICK PEOPLE.

THE NADIR OF MY VOYAGE THROUGH THE WORLD OF SELF-HELP AND ALTERNATIVE THERAPIES CAME WHEN I TRIED COLONIC IRRIGATION.

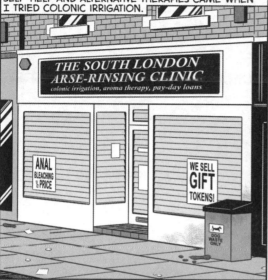

THE SOUTH LONDON ARSE-RINSING CLINIC
colonic irrigation, aroma therapy, pay-day loans

ANAL BLEACHING ½ PRICE

WE SELL GIFT TOKENS!

DOG WASTE ONLY

I'D BEEN READING ABOUT THE SUPPOSED BENEFITS OF COLONIC IRRIGATION ON THE INTERNET FOR QUITE SOME TIME, AND ON ONE OCCASION I'D EVEN ORDERED AN ENEMA BAG FROM AN ONLINE CHEMIST.

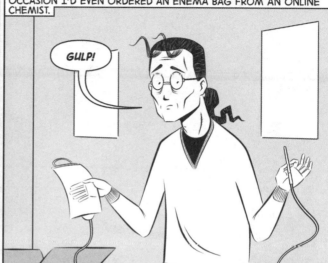

GULP!

I TRIED TO USE IT ONCE BUT STRUGGLED TO INSERT THE TUBE MORE THAN A CENTIMETRE OR SO INTO MY OWN ANUS, CHICKENED OUT AND EVENTUALLY THREW IT AWAY, MORE OR LESS UNUSED.

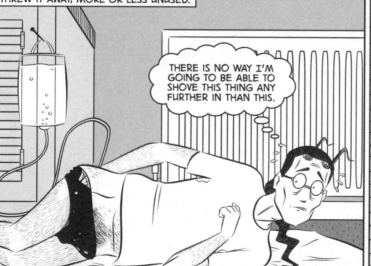

THERE IS NO WAY I'M GOING TO BE ABLE TO SHOVE THIS THING ANY FURTHER IN THAN THIS.

BUT WHILE MY HEALTH PROBLEMS DRAGGED ON, THE IDEA OF TRYING COLONIC IRRIGATION LINGERED IN MY MIND, AND EVENTUALLY I BECAME DESPERATE ENOUGH TO BOOK AN APPOINTMENT AT A 'NATURAL HEALTH' CLINIC.

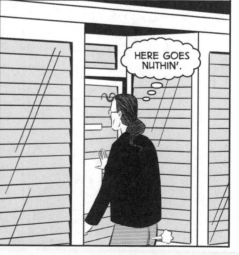

HERE GOES NUTHIN'.

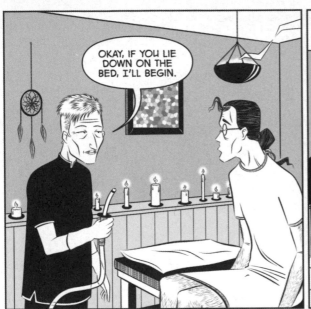

OKAY, IF YOU LIE DOWN ON THE BED, I'LL BEGIN.

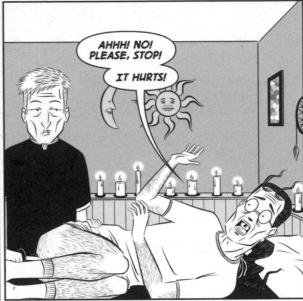

AHHH! NO! PLEASE, STOP!

IT HURTS!

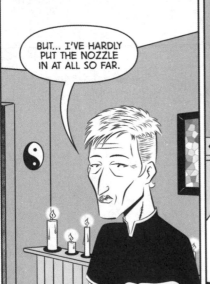

BUT... I'VE HARDLY PUT THE NOZZLE IN AT ALL SO FAR.

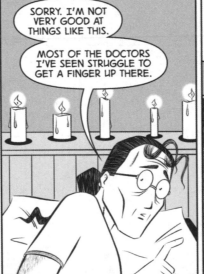

SORRY. I'M NOT VERY GOOD AT THINGS LIKE THIS.

MOST OF THE DOCTORS I'VE SEEN STRUGGLE TO GET A FINGER UP THERE.

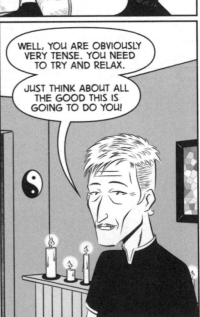

WELL, YOU ARE OBVIOUSLY VERY TENSE. YOU NEED TO TRY AND RELAX.

JUST THINK ABOUT ALL THE GOOD THIS IS GOING TO DO YOU!

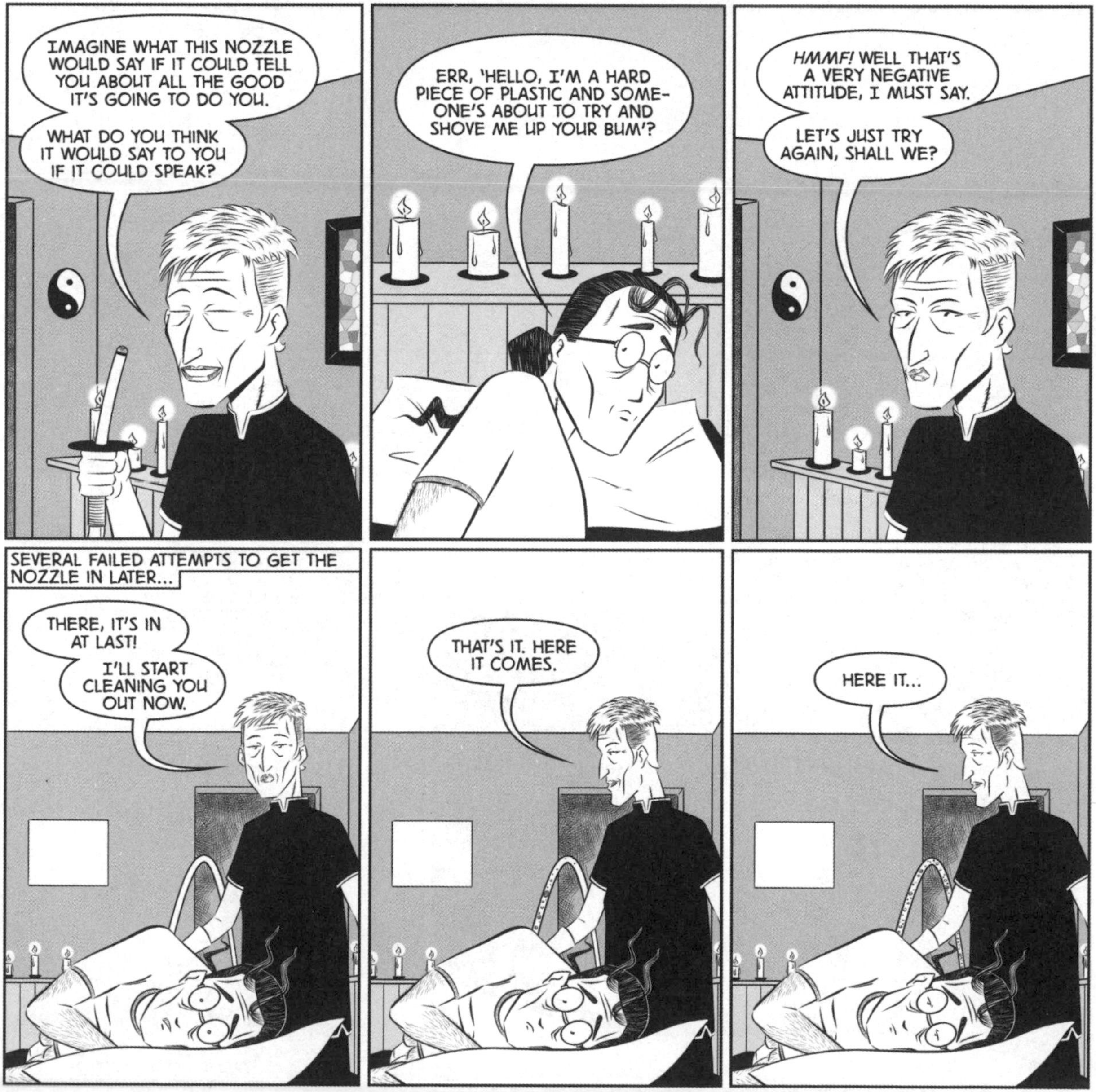
IMAGINE WHAT THIS NOZZLE WOULD SAY IF IT COULD TELL YOU ABOUT ALL THE GOOD IT'S GOING TO DO YOU.
WHAT DO YOU THINK IT WOULD SAY TO YOU IF IT COULD SPEAK?
ERR, 'HELLO, I'M A HARD PIECE OF PLASTIC AND SOMEONE'S ABOUT TO TRY AND SHOVE ME UP YOUR BUM'?
HMMF! WELL THAT'S A VERY NEGATIVE ATTITUDE, I MUST SAY.
LET'S JUST TRY AGAIN, SHALL WE?
SEVERAL FAILED ATTEMPTS TO GET THE NOZZLE IN LATER...
THERE, IT'S IN AT LAST!
I'LL START CLEANING YOU OUT NOW.
THAT'S IT. HERE IT COMES.
HERE IT...

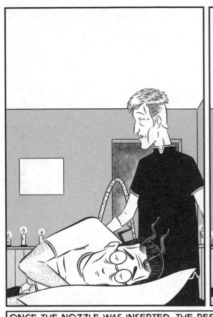

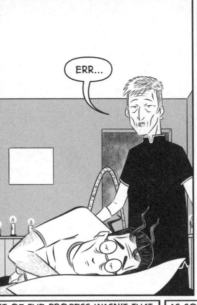

ERR...

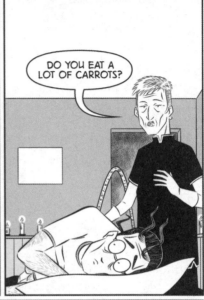

DO YOU EAT A LOT OF CARROTS?

ONCE THE NOZZLE WAS INSERTED, THE REST OF THE PROCESS WASN'T THAT UNCOMFORTABLE AT ALL. IN FACT, I FELL ASLEEP DURING IT. AND WHEN IT WAS ALL OVER, I WOKE UP FEELING EXHAUSTED, GOT DRESSED, AND LEFT FEELING MORE THAN A LITTLE BIT EMBARRASSED.

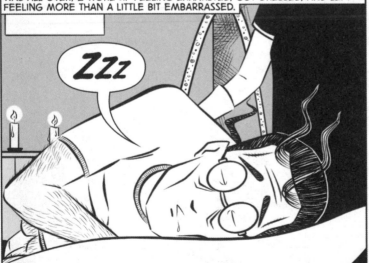

ZZz

AS SOON AS I GOT HOME, I ATE SOME LUNCH, AND ALMOST IMMEDIATELY STARTED TO GET A STOMACH ACHE, SO I NEVER TRIED COLONIC IRRIGATION AGAIN.

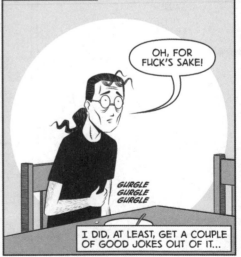

OH, FOR FUCK'S SAKE!

GURGLE GURGLE GURGLE

I DID, AT LEAST, GET A COUPLE OF GOOD JOKES OUT OF IT...

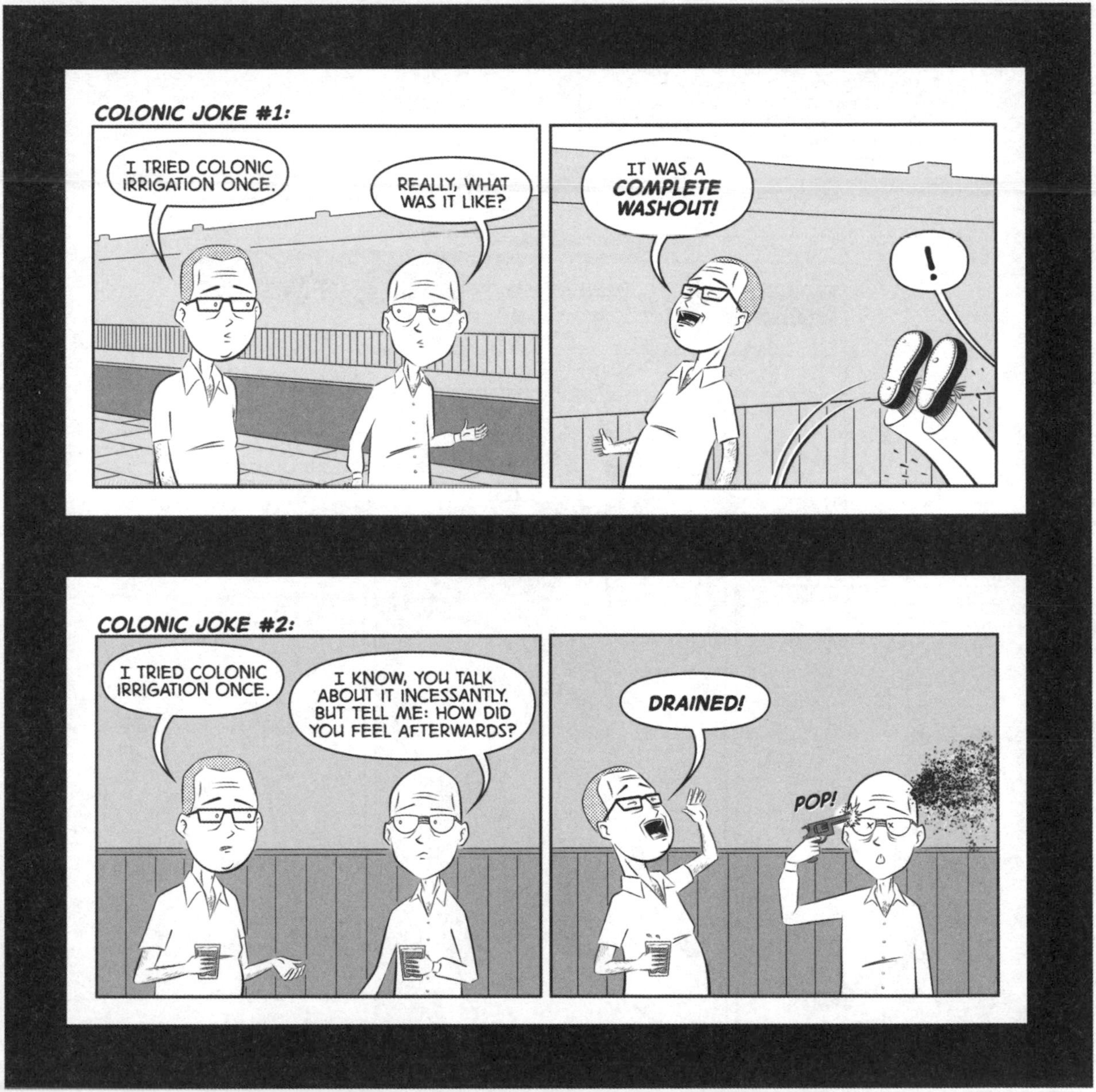
COLONIC JOKE #1:
I TRIED COLONIC IRRIGATION ONCE.
REALLY, WHAT WAS IT LIKE?
IT WAS A COMPLETE WASHOUT!
!
COLONIC JOKE #2:
I TRIED COLONIC IRRIGATION ONCE.
I KNOW, YOU TALK ABOUT IT INCESSANTLY. BUT TELL ME: HOW DID YOU FEEL AFTERWARDS?
DRAINED!
POP!

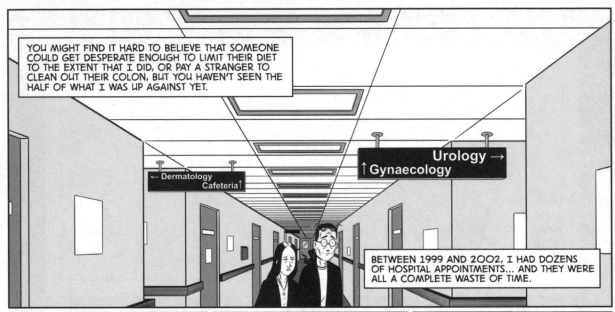

YOU MIGHT FIND IT HARD TO BELIEVE THAT SOMEONE COULD GET DESPERATE ENOUGH TO LIMIT THEIR DIET TO THE EXTENT THAT I DID, OR PAY A STRANGER TO CLEAN OUT THEIR COLON, BUT YOU HAVEN'T SEEN THE HALF OF WHAT I WAS UP AGAINST YET.

Urology →
↑Gynaecology

← Dermatology
Cafeteria↑

BETWEEN 1999 AND 2002, I HAD DOZENS OF HOSPITAL APPOINTMENTS... AND THEY WERE ALL A COMPLETE WASTE OF TIME.

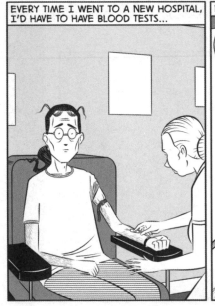

EVERY TIME I WENT TO A NEW HOSPITAL, I'D HAVE TO HAVE BLOOD TESTS...

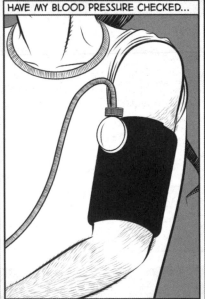

HAVE MY BLOOD PRESSURE CHECKED...

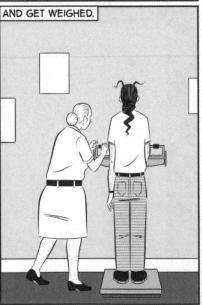

AND GET WEIGHED.

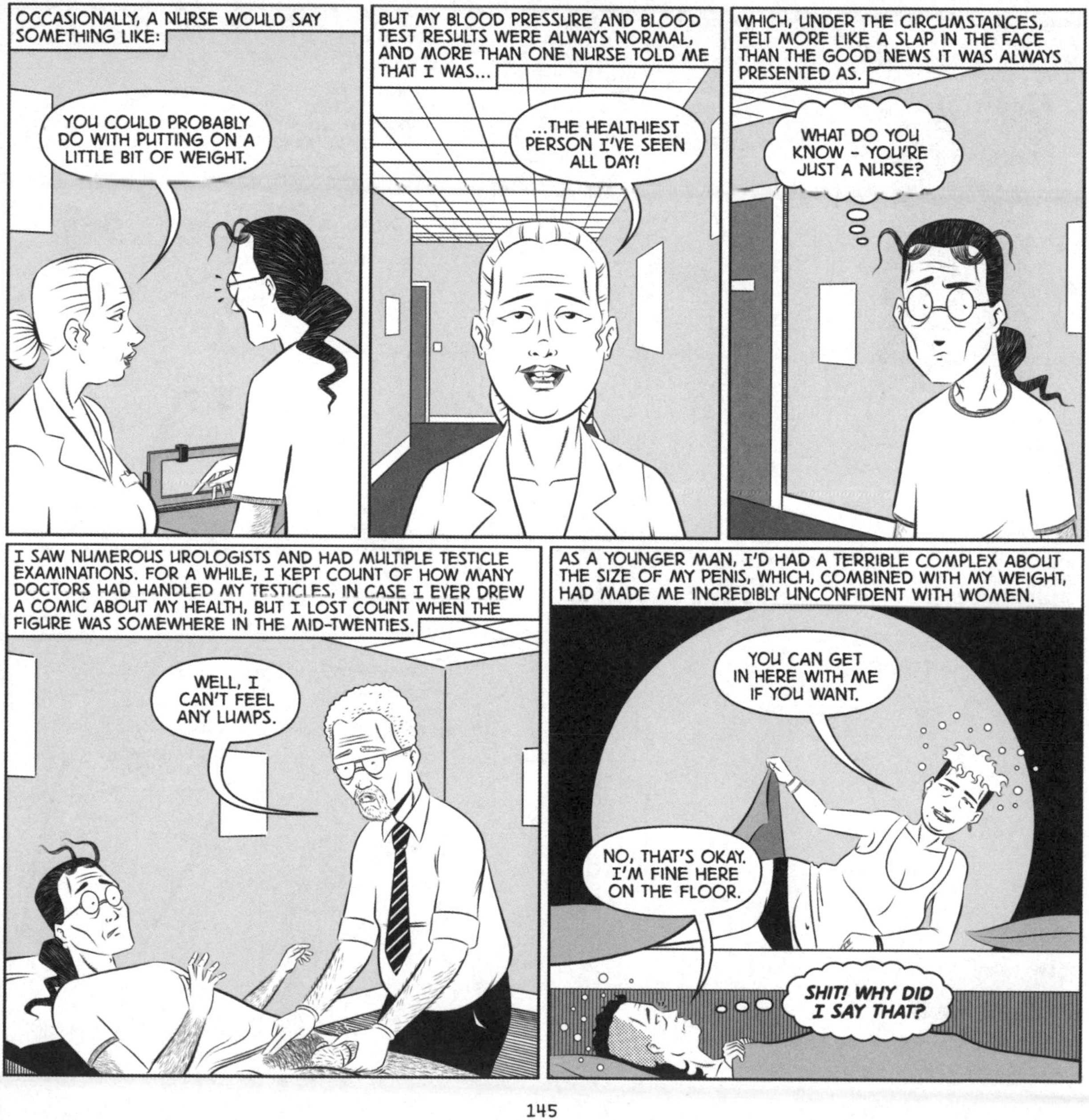
OCCASIONALLY, A NURSE WOULD SAY SOMETHING LIKE:
YOU COULD PROBABLY DO WITH PUTTING ON A LITTLE BIT OF WEIGHT.
BUT MY BLOOD PRESSURE AND BLOOD TEST RESULTS WERE ALWAYS NORMAL, AND MORE THAN ONE NURSE TOLD ME THAT I WAS...
...THE HEALTHIEST PERSON I'VE SEEN ALL DAY!
WHICH, UNDER THE CIRCUMSTANCES, FELT MORE LIKE A SLAP IN THE FACE THAN THE GOOD NEWS IT WAS ALWAYS PRESENTED AS.
WHAT DO YOU KNOW - YOU'RE JUST A NURSE?
I SAW NUMEROUS UROLOGISTS AND HAD MULTIPLE TESTICLE EXAMINATIONS. FOR A WHILE, I KEPT COUNT OF HOW MANY DOCTORS HAD HANDLED MY TESTICLES, IN CASE I EVER DREW A COMIC ABOUT MY HEALTH, BUT I LOST COUNT WHEN THE FIGURE WAS SOMEWHERE IN THE MID-TWENTIES.
WELL, I CAN'T FEEL ANY LUMPS.
AS A YOUNGER MAN, I'D HAD A TERRIBLE COMPLEX ABOUT THE SIZE OF MY PENIS, WHICH, COMBINED WITH MY WEIGHT, HAD MADE ME INCREDIBLY UNCONFIDENT WITH WOMEN.
YOU CAN GET IN HERE WITH ME IF YOU WANT.
NO, THAT'S OKAY. I'M FINE HERE ON THE FLOOR.
SHIT! WHY DID I SAY THAT?

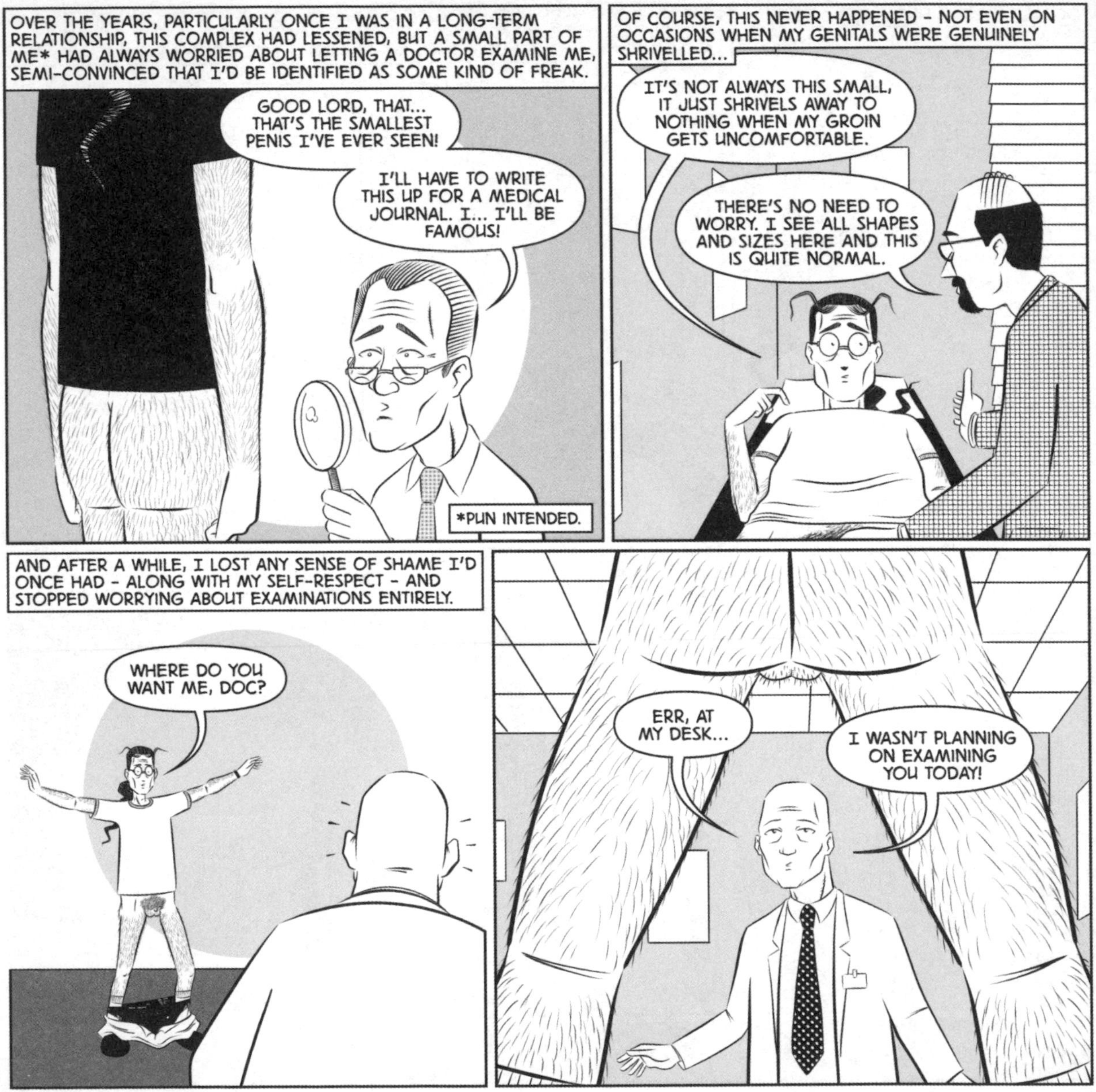
OVER THE YEARS, PARTICULARLY ONCE I WAS IN A LONG-TERM RELATIONSHIP, THIS COMPLEX HAD LESSENED, BUT A SMALL PART OF ME* HAD ALWAYS WORRIED ABOUT LETTING A DOCTOR EXAMINE ME, SEMI-CONVINCED THAT I'D BE IDENTIFIED AS SOME KIND OF FREAK.
GOOD LORD, THAT... THAT'S THE SMALLEST PENIS I'VE EVER SEEN!
I'LL HAVE TO WRITE THIS UP FOR A MEDICAL JOURNAL. I... I'LL BE FAMOUS!
*PUN INTENDED.
OF COURSE, THIS NEVER HAPPENED - NOT EVEN ON OCCASIONS WHEN MY GENITALS WERE GENUINELY SHRIVELLED...
IT'S NOT ALWAYS THIS SMALL, IT JUST SHRIVELS AWAY TO NOTHING WHEN MY GROIN GETS UNCOMFORTABLE.
THERE'S NO NEED TO WORRY. I SEE ALL SHAPES AND SIZES HERE AND THIS IS QUITE NORMAL.
AND AFTER A WHILE, I LOST ANY SENSE OF SHAME I'D ONCE HAD - ALONG WITH MY SELF-RESPECT - AND STOPPED WORRYING ABOUT EXAMINATIONS ENTIRELY.
WHERE DO YOU WANT ME, DOC?
ERR, AT MY DESK...
I WASN'T PLANNING ON EXAMINING YOU TODAY!

AS WELL AS THE PHYSICAL EXAMINATIONS, I HAD TWO MORE TESTICULAR ULTRASOUNDS. BOTH REVEALED VARICOSE VEINS AND ONE REVEALED A CYST ABOVE ONE OF MY TESTICLES.

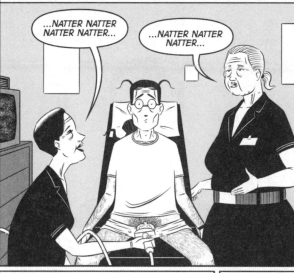

...NATTER NATTER NATTER NATTER...

...NATTER NATTER NATTER...

HOWEVER:

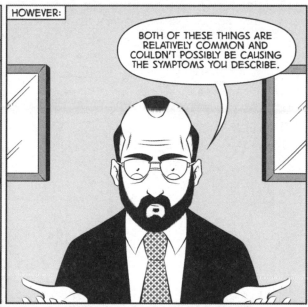

BOTH OF THESE THINGS ARE RELATIVELY COMMON AND COULDN'T POSSIBLY BE CAUSING THE SYMPTOMS YOU DESCRIBE.

ON ONE OCCASION, I WAS TESTED FOR SEXUALLY TRANSMITTED DISEASES, JUST IN CASE.

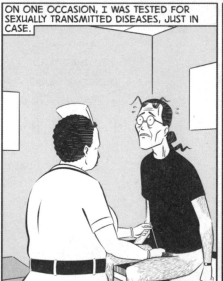

THIS INVOLVED A NURSE STICKING WHAT APPEARED TO BE A LONG TOOTHPICK WITH SOME COTTON WOOL ON THE END OF IT DOWN THE END OF MY PENIS AND TWISTING IT AROUND TO OBTAIN A SWAB.

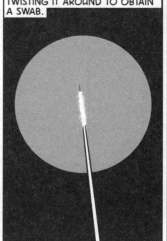

OF COURSE, I DIDN'T HAVE A SEXUALLY TRANSMITTED DISEASE – THERE WAS NO SIGN OF ANY SORT OF INFECTION – AND THE CHANCES OF ME EVER HAVING CONTRACTED A SEXUALLY TRANSMITTED DISEASE WERE ALMOST DEPRESSINGLY SLIM.

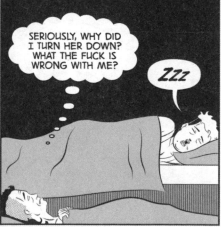

SERIOUSLY, WHY DID I TURN HER DOWN? WHAT THE FUCK IS WRONG WITH ME?

Zzz

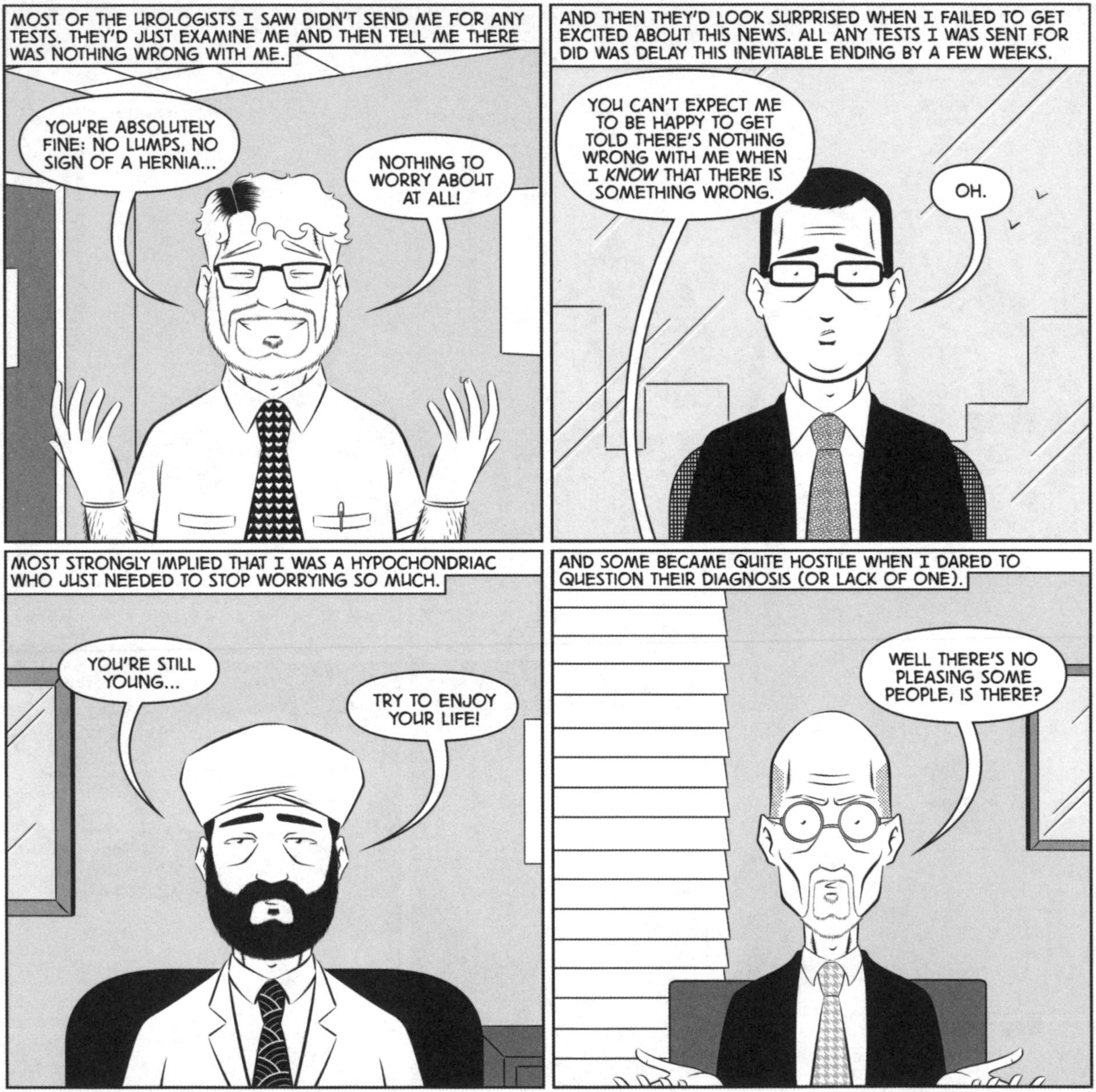
MOST OF THE UROLOGISTS I SAW DIDN'T SEND ME FOR ANY TESTS. THEY'D JUST EXAMINE ME AND THEN TELL ME THERE WAS NOTHING WRONG WITH ME.
YOU'RE ABSOLUTELY FINE: NO LUMPS, NO SIGN OF A HERNIA...
NOTHING TO WORRY ABOUT AT ALL!
AND THEN THEY'D LOOK SURPRISED WHEN I FAILED TO GET EXCITED ABOUT THIS NEWS. ALL ANY TESTS I WAS SENT FOR DID WAS DELAY THIS INEVITABLE ENDING BY A FEW WEEKS.
YOU CAN'T EXPECT ME TO BE HAPPY TO GET TOLD THERE'S NOTHING WRONG WITH ME WHEN I *KNOW* THAT THERE IS SOMETHING WRONG.
OH.
MOST STRONGLY IMPLIED THAT I WAS A HYPOCHONDRIAC WHO JUST NEEDED TO STOP WORRYING SO MUCH.
YOU'RE STILL YOUNG...
TRY TO ENJOY YOUR LIFE!
AND SOME BECAME QUITE HOSTILE WHEN I DARED TO QUESTION THEIR DIAGNOSIS (OR LACK OF ONE).
WELL THERE'S NO PLEASING SOME PEOPLE, IS THERE?

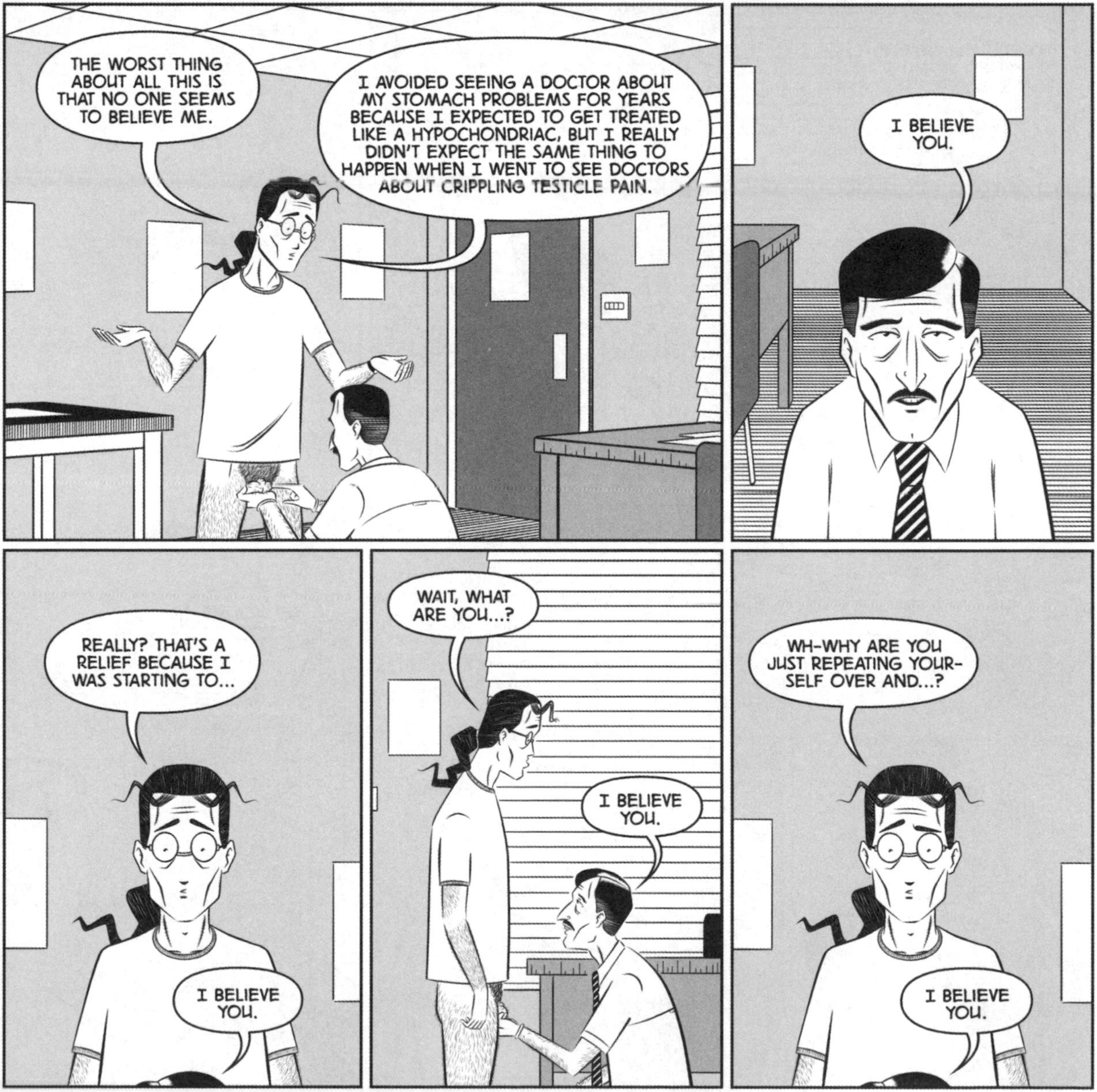
THE WORST THING ABOUT ALL THIS IS THAT NO ONE SEEMS TO BELIEVE ME.
I AVOIDED SEEING A DOCTOR ABOUT MY STOMACH PROBLEMS FOR YEARS BECAUSE I EXPECTED TO GET TREATED LIKE A HYPOCHONDRIAC, BUT I REALLY DIDN'T EXPECT THE SAME THING TO HAPPEN WHEN I WENT TO SEE DOCTORS ABOUT CRIPPLING TESTICLE PAIN.
I BELIEVE YOU.
REALLY? THAT'S A RELIEF BECAUSE I WAS STARTING TO...
I BELIEVE YOU.
WAIT, WHAT ARE YOU...?
I BELIEVE YOU.
WH-WHY ARE YOU JUST REPEATING YOURSELF OVER AND...?
I BELIEVE YOU.

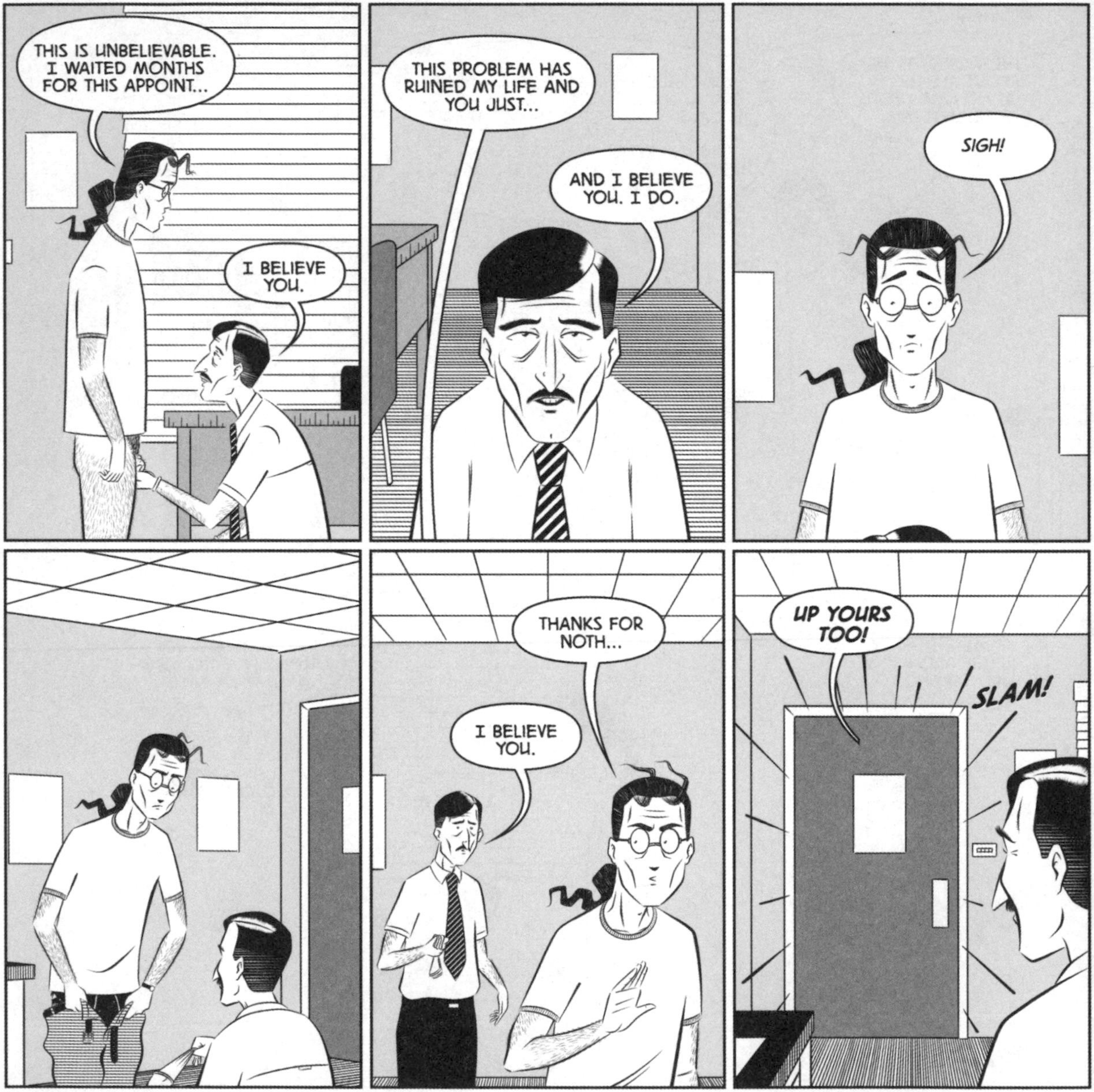
THIS IS UNBELIEVABLE. I WAITED MONTHS FOR THIS APPOINT...
I BELIEVE YOU.
THIS PROBLEM HAS RUINED MY LIFE AND YOU JUST...
AND I BELIEVE YOU. I DO.
SIGH!
THANKS FOR NOTH...
I BELIEVE YOU.
UP YOURS TOO!
SLAM!

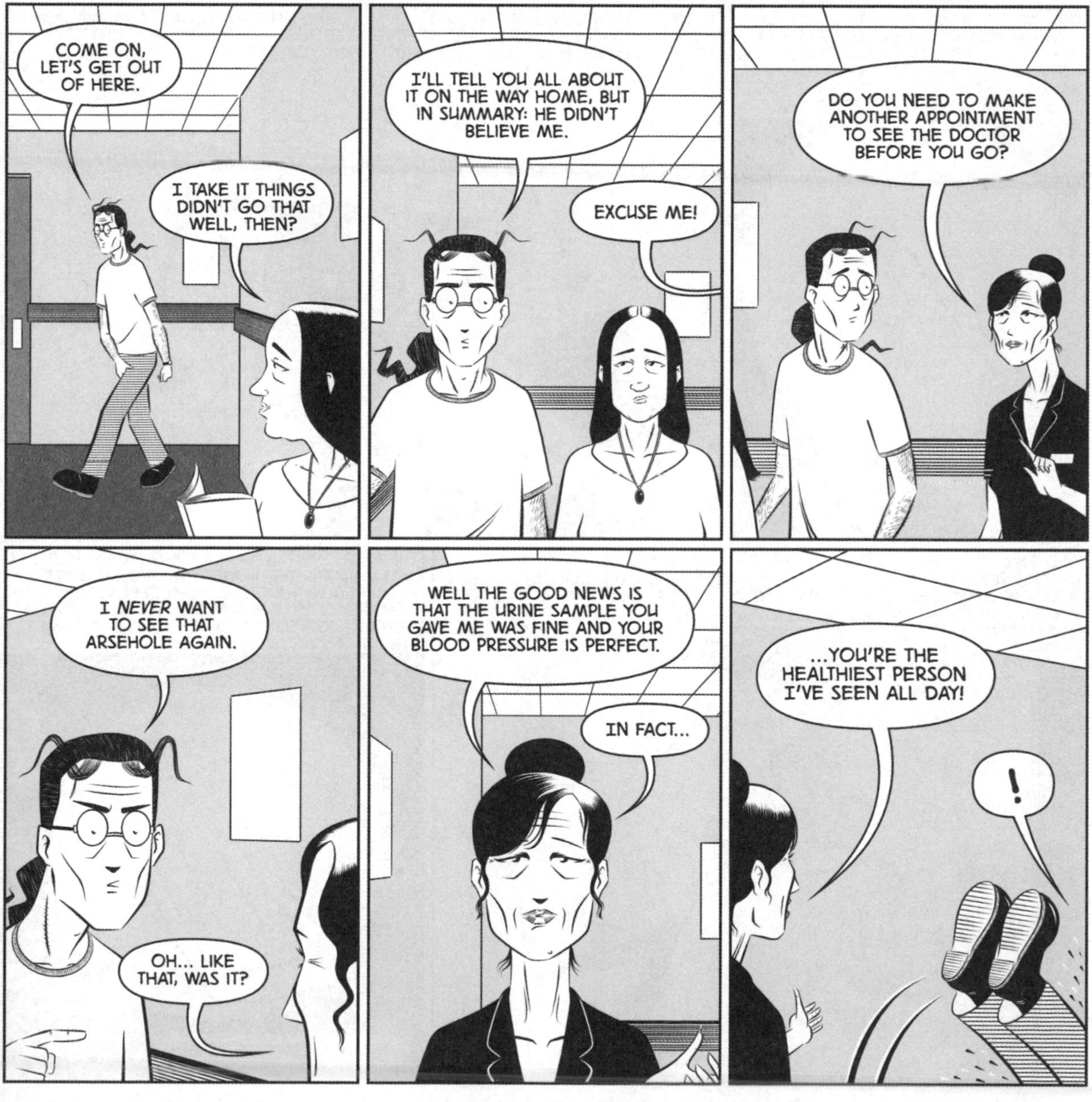
COME ON, LET'S GET OUT OF HERE.
I TAKE IT THINGS DIDN'T GO THAT WELL, THEN?
I'LL TELL YOU ALL ABOUT IT ON THE WAY HOME, BUT IN SUMMARY: HE DIDN'T BELIEVE ME.
EXCUSE ME!
DO YOU NEED TO MAKE ANOTHER APPOINTMENT TO SEE THE DOCTOR BEFORE YOU GO?
I *NEVER* WANT TO SEE THAT ARSEHOLE AGAIN.
OH... LIKE THAT, WAS IT?
WELL THE GOOD NEWS IS THAT THE URINE SAMPLE YOU GAVE ME WAS FINE AND YOUR BLOOD PRESSURE IS PERFECT.
IN FACT...
...YOU'RE THE HEALTHIEST PERSON I'VE SEEN ALL DAY!
!

DURING THE SAME PERIOD, I ALSO SAW SEVERAL GASTROENTEROLOGISTS AND HAD MULTIPLE RECTAL EXAMINATIONS. NONE OF THEM WERE ANYWHERE NEAR AS BAD AS THE ONE I'D HAD THE FIRST TIME I SAW A GASTROENTEROLOGIST.

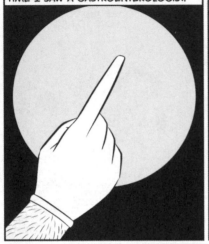

EITHER GASTROENTEROLOGY HAD COME A LONG WAY SINCE 1991 OR THE FIRST GASTROENTEROLOGIST I'D SEEN HAD BEEN A SADIST.

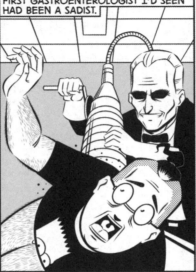

I HAD AN ENDOSCOPY (CAMERA DOWN THE THROAT)...

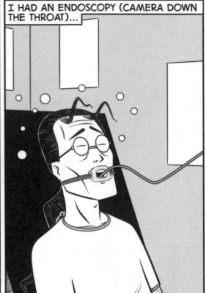

AND *TWO* COLONOSCOPIES (CAMERAS UP THE BUM). BECAUSE OF MY EXPERIENCES IN THE EARLY '90S, I WORRIED ABOUT THE COLONOSCOPIES *A LOT* IN ADVANCE, BUT BOTH WERE DONE UNDER ANAESTHETIC - AS WAS THE ENDOSCOPY - AND WERE RELATIVELY PAINLESS.

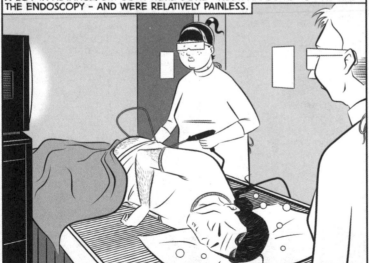

THE WORST THING WAS GETTING TO THE HOSPITAL AFTER TAKING THE POWERFUL LAXATIVE I WAS REQUIRED TO HAVE THE NIGHT BEFORE THE COLONOSCOPY. ON ONE OCCASION, I WORE A SANITARY TOWEL IN MY UNDERPANTS, IN CASE I HAD AN *ACCIDENT* ON THE WAY THERE.*

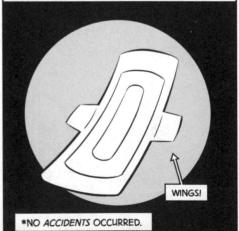

WINGS!

*NO *ACCIDENTS* OCCURRED.

MOST OF THESE EXAMINATIONS / TESTS FOUND NOTHING WRONG AND I WAS TREATED PRETTY MUCH THE WAY I EXPECTED TO GET TREATED.

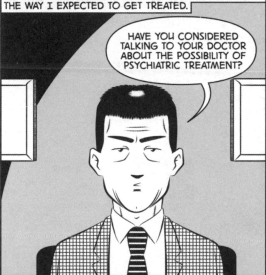

HAVE YOU CONSIDERED TALKING TO YOUR DOCTOR ABOUT THE POSSIBILITY OF PSYCHIATRIC TREATMENT?

THE SECOND COLONOSCOPY DID REVEAL SOME MILD INFLAMATION IN MY BOWEL AND AN X-RAY OF MY SMALL INTESTINE* APPEARED TO REVEAL SOME ABNORMALITIES. THIS LED THE GASTROENTEROLOGIST WHO ORDERED THESE TESTS TO DIAGNOSE ME WITH MILD *CROHN'S DISEASE* AND PRESCRIBE ME SOME APPROPRIATE MEDICATION.

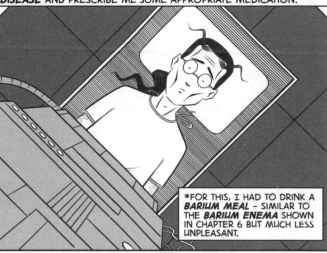

*FOR THIS, I HAD TO DRINK A *BARIUM MEAL* – SIMILAR TO THE *BARIUM ENEMA* SHOWN IN CHAPTER 6 BUT MUCH LESS UNPLEASANT.

I WAS OVER THE MOON. I MEAN, I WAS ALREADY ILL, AND IF I HAD TO BE ILL, I'D RATHER HAVE SOMETHING WITH A COOLER NAME THAN *IRRITABLE BOWEL SYNDROME* – SOMETHING THAT I COULD TELL PEOPLE ABOUT WITHOUT WANTING TO DIE OF EMBARRASSMENT.

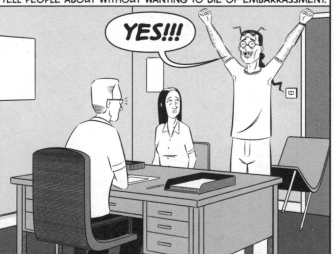

YES!!!

HOWEVER, THE MEDICATION DIDN'T HELP AT ALL AND THE NEXT TIME I SAW THIS GASTROENTEROLOGIST, HE DECIDED THAT THE X-RAY OF MY SMALL INTESTINE HAD BEEN MISINTERPRETED AND REVISED HIS DIAGNOSIS TO:

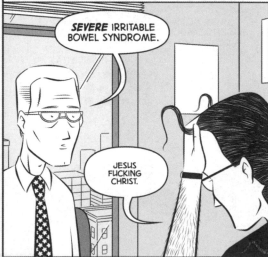

SEVERE IRRITABLE BOWEL SYNDROME.

JESUS FUCKING CHRIST.

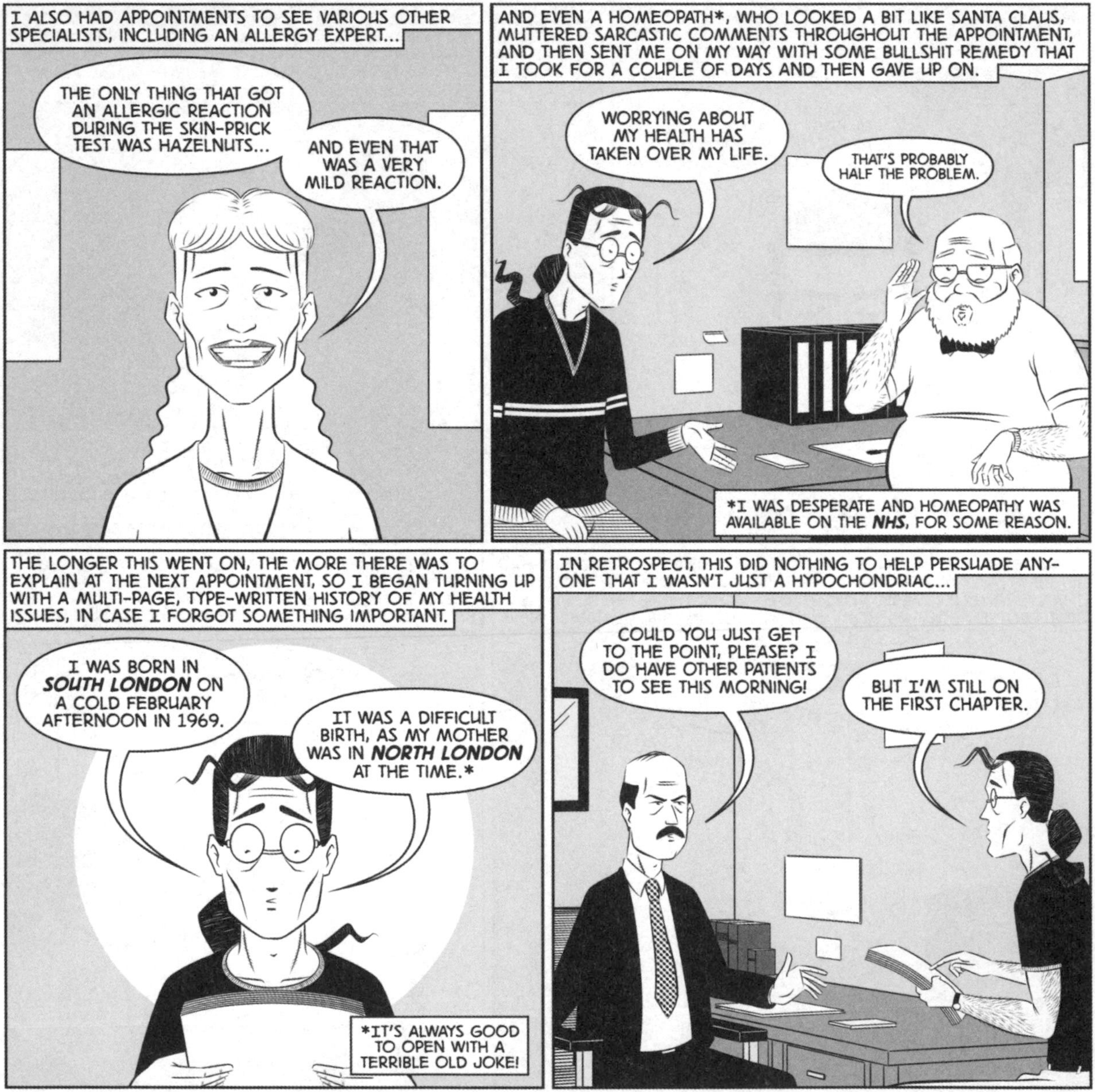
I ALSO HAD APPOINTMENTS TO SEE VARIOUS OTHER SPECIALISTS, INCLUDING AN ALLERGY EXPERT...
THE ONLY THING THAT GOT AN ALLERGIC REACTION DURING THE SKIN-PRICK TEST WAS HAZELNUTS...
AND EVEN THAT WAS A VERY MILD REACTION.
AND EVEN A HOMEOPATH*, WHO LOOKED A BIT LIKE SANTA CLAUS, MUTTERED SARCASTIC COMMENTS THROUGHOUT THE APPOINTMENT, AND THEN SENT ME ON MY WAY WITH SOME BULLSHIT REMEDY THAT I TOOK FOR A COUPLE OF DAYS AND THEN GAVE UP ON.
WORRYING ABOUT MY HEALTH HAS TAKEN OVER MY LIFE.
THAT'S PROBABLY HALF THE PROBLEM.
*I WAS DESPERATE AND HOMEOPATHY WAS AVAILABLE ON THE **NHS**, FOR SOME REASON.
THE LONGER THIS WENT ON, THE MORE THERE WAS TO EXPLAIN AT THE NEXT APPOINTMENT, SO I BEGAN TURNING UP WITH A MULTI-PAGE, TYPE-WRITTEN HISTORY OF MY HEALTH ISSUES, IN CASE I FORGOT SOMETHING IMPORTANT.
I WAS BORN IN **SOUTH LONDON** ON A COLD FEBRUARY AFTERNOON IN 1969.
IT WAS A DIFFICULT BIRTH, AS MY MOTHER WAS IN **NORTH LONDON** AT THE TIME.*
*IT'S ALWAYS GOOD TO OPEN WITH A TERRIBLE OLD JOKE!
IN RETROSPECT, THIS DID NOTHING TO HELP PERSUADE ANY-ONE THAT I WASN'T JUST A HYPOCHONDRIAC...
COULD YOU JUST GET TO THE POINT, PLEASE? I DO HAVE OTHER PATIENTS TO SEE THIS MORNING!
BUT I'M STILL ON THE FIRST CHAPTER.

AND ME OCCASIONALLY LOSING MY COOL DIDN'T HELP MY CASE MUCH, EITHER.

I KNOW THIS ISN'T WHAT YOU WANT TO HEAR, BUT I'D LIKE TO REFER YOU TO A COLLEAGUE OF MINE WHO IS AN EXPERT ON IRRITABLE BOWEL SYNDROME.

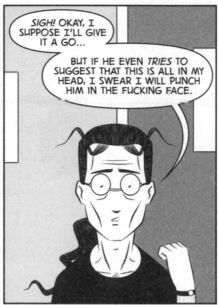

SIGH! OKAY, I SUPPOSE I'LL GIVE IT A GO...

BUT IF HE EVEN *TRIES* TO SUGGEST THAT THIS IS ALL IN MY HEAD, I SWEAR I WILL PUNCH HIM IN THE FUCKING FACE.

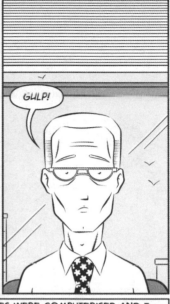

GULP!

THE FOLDER CONTAINING MY MEDICAL NOTES THAT WAS KEPT BY MY DOCTOR GOT THICKER AND THICKER. THE LAST TIME I SAW IT, THERE WERE TWO THICK FOLDERS, HELD TOGETHER WITH ELASTIC BANDS, AND I OFTEN THOUGHT ABOUT STEALING THEM SO THAT I COULD SEE EXACTLY WHAT ALL THESE SPECIALISTS HAD SAID ABOUT ME.

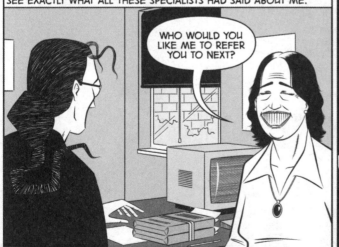

WHO WOULD YOU LIKE ME TO REFER YOU TO NEXT?

EVENTUALLY, THE NOTES WERE COMPUTERISED AND I LOST MY CHANCE, BUT I HAD A PRETTY GOOD IDEA OF THE SORT OF THING THAT WOULD HAVE BEEN IN THERE.

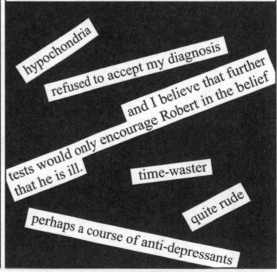

hypochondria

refused to accept my diagnosis

and I believe that further tests would only encourage Robert in the belief that he is ill.

time-waster

quite rude

perhaps a course of anti-depressants

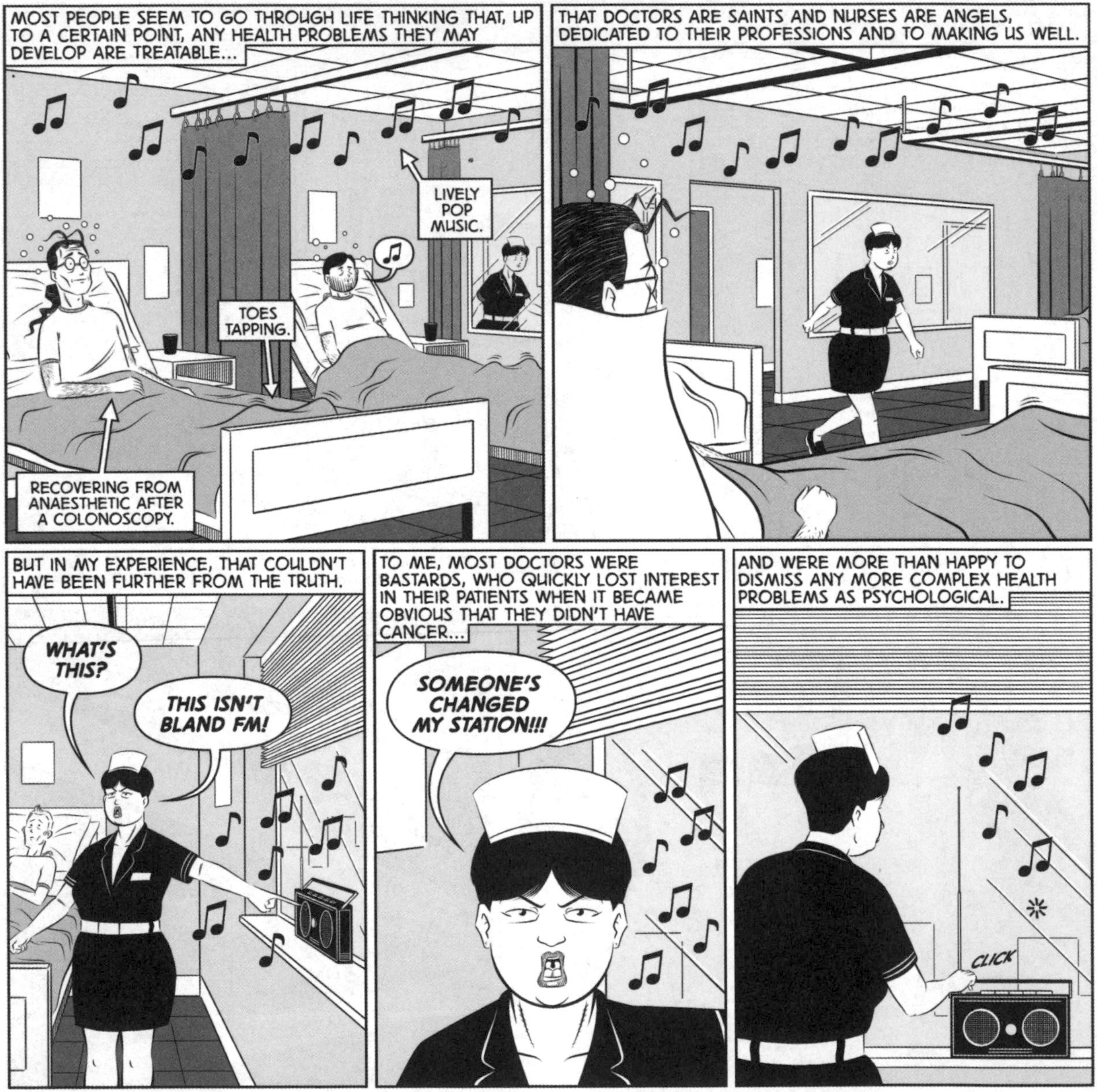
MOST PEOPLE SEEM TO GO THROUGH LIFE THINKING THAT, UP TO A CERTAIN POINT, ANY HEALTH PROBLEMS THEY MAY DEVELOP ARE TREATABLE...
LIVELY POP MUSIC.
TOES TAPPING.
RECOVERING FROM ANAESTHETIC AFTER A COLONOSCOPY.
THAT DOCTORS ARE SAINTS AND NURSES ARE ANGELS, DEDICATED TO THEIR PROFESSIONS AND TO MAKING US WELL.
BUT IN MY EXPERIENCE, THAT COULDN'T HAVE BEEN FURTHER FROM THE TRUTH.
WHAT'S THIS?
THIS ISN'T BLAND FM!
TO ME, MOST DOCTORS WERE BASTARDS, WHO QUICKLY LOST INTEREST IN THEIR PATIENTS WHEN IT BECAME OBVIOUS THAT THEY DIDN'T HAVE CANCER...
SOMEONE'S CHANGED MY STATION!!!
AND WERE MORE THAN HAPPY TO DISMISS ANY MORE COMPLEX HEALTH PROBLEMS AS PSYCHOLOGICAL.
CLICK

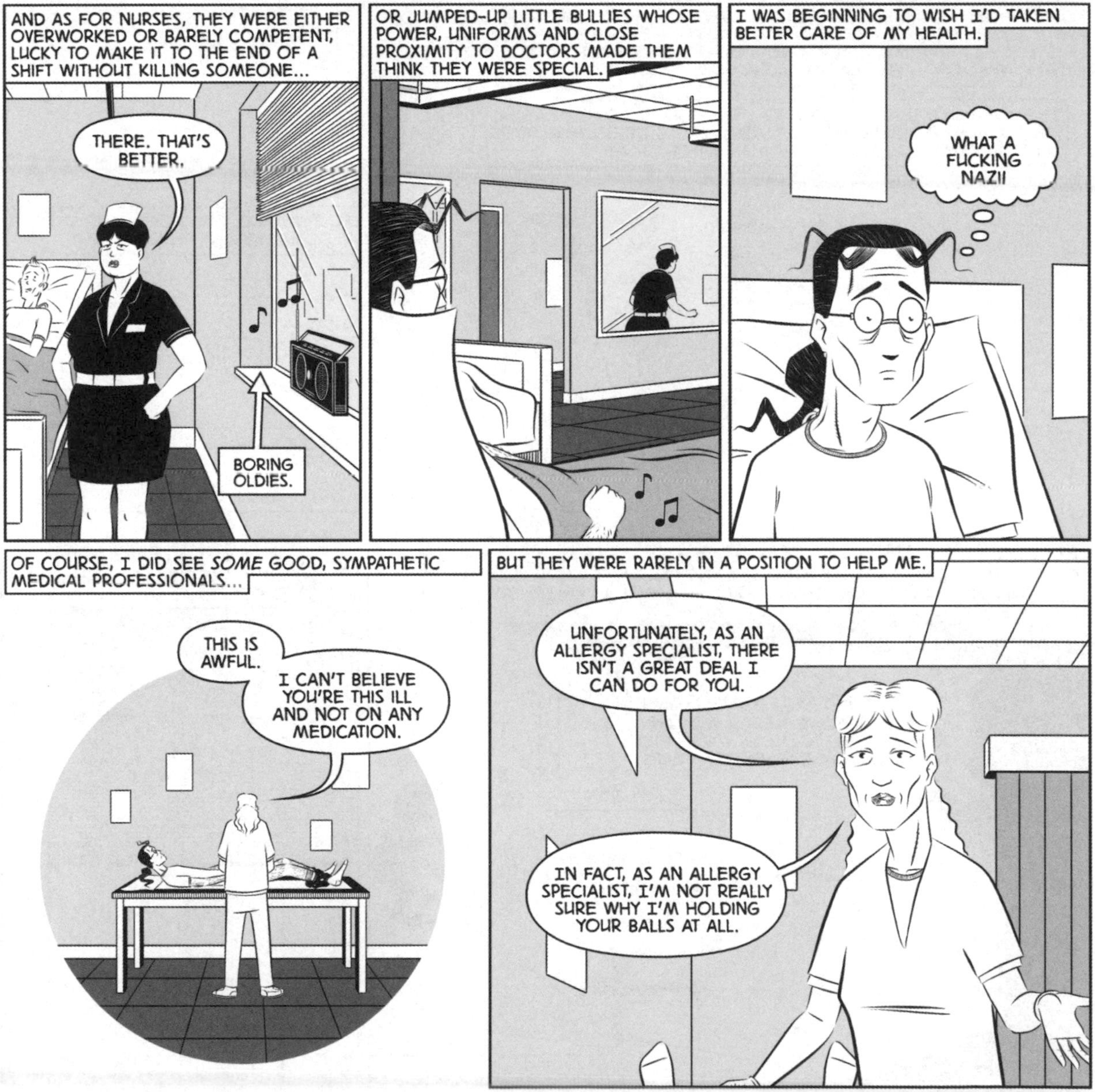
AND AS FOR NURSES, THEY WERE EITHER OVERWORKED OR BARELY COMPETENT, LUCKY TO MAKE IT TO THE END OF A SHIFT WITHOUT KILLING SOMEONE...
THERE. THAT'S BETTER.
BORING OLDIES.
OR JUMPED-UP LITTLE BULLIES WHOSE POWER, UNIFORMS AND CLOSE PROXIMITY TO DOCTORS MADE THEM THINK THEY WERE SPECIAL.
I WAS BEGINNING TO WISH I'D TAKEN BETTER CARE OF MY HEALTH.
WHAT A FUCKING NAZI!
OF COURSE, I DID SEE *SOME* GOOD, SYMPATHETIC MEDICAL PROFESSIONALS...
THIS IS AWFUL.
I CAN'T BELIEVE YOU'RE THIS ILL AND NOT ON ANY MEDICATION.
BUT THEY WERE RARELY IN A POSITION TO HELP ME.
UNFORTUNATELY, AS AN ALLERGY SPECIALIST, THERE ISN'T A GREAT DEAL I CAN DO FOR YOU.
IN FACT, AS AN ALLERGY SPECIALIST, I'M NOT REALLY SURE WHY I'M HOLDING YOUR BALLS AT ALL.

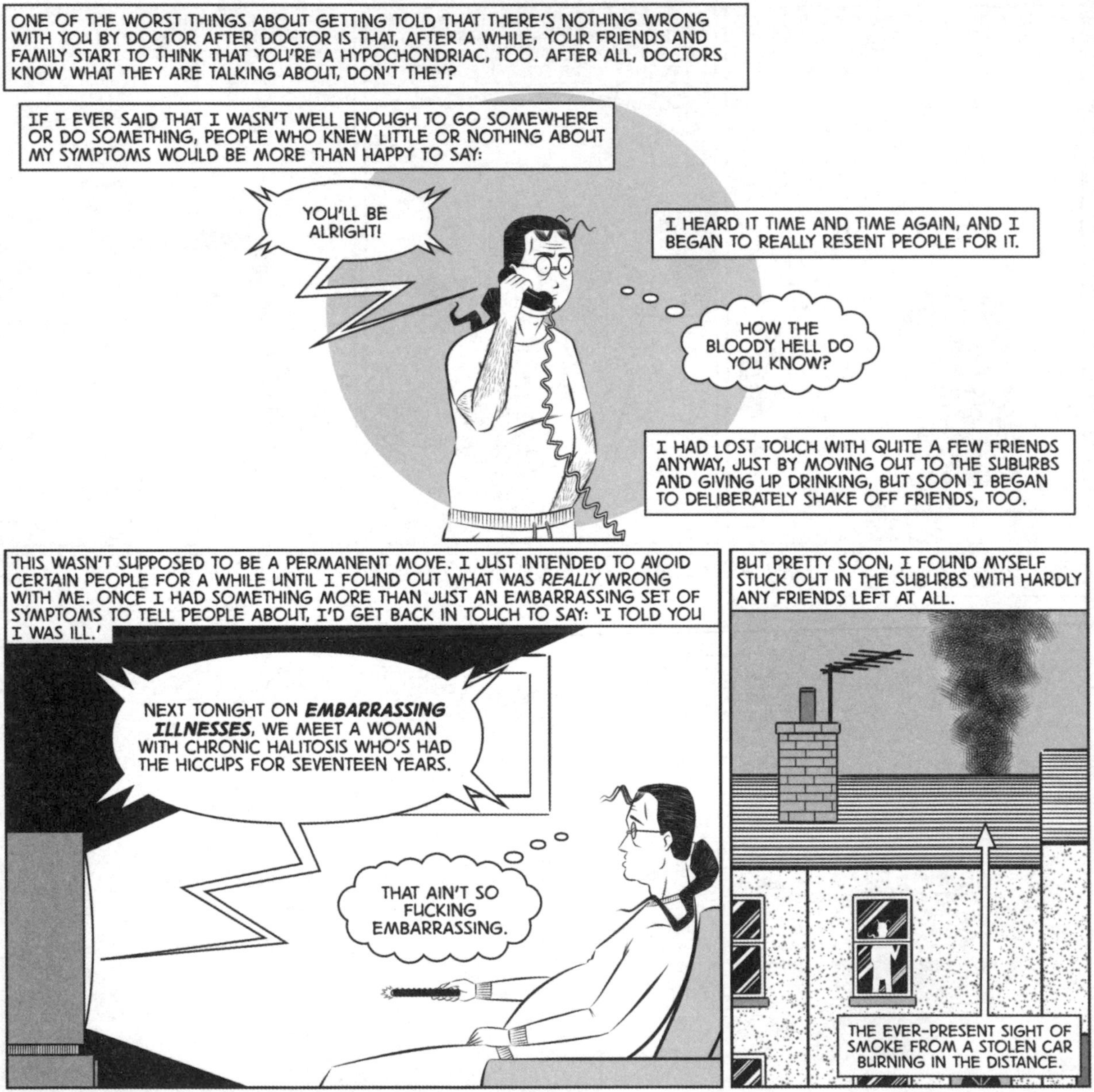
ONE OF THE WORST THINGS ABOUT GETTING TOLD THAT THERE'S NOTHING WRONG WITH YOU BY DOCTOR AFTER DOCTOR IS THAT, AFTER A WHILE, YOUR FRIENDS AND FAMILY START TO THINK THAT YOU'RE A HYPOCHONDRIAC, TOO. AFTER ALL, DOCTORS KNOW WHAT THEY ARE TALKING ABOUT, DON'T THEY?
IF I EVER SAID THAT I WASN'T WELL ENOUGH TO GO SOMEWHERE OR DO SOMETHING, PEOPLE WHO KNEW LITTLE OR NOTHING ABOUT MY SYMPTOMS WOULD BE MORE THAN HAPPY TO SAY:
YOU'LL BE ALRIGHT!
I HEARD IT TIME AND TIME AGAIN, AND I BEGAN TO REALLY RESENT PEOPLE FOR IT.
HOW THE BLOODY HELL DO YOU KNOW?
I HAD LOST TOUCH WITH QUITE A FEW FRIENDS ANYWAY, JUST BY MOVING OUT TO THE SUBURBS AND GIVING UP DRINKING, BUT SOON I BEGAN TO DELIBERATELY SHAKE OFF FRIENDS, TOO.
THIS WASN'T SUPPOSED TO BE A PERMANENT MOVE. I JUST INTENDED TO AVOID CERTAIN PEOPLE FOR A WHILE UNTIL I FOUND OUT WHAT WAS *REALLY* WRONG WITH ME. ONCE I HAD SOMETHING MORE THAN JUST AN EMBARRASSING SET OF SYMPTOMS TO TELL PEOPLE ABOUT, I'D GET BACK IN TOUCH TO SAY: 'I TOLD YOU I WAS ILL.'
NEXT TONIGHT ON ***EMBARRASSING ILLNESSES***, WE MEET A WOMAN WITH CHRONIC HALITOSIS WHO'S HAD THE HICCUPS FOR SEVENTEEN YEARS.
THAT AIN'T SO FUCKING EMBARRASSING.
BUT PRETTY SOON, I FOUND MYSELF STUCK OUT IN THE SUBURBS WITH HARDLY ANY FRIENDS LEFT AT ALL.
THE EVER-PRESENT SIGHT OF SMOKE FROM A STOLEN CAR BURNING IN THE DISTANCE.

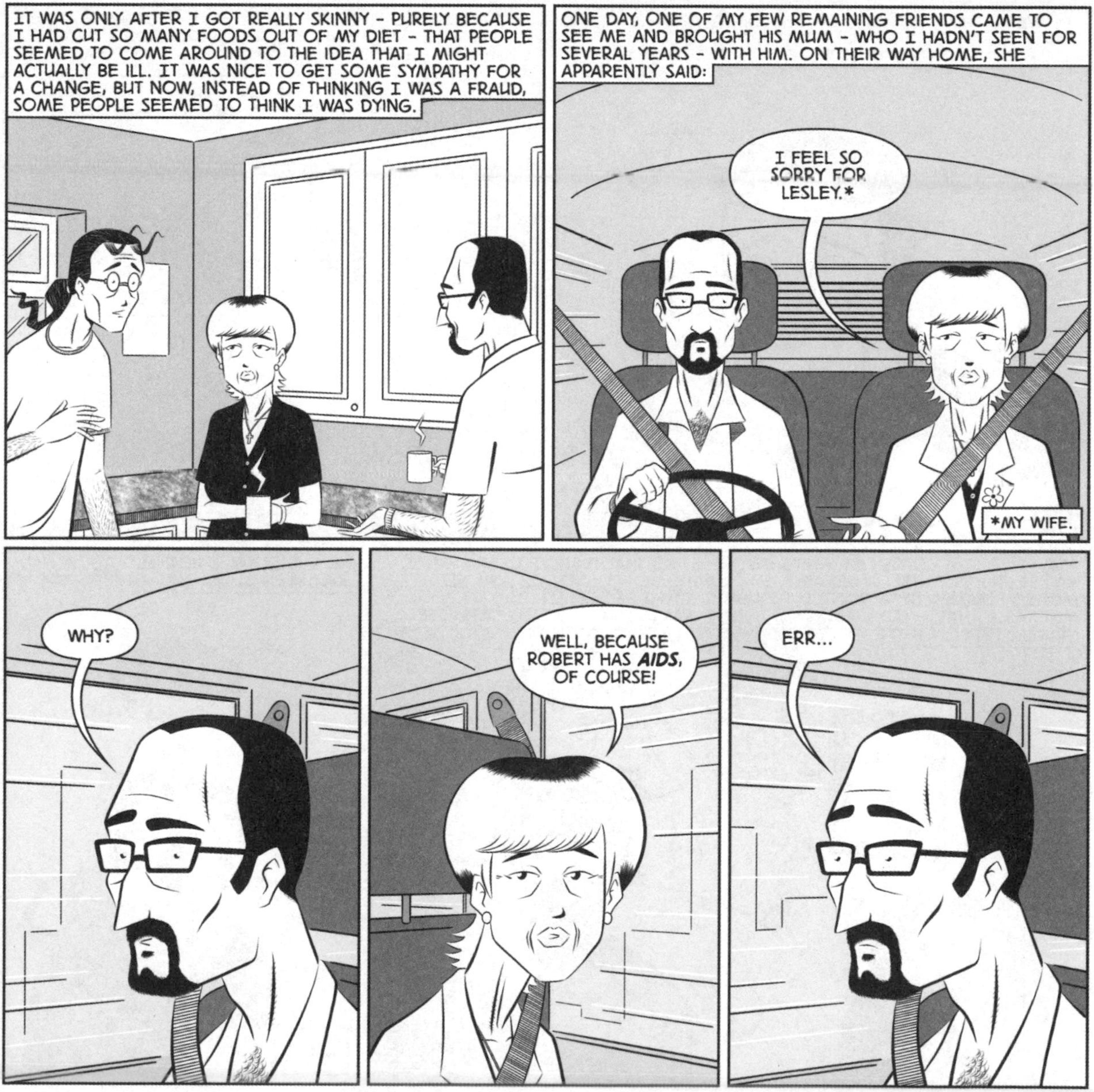

IT WAS ONLY AFTER I GOT REALLY SKINNY - PURELY BECAUSE I HAD CUT SO MANY FOODS OUT OF MY DIET - THAT PEOPLE SEEMED TO COME AROUND TO THE IDEA THAT I MIGHT ACTUALLY BE ILL. IT WAS NICE TO GET SOME SYMPATHY FOR A CHANGE, BUT NOW, INSTEAD OF THINKING I WAS A FRAUD, SOME PEOPLE SEEMED TO THINK I WAS DYING.
ONE DAY, ONE OF MY FEW REMAINING FRIENDS CAME TO SEE ME AND BROUGHT HIS MUM - WHO I HADN'T SEEN FOR SEVERAL YEARS - WITH HIM. ON THEIR WAY HOME, SHE APPARENTLY SAID:
I FEEL SO SORRY FOR LESLEY.*
*MY WIFE.
WHY?
WELL, BECAUSE ROBERT HAS ***AIDS***, OF COURSE!
ERR...

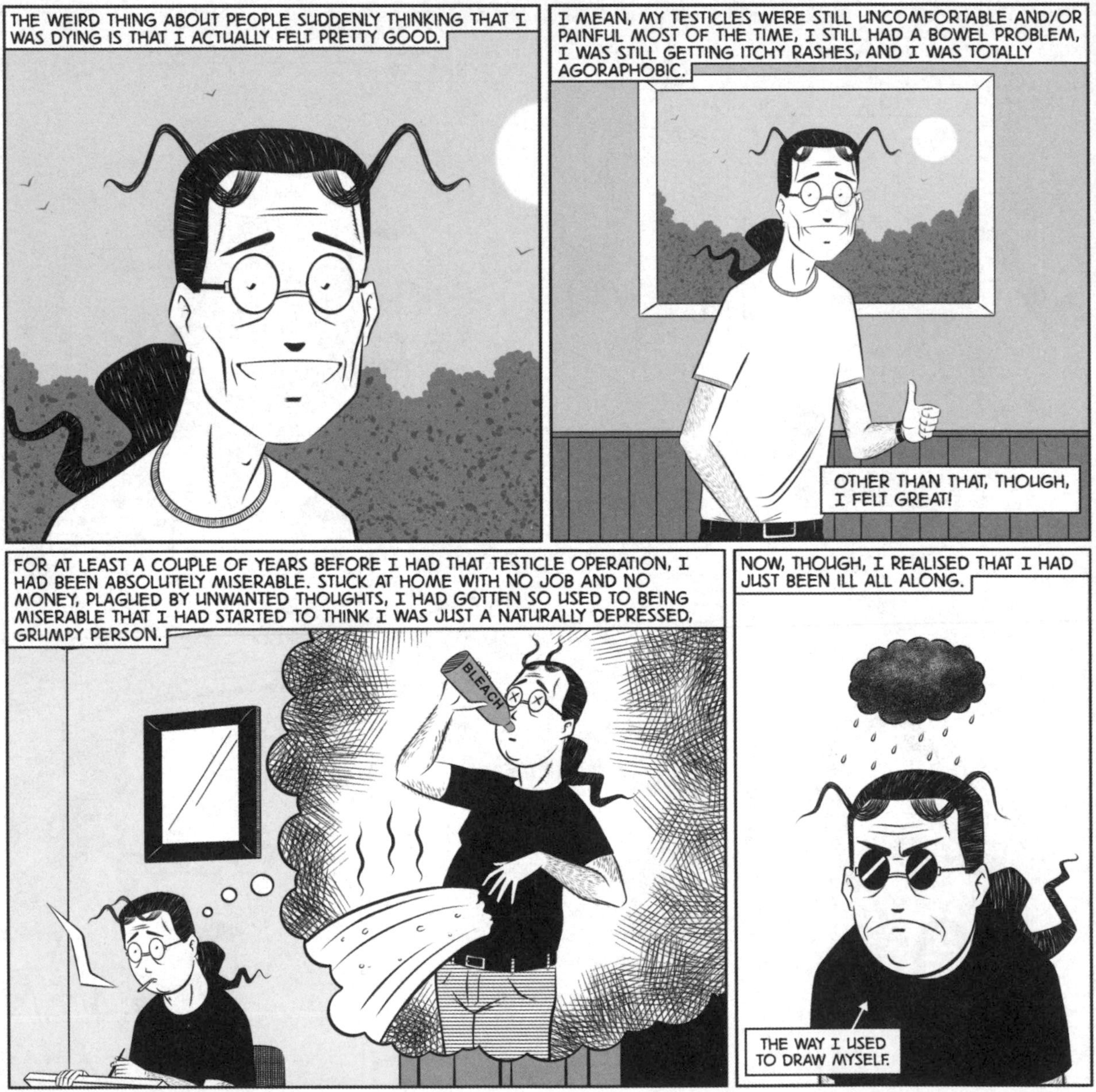
THE WEIRD THING ABOUT PEOPLE SUDDENLY THINKING THAT I WAS DYING IS THAT I ACTUALLY FELT PRETTY GOOD.
I MEAN, MY TESTICLES WERE STILL UNCOMFORTABLE AND/OR PAINFUL MOST OF THE TIME, I STILL HAD A BOWEL PROBLEM, I WAS STILL GETTING ITCHY RASHES, AND I WAS TOTALLY AGORAPHOBIC.
OTHER THAN THAT, THOUGH, I FELT GREAT!
FOR AT LEAST A COUPLE OF YEARS BEFORE I HAD THAT TESTICLE OPERATION, I HAD BEEN ABSOLUTELY MISERABLE. STUCK AT HOME WITH NO JOB AND NO MONEY, PLAGUED BY UNWANTED THOUGHTS, I HAD GOTTEN SO USED TO BEING MISERABLE THAT I HAD STARTED TO THINK I WAS JUST A NATURALLY DEPRESSED, GRUMPY PERSON.
BLEACH
NOW, THOUGH, I REALISED THAT I HAD JUST BEEN ILL ALL ALONG.
THE WAY I USED TO DRAW MYSELF.

MAYBE I HAD MANAGED TO REVERSE SOME CHEMICAL IMBALANCE IN MY BRAIN BY GIVING UP DRINKING, GIVING UP SMOKING, LOSING SO MUCH WEIGHT, OR SOME COMBINATION OF THESE FACTORS?

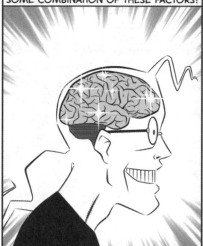

MAYBE I HAD FINALLY REALISED THAT THE THINGS I HAD WASTED SO MUCH TIME WORRYING ABOUT BEFORE REALLY WEREN'T THAT IMPORTANT?

CHRONIC TESTICLE PAIN TENDS TO PUT OTHER THINGS INTO PERSPECTIVE.

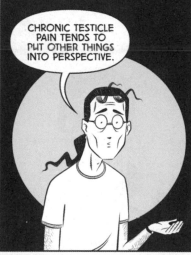

ALL I KNOW FOR SURE IS THAT I HAD MORE REASON TO BE DEPRESSED THAN EVER, BUT FOR THE FIRST TIME IN YEARS, POSSIBLY EVEN SINCE CHILDHOOD, I DIDN'T FEEL DEPRESSED AT ALL.

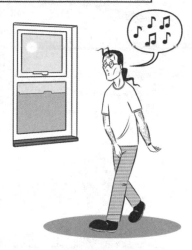

I WOULD STILL LEAVE HOSPITAL APPOINTMENTS FEELING DESPONDENT BUT THIS WOULD USUALLY PASS BEFORE I EVEN GOT HOME.

FUCKING DOCTORS! I CAN'T TAKE ANOTHER FUCKING MINUTE OF THIS. I'M JUST GOING TO HAVE TO KILL MYSELF!

WELL, MAYBE NOT LITERALLY KILL MYSELF. MAYBE I JUST NEED TO TRY EVEN HARDER TO SORT THIS OUT MYSELF?

ANY IDEA WHAT'S ON THE TELLY TONIGHT?

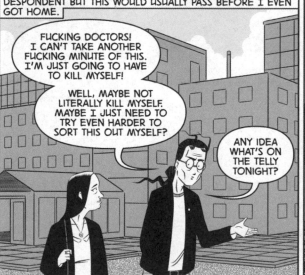

I HAD NO JOB BUT, AS I WAS ILL, I WASN'T UNDER ANY PRESSURE TO GET A JOB. I HAD NO INCOME OF MY OWN AT ALL, AS I WAS UNABLE TO CLAIM BENEFITS, BUT AS I HAD NO BAD HABITS, NO SOCIAL LIFE, AND I DIDN'T EVEN EAT THAT MUCH, I WAS ALMOST AS CHEAP TO KEEP AS A HAMSTER.

THERE IS NO WAY I'M RUNNING AROUND IN THAT THING WHILE MY BALLS FEEL LIKE THIS.

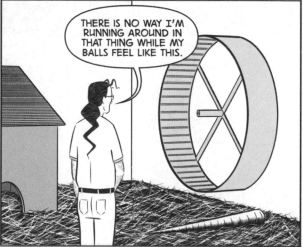

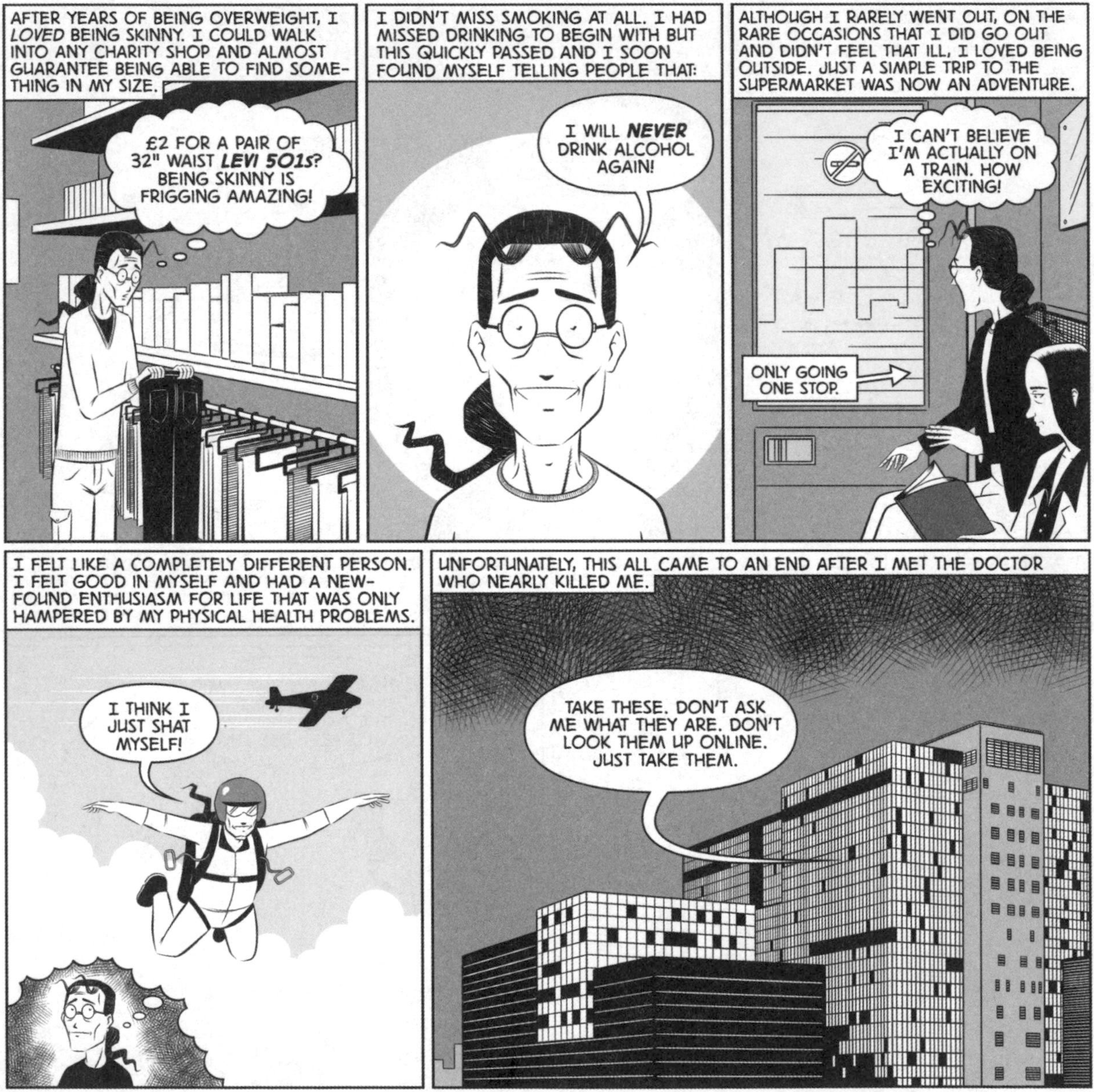
AFTER YEARS OF BEING OVERWEIGHT, I LOVED BEING SKINNY. I COULD WALK INTO ANY CHARITY SHOP AND ALMOST GUARANTEE BEING ABLE TO FIND SOMETHING IN MY SIZE.
£2 FOR A PAIR OF 32" WAIST LEVI 501s? BEING SKINNY IS FRIGGING AMAZING!
I DIDN'T MISS SMOKING AT ALL. I HAD MISSED DRINKING TO BEGIN WITH BUT THIS QUICKLY PASSED AND I SOON FOUND MYSELF TELLING PEOPLE THAT:
I WILL NEVER DRINK ALCOHOL AGAIN!
ALTHOUGH I RARELY WENT OUT, ON THE RARE OCCASIONS THAT I DID GO OUT AND DIDN'T FEEL THAT ILL, I LOVED BEING OUTSIDE. JUST A SIMPLE TRIP TO THE SUPERMARKET WAS NOW AN ADVENTURE.
I CAN'T BELIEVE I'M ACTUALLY ON A TRAIN. HOW EXCITING!
ONLY GOING ONE STOP.
I FELT LIKE A COMPLETELY DIFFERENT PERSON. I FELT GOOD IN MYSELF AND HAD A NEW-FOUND ENTHUSIASM FOR LIFE THAT WAS ONLY HAMPERED BY MY PHYSICAL HEALTH PROBLEMS.
I THINK I JUST SHAT MYSELF!
UNFORTUNATELY, THIS ALL CAME TO AN END AFTER I MET THE DOCTOR WHO NEARLY KILLED ME.
TAKE THESE. DON'T ASK ME WHAT THEY ARE. DON'T LOOK THEM UP ONLINE. JUST TAKE THEM.

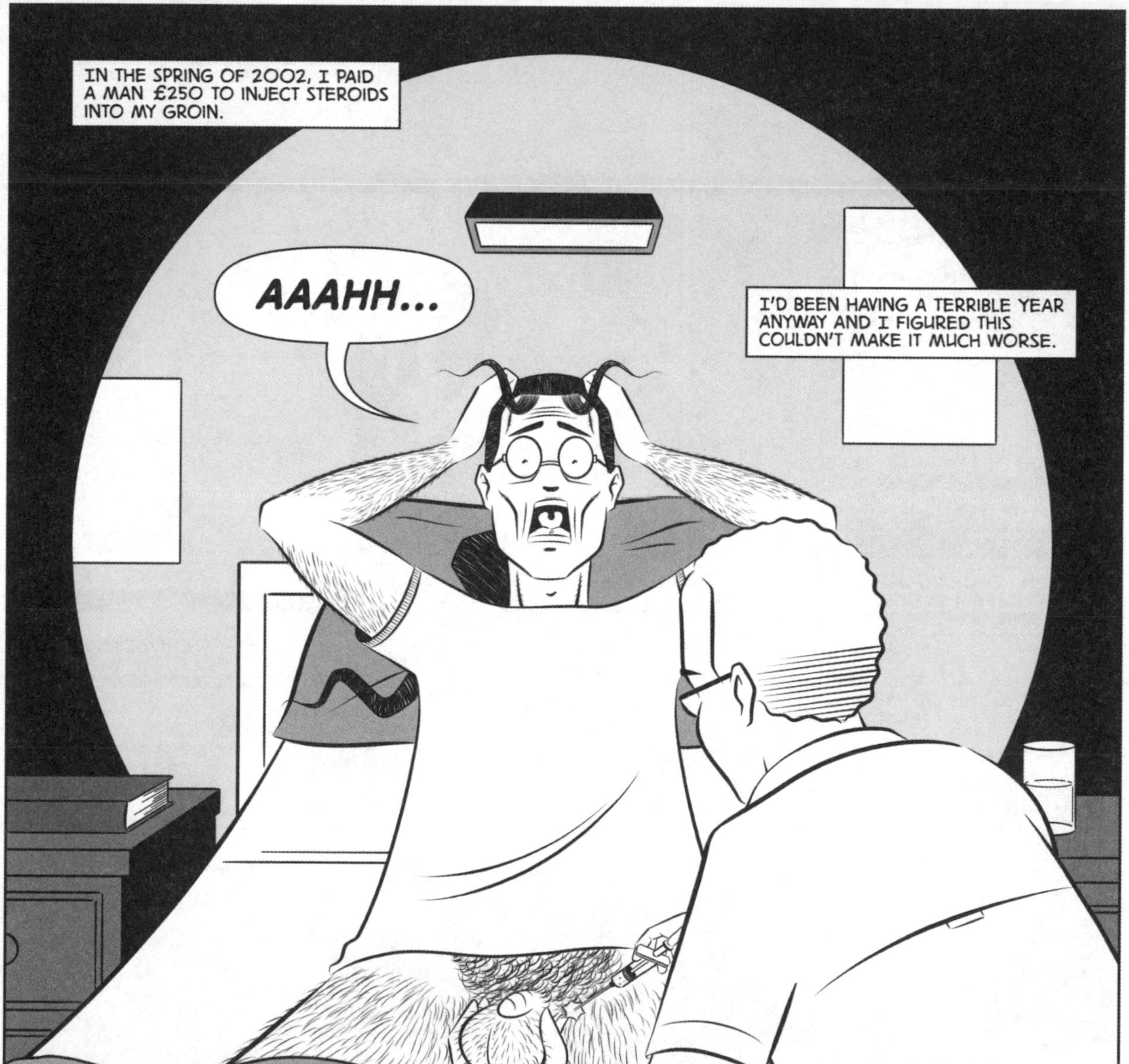
IN THE SPRING OF 2002, I PAID A MAN £250 TO INJECT STEROIDS INTO MY GROIN.
AAAHH...
I'D BEEN HAVING A TERRIBLE YEAR ANYWAY AND I FIGURED THIS COULDN'T MAKE IT MUCH WORSE.

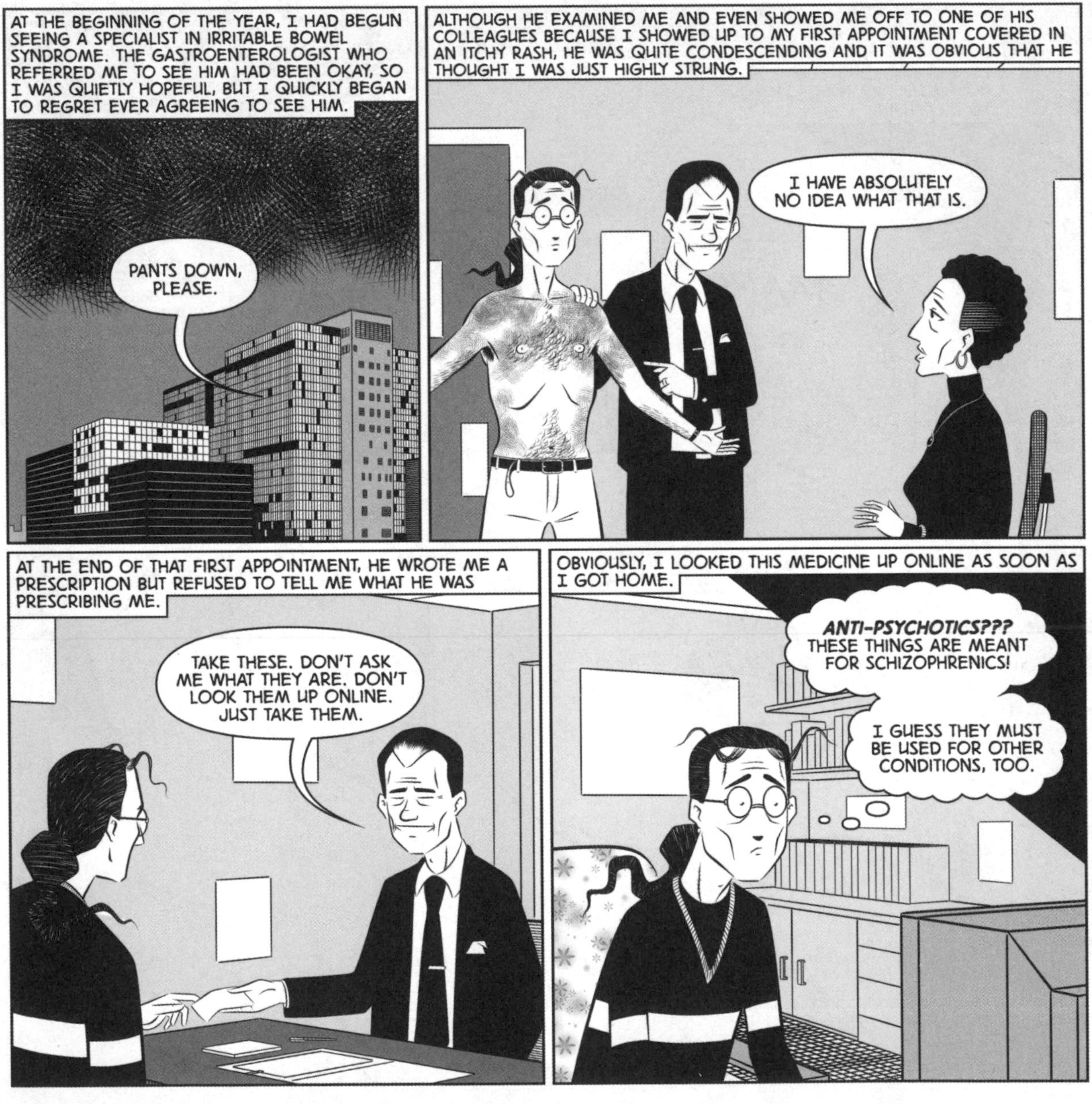
AT THE BEGINNING OF THE YEAR, I HAD BEGUN SEEING A SPECIALIST IN IRRITABLE BOWEL SYNDROME. THE GASTROENTEROLOGIST WHO REFERRED ME TO SEE HIM HAD BEEN OKAY, SO I WAS QUIETLY HOPEFUL, BUT I QUICKLY BEGAN TO REGRET EVER AGREEING TO SEE HIM.
PANTS DOWN, PLEASE.
ALTHOUGH HE EXAMINED ME AND EVEN SHOWED ME OFF TO ONE OF HIS COLLEAGUES BECAUSE I SHOWED UP TO MY FIRST APPOINTMENT COVERED IN AN ITCHY RASH, HE WAS QUITE CONDESCENDING AND IT WAS OBVIOUS THAT HE THOUGHT I WAS JUST HIGHLY STRUNG.
I HAVE ABSOLUTELY NO IDEA WHAT THAT IS.
AT THE END OF THAT FIRST APPOINTMENT, HE WROTE ME A PRESCRIPTION BUT REFUSED TO TELL ME WHAT HE WAS PRESCRIBING ME.
TAKE THESE. DON'T ASK ME WHAT THEY ARE. DON'T LOOK THEM UP ONLINE. JUST TAKE THEM.
OBVIOUSLY, I LOOKED THIS MEDICINE UP ONLINE AS SOON AS I GOT HOME.
ANTI-PSYCHOTICS??? THESE THINGS ARE MEANT FOR SCHIZOPHRENICS!
I GUESS THEY MUST BE USED FOR OTHER CONDITIONS, TOO.

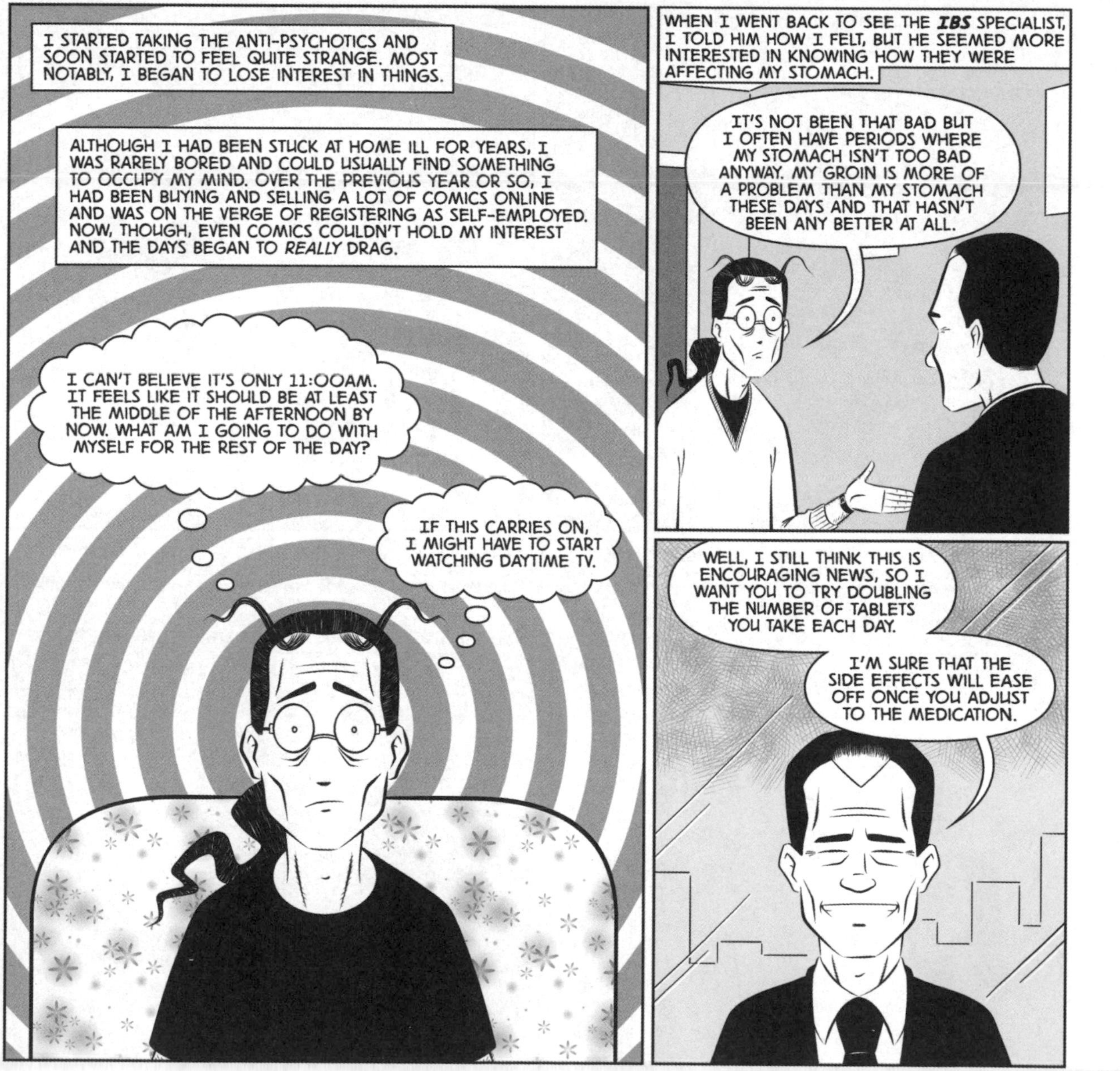
I STARTED TAKING THE ANTI-PSYCHOTICS AND SOON STARTED TO FEEL QUITE STRANGE. MOST NOTABLY, I BEGAN TO LOSE INTEREST IN THINGS.
ALTHOUGH I HAD BEEN STUCK AT HOME ILL FOR YEARS, I WAS RARELY BORED AND COULD USUALLY FIND SOMETHING TO OCCUPY MY MIND. OVER THE PREVIOUS YEAR OR SO, I HAD BEEN BUYING AND SELLING A LOT OF COMICS ONLINE AND WAS ON THE VERGE OF REGISTERING AS SELF-EMPLOYED. NOW, THOUGH, EVEN COMICS COULDN'T HOLD MY INTEREST AND THE DAYS BEGAN TO *REALLY* DRAG.
I CAN'T BELIEVE IT'S ONLY 11:00AM. IT FEELS LIKE IT SHOULD BE AT LEAST THE MIDDLE OF THE AFTERNOON BY NOW. WHAT AM I GOING TO DO WITH MYSELF FOR THE REST OF THE DAY?
IF THIS CARRIES ON, I MIGHT HAVE TO START WATCHING DAYTIME TV.
WHEN I WENT BACK TO SEE THE ***IBS*** SPECIALIST, I TOLD HIM HOW I FELT, BUT HE SEEMED MORE INTERESTED IN KNOWING HOW THEY WERE AFFECTING MY STOMACH.
IT'S NOT BEEN THAT BAD BUT I OFTEN HAVE PERIODS WHERE MY STOMACH ISN'T TOO BAD ANYWAY. MY GROIN IS MORE OF A PROBLEM THAN MY STOMACH THESE DAYS AND THAT HASN'T BEEN ANY BETTER AT ALL.
WELL, I STILL THINK THIS IS ENCOURAGING NEWS, SO I WANT YOU TO TRY DOUBLING THE NUMBER OF TABLETS YOU TAKE EACH DAY.
I'M SURE THAT THE SIDE EFFECTS WILL EASE OFF ONCE YOU ADJUST TO THE MEDICATION.

AS SUGGESTED, I DOUBLED THE DOSE OF ANTI-PSYCHOTICS I WAS TAKING AND QUICKLY BEGAN TO FEEL EVEN WORSE. SOON, THE DAYS *AND* THE NIGHTS WERE DRAGGING, AS I STARTED TO HAVE A LOT OF TROUBLE SLEEPING.

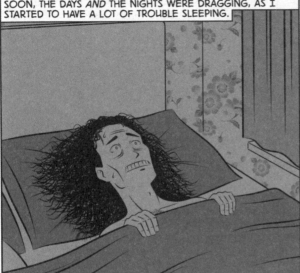

I ALSO STARTED TO EXPERIENCE SUICIDAL THOUGHTS, AND BEGAN TO DREAD BEING AT HOME ON MY OWN IN CASE I ACTED ON THEM.

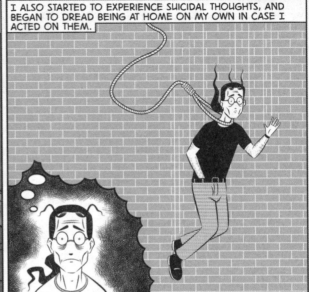

AROUND THE SAME TIME, MY WIFE ANNOUNCED THAT SHE WOULD SOON BE GOING AWAY ON A TEN-DAY BUSINESS TRIP. OVER THE PREVIOUS FEW YEARS, I HAD BECOME COMPLETELY DEPENDENT ON HER - I LITERALLY DIDN'T GO ANYWHERE ON MY OWN ANYMORE - AND IN MY DRUGGED-UP STATE, TEN DAYS SEEMED LIKE A *VERY* LONG TIME.

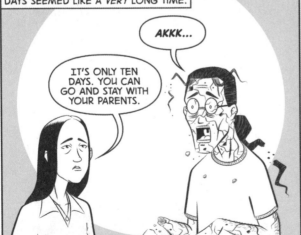

AKKK...

IT'S ONLY TEN DAYS. YOU CAN GO AND STAY WITH YOUR PARENTS.

IGNORING THE ADVICE THAT CAME WITH THE MEDICATION, I SUDDENLY STOPPED TAKING THE ANTI-PSYCHOTICS - EVEN IF I STAYED WITH MY PARENTS WHILE MY WIFE WAS AWAY, I DIDN'T WANT TO FEEL SUICIDAL WHILE I WAS THERE - BUT THE DAYS CONTINUED TO DRAG, I HAD EVEN MORE TROUBLE SLEEPING, AND THE SUICIDAL THOUGHTS PERSISTED.

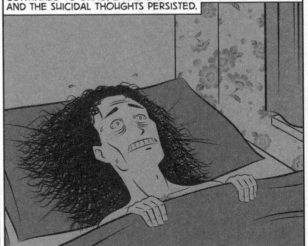

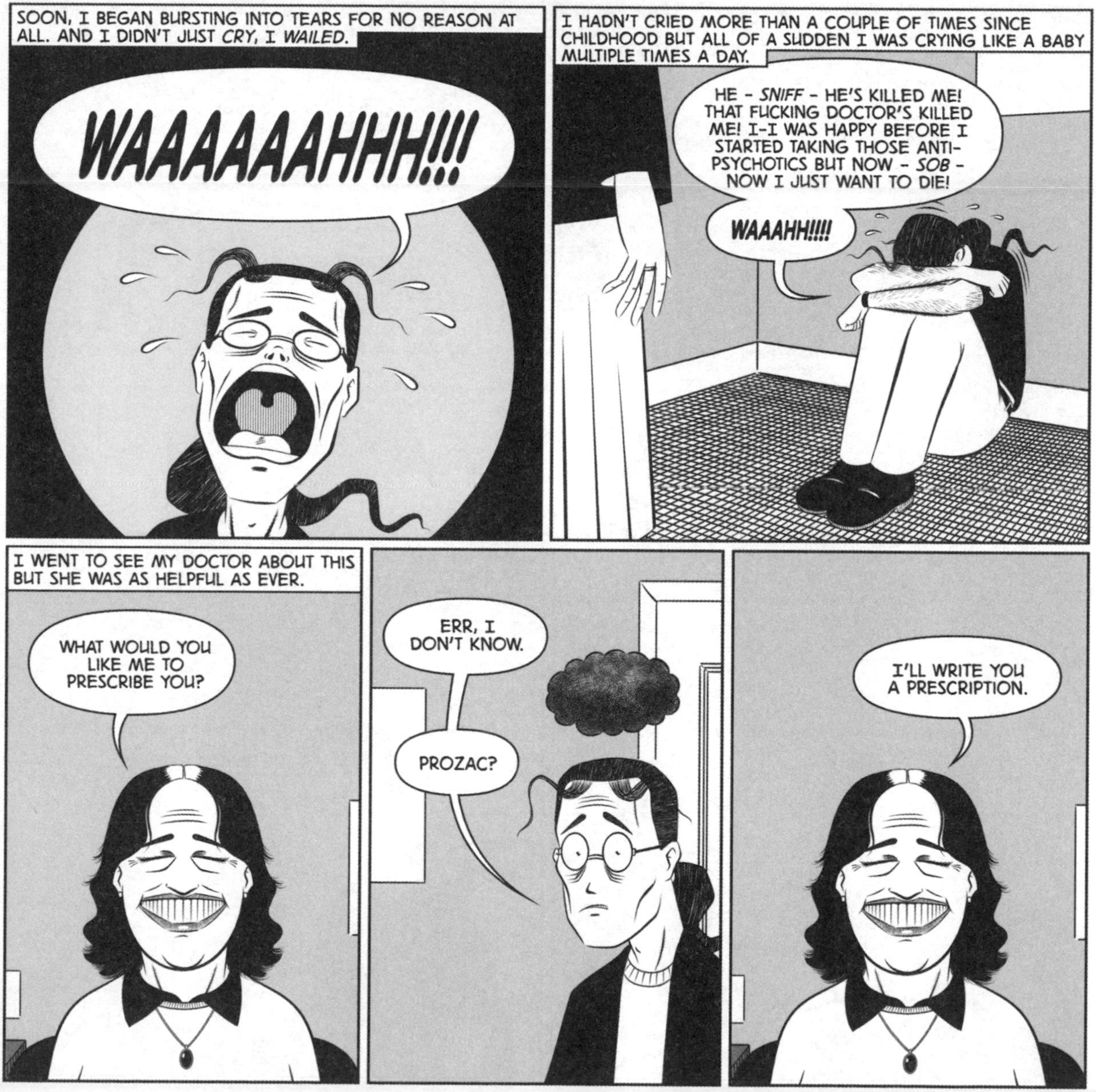

SOON, I BEGAN BURSTING INTO TEARS FOR NO REASON AT ALL. AND I DIDN'T JUST *CRY*, I *WAILED*.
WAAAAAAAHHH!!!
I HADN'T CRIED MORE THAN A COUPLE OF TIMES SINCE CHILDHOOD BUT ALL OF A SUDDEN I WAS CRYING LIKE A BABY MULTIPLE TIMES A DAY.
HE - *SNIFF* - HE'S KILLED ME! THAT FUCKING DOCTOR'S KILLED ME! I-I WAS HAPPY BEFORE I STARTED TAKING THOSE ANTI-PSYCHOTICS BUT NOW - *SOB* - NOW I JUST WANT TO DIE!
WAAAHH!!!!
I WENT TO SEE MY DOCTOR ABOUT THIS BUT SHE WAS AS HELPFUL AS EVER.
WHAT WOULD YOU LIKE ME TO PRESCRIBE YOU?
ERR, I DON'T KNOW.
PROZAC?
I'LL WRITE YOU A PRESCRIPTION.

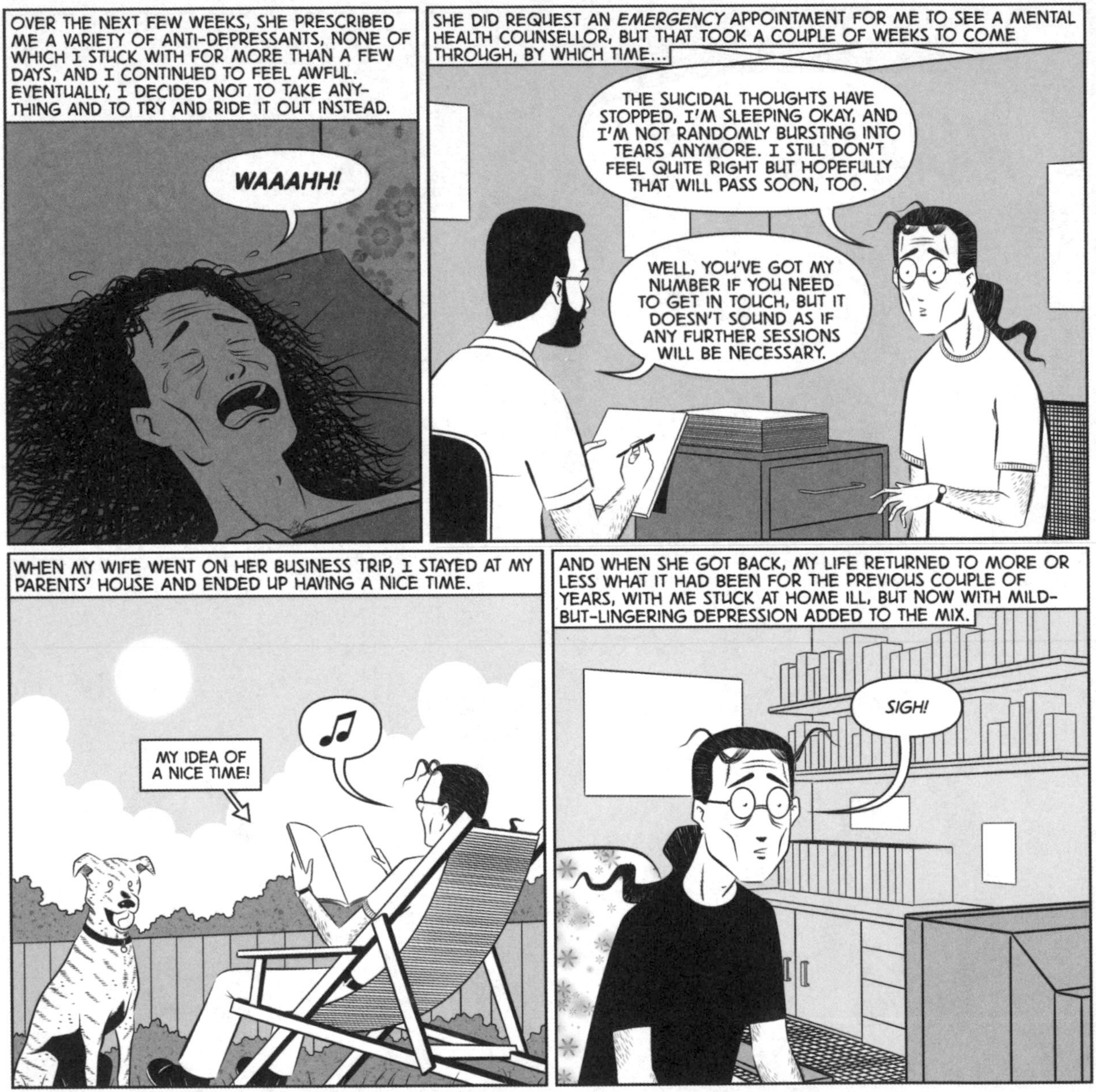
OVER THE NEXT FEW WEEKS, SHE PRESCRIBED ME A VARIETY OF ANTI-DEPRESSANTS, NONE OF WHICH I STUCK WITH FOR MORE THAN A FEW DAYS, AND I CONTINUED TO FEEL AWFUL. EVENTUALLY, I DECIDED NOT TO TAKE ANYTHING AND TO TRY AND RIDE IT OUT INSTEAD.
WAAAHH!
SHE DID REQUEST AN *EMERGENCY* APPOINTMENT FOR ME TO SEE A MENTAL HEALTH COUNSELLOR, BUT THAT TOOK A COUPLE OF WEEKS TO COME THROUGH, BY WHICH TIME...
THE SUICIDAL THOUGHTS HAVE STOPPED, I'M SLEEPING OKAY, AND I'M NOT RANDOMLY BURSTING INTO TEARS ANYMORE. I STILL DON'T FEEL QUITE RIGHT BUT HOPEFULLY THAT WILL PASS SOON, TOO.
WELL, YOU'VE GOT MY NUMBER IF YOU NEED TO GET IN TOUCH, BUT IT DOESN'T SOUND AS IF ANY FURTHER SESSIONS WILL BE NECESSARY.
WHEN MY WIFE WENT ON HER BUSINESS TRIP, I STAYED AT MY PARENTS' HOUSE AND ENDED UP HAVING A NICE TIME.
MY IDEA OF A NICE TIME!
AND WHEN SHE GOT BACK, MY LIFE RETURNED TO MORE OR LESS WHAT IT HAD BEEN FOR THE PREVIOUS COUPLE OF YEARS, WITH ME STUCK AT HOME ILL, BUT NOW WITH MILD-BUT-LINGERING DEPRESSION ADDED TO THE MIX.
SIGH!

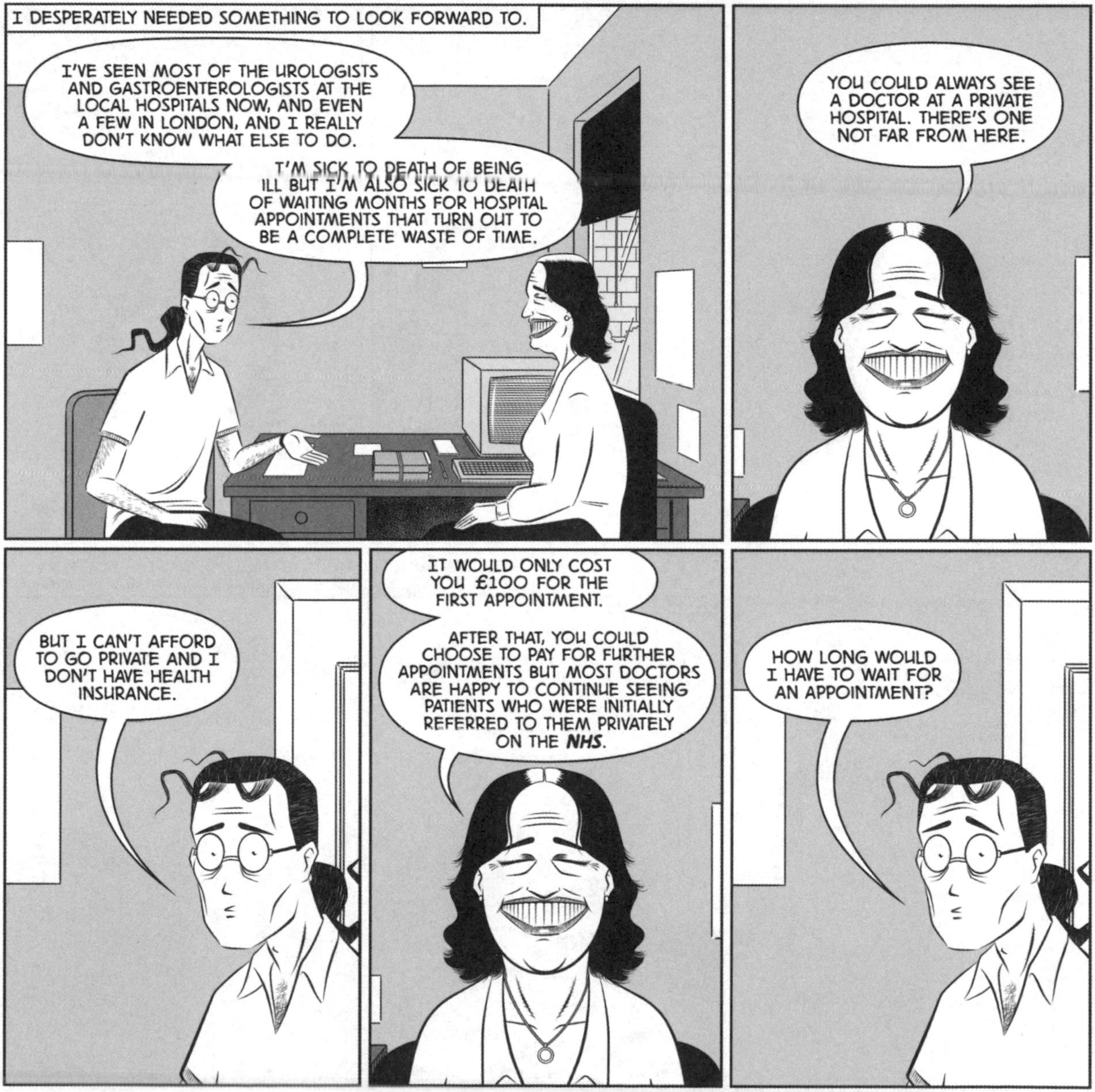
I DESPERATELY NEEDED SOMETHING TO LOOK FORWARD TO.
I'VE SEEN MOST OF THE UROLOGISTS AND GASTROENTEROLOGISTS AT THE LOCAL HOSPITALS NOW, AND EVEN A FEW IN LONDON, AND I REALLY DON'T KNOW WHAT ELSE TO DO.
I'M SICK TO DEATH OF BEING ILL BUT I'M ALSO SICK TO DEATH OF WAITING MONTHS FOR HOSPITAL APPOINTMENTS THAT TURN OUT TO BE A COMPLETE WASTE OF TIME.
YOU COULD ALWAYS SEE A DOCTOR AT A PRIVATE HOSPITAL. THERE'S ONE NOT FAR FROM HERE.
BUT I CAN'T AFFORD TO GO PRIVATE AND I DON'T HAVE HEALTH INSURANCE.
IT WOULD ONLY COST YOU £100 FOR THE FIRST APPOINTMENT.
AFTER THAT, YOU COULD CHOOSE TO PAY FOR FURTHER APPOINTMENTS BUT MOST DOCTORS ARE HAPPY TO CONTINUE SEEING PATIENTS WHO WERE INITIALLY REFERRED TO THEM PRIVATELY ON THE ***NHS***.
HOW LONG WOULD I HAVE TO WAIT FOR AN APPOINTMENT?

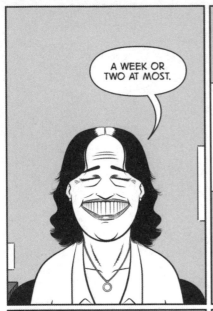

A WEEK OR TWO AT MOST.

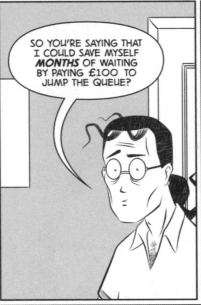

SO YOU'RE SAYING THAT I COULD SAVE MYSELF *MONTHS* OF WAITING BY PAYING £100 TO JUMP THE QUEUE?

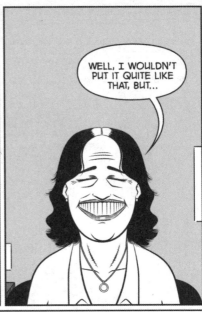

WELL, I WOULDN'T PUT IT QUITE LIKE THAT, BUT...

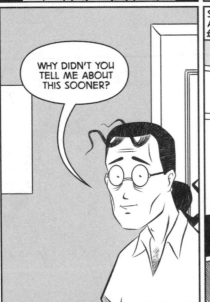

WHY DIDN'T YOU TELL ME ABOUT THIS SOONER?

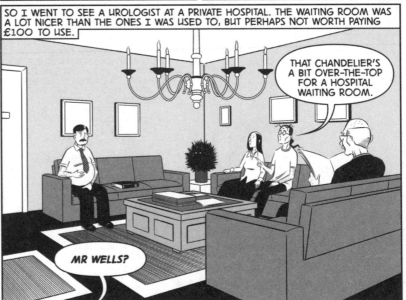

SO I WENT TO SEE A UROLOGIST AT A PRIVATE HOSPITAL. THE WAITING ROOM WAS A LOT NICER THAN THE ONES I WAS USED TO, BUT PERHAPS NOT WORTH PAYING £100 TO USE.

THAT CHANDELIER'S A BIT OVER-THE-TOP FOR A HOSPITAL WAITING ROOM.

MR WELLS?

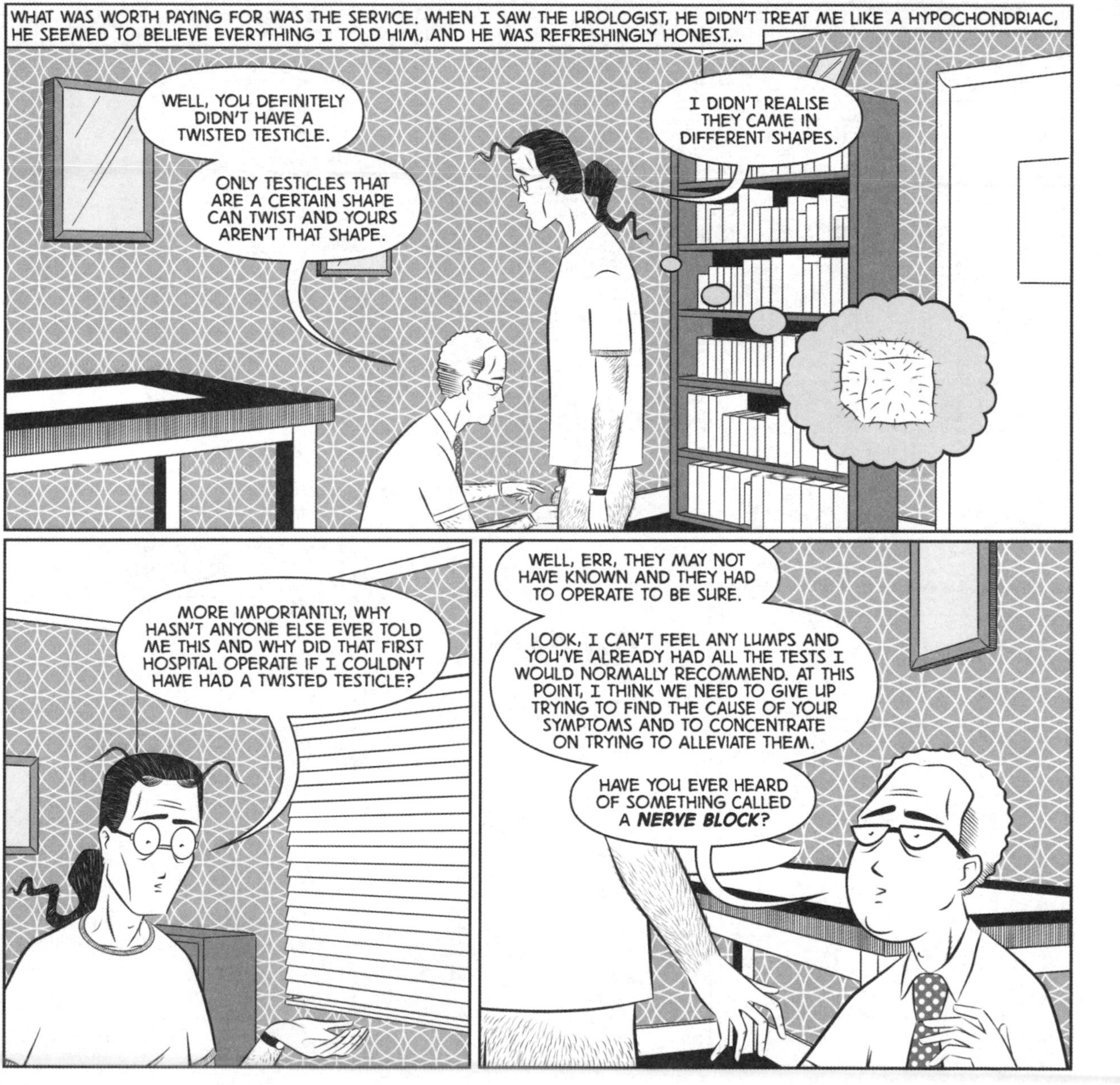
WHAT WAS WORTH PAYING FOR WAS THE SERVICE. WHEN I SAW THE UROLOGIST, HE DIDN'T TREAT ME LIKE A HYPOCHONDRIAC, HE SEEMED TO BELIEVE EVERYTHING I TOLD HIM, AND HE WAS REFRESHINGLY HONEST...
WELL, YOU DEFINITELY DIDN'T HAVE A TWISTED TESTICLE.
ONLY TESTICLES THAT ARE A CERTAIN SHAPE CAN TWIST AND YOURS AREN'T THAT SHAPE.
I DIDN'T REALISE THEY CAME IN DIFFERENT SHAPES.
MORE IMPORTANTLY, WHY HASN'T ANYONE ELSE EVER TOLD ME THIS AND WHY DID THAT FIRST HOSPITAL OPERATE IF I COULDN'T HAVE HAD A TWISTED TESTICLE?
WELL, ERR, THEY MAY NOT HAVE KNOWN AND THEY HAD TO OPERATE TO BE SURE.
LOOK, I CAN'T FEEL ANY LUMPS AND YOU'VE ALREADY HAD ALL THE TESTS I WOULD NORMALLY RECOMMEND. AT THIS POINT, I THINK WE NEED TO GIVE UP TRYING TO FIND THE CAUSE OF YOUR SYMPTOMS AND TO CONCENTRATE ON TRYING TO ALLEVIATE THEM.
HAVE YOU EVER HEARD OF SOMETHING CALLED A ***NERVE BLOCK***?

A 'NERVE BLOCK' IS AN INJECTION OF STEROIDS THAT IS USED TO BLOCK PAIN SIGNALS IN PATIENTS SUFFERING FROM CHRONIC PAIN. IF SUCCESSFUL, IT CAN ALLEVIATE PAIN FOR A PERIOD OF MONTHS, YEARS, OR EVEN PERMANENTLY.

A FEW DAYS AFTER MY INITIAL APPOINTMENT, I WAS BACK AT THE PRIVATE HOSPITAL, WHERE I PAID £250 FOR NERVE BLOCK INJECTIONS IN MY GROIN.

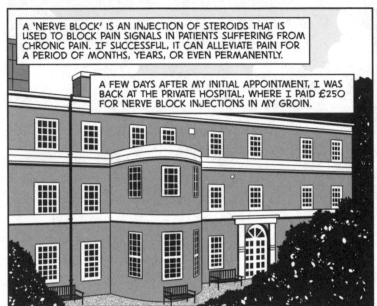

AS SOON AS I ARRIVED AT THE HOSPITAL, I WAS SHOWN TO A PRIVATE ROOM, AND SHORTLY AFTER THAT, THE UROLOGIST CAME IN HOLDING A RATHER LARGE SYRINGE.

GULP!

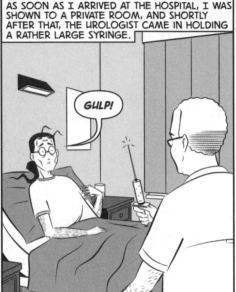

HE ASKED ME TO TAKE OFF MY UNDER-WEAR, PULLED MY TESTICLES TO ONE SIDE, AND PLUNGED THE NEEDLE DEEP INTO THE SIDE OF MY GROIN.

AAAHH...

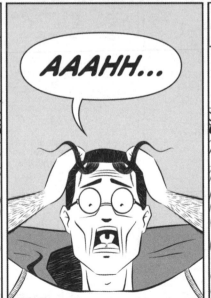

THEN HE PULLED MY TESTICLES THE OTHER WAY AND PLUNGED THE NEEDLE DEEP INTO THE OTHER SIDE OF MY GROIN.

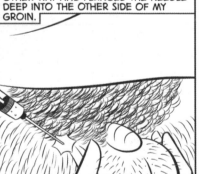

THE PROCEDURE WAS OVER AND DONE WITH VERY QUICKLY, BUT I THEN HAD TO SPEND THE REST OF THE MORNING IN HOSPITAL, IN CASE THERE WERE ANY UNPLEASANT SIDE-EFFECTS. I HAD A NICE ROOM WITH A TELEVISION AND AN EN-SUITE BATHROOM...

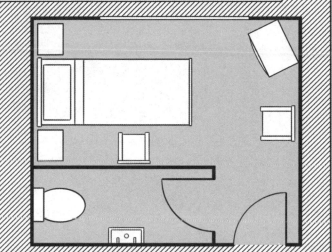

WHICH WAS JUST AS WELL, BECAUSE NOT LONG AFTER I'D HAD THE INJECTIONS:

BLOODY HELL! I REALLY NEED A WEE!

THANKS FOR LETTING ME KNOW.

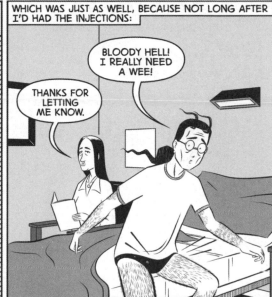

TEN MINUTES LATER...

BLIMEY. THREE WEES IN TEN MINUTES!

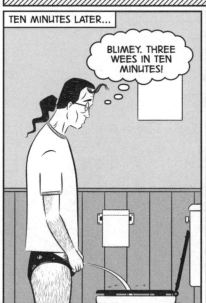

ANOTHER TEN MINUTES LATER...

I'M BURSTING AGAIN ALREADY!

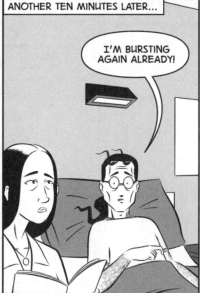

YET ANOTHER TEN MINUTES LATER...

SIX WEES IN A ROW AND THE FLOW'S STILL GAINING POWER!

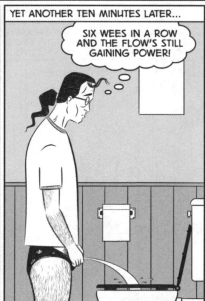

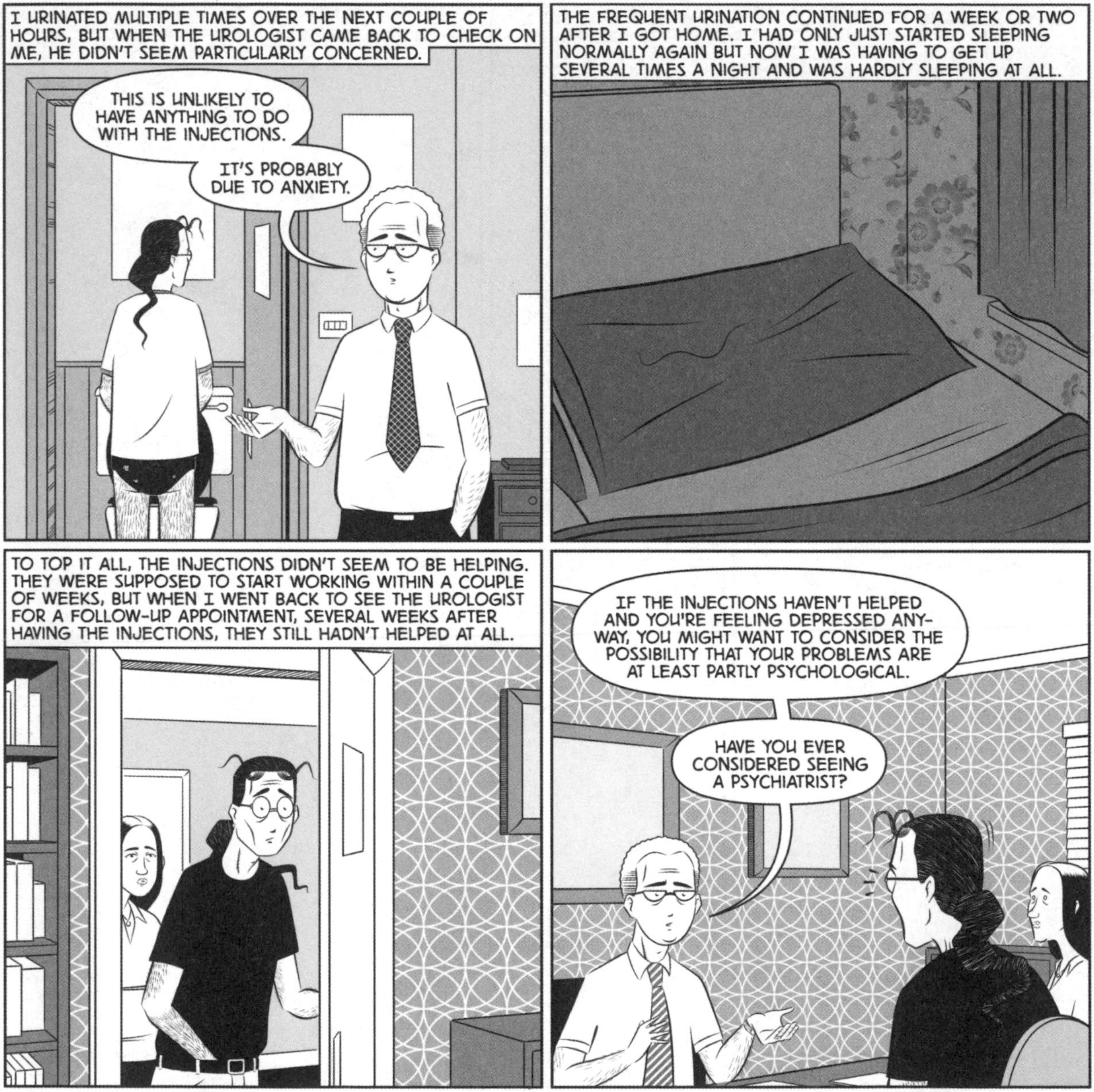
I URINATED MULTIPLE TIMES OVER THE NEXT COUPLE OF HOURS, BUT WHEN THE UROLOGIST CAME BACK TO CHECK ON ME, HE DIDN'T SEEM PARTICULARLY CONCERNED.
THIS IS UNLIKELY TO HAVE ANYTHING TO DO WITH THE INJECTIONS.
IT'S PROBABLY DUE TO ANXIETY.
THE FREQUENT URINATION CONTINUED FOR A WEEK OR TWO AFTER I GOT HOME. I HAD ONLY JUST STARTED SLEEPING NORMALLY AGAIN BUT NOW I WAS HAVING TO GET UP SEVERAL TIMES A NIGHT AND WAS HARDLY SLEEPING AT ALL.
TO TOP IT ALL, THE INJECTIONS DIDN'T SEEM TO BE HELPING. THEY WERE SUPPOSED TO START WORKING WITHIN A COUPLE OF WEEKS, BUT WHEN I WENT BACK TO SEE THE UROLOGIST FOR A FOLLOW-UP APPOINTMENT, SEVERAL WEEKS AFTER HAVING THE INJECTIONS, THEY STILL HADN'T HELPED AT ALL.
IF THE INJECTIONS HAVEN'T HELPED AND YOU'RE FEELING DEPRESSED ANY-WAY, YOU MIGHT WANT TO CONSIDER THE POSSIBILITY THAT YOUR PROBLEMS ARE AT LEAST PARTLY PSYCHOLOGICAL.
HAVE YOU EVER CONSIDERED SEEING A PSYCHIATRIST?

I DIDN'T BOTHER SEEING A PSYCHIATRIST. IN FACT, NOT FOR THE FIRST TIME, I DECIDED TO STOP SEEING DOCTORS ALTOGETHER.

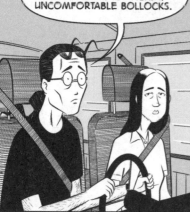

OH WELL. I GUESS THAT'S IT FOR ME. I'M DOOMED TO A LIFETIME OF ACHEY, UNCOMFORTABLE BOLLOCKS.

I'D EXHAUSTED MOST OF THE OPTIONS AVAILABLE TO ME AND I WAS SO SICK OF WAITING FOR HOSPITAL APPOINTMENTS THAT I FIGURED I'D BE HAPPIER IF I JUST ACCEPTED THE FACT THAT I WAS ILL FOR A WHILE.

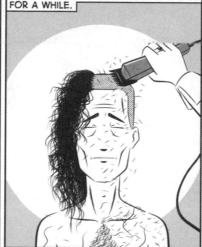

I STILL SPENT SOME TIME RESEARCHING HEALTH PROBLEMS ONLINE AND STILL BOUGHT THE ODD SELF-HELP BOOK, BUT MOSTLY I JUST THREW MYSELF INTO MY NEW MAIL ORDER BUSINESS AND TRIED NOT TO THINK ABOUT MY PREDICAMENT TOO MUCH.

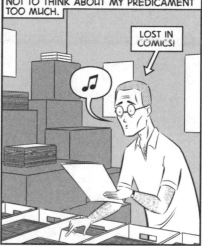

LOST IN COMICS!

BUT IN THE MONTHS AFTER I'D HAD THOSE INJECTIONS, THE PAIN AND DISCOMFORT IN MY GROIN DID SLOWLY, UNEXPECTEDLY, BEGIN TO EASE OFF.

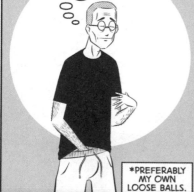

THERE IS NOTHING MORE SATISFYING THAN JUGGLING A PAIR OF LOOSE BALLS.*

*PREFERABLY MY OWN LOOSE BALLS.

BEFORE, I FELT TERRIBLE MOST OF THE TIME AND WAS LUCKY IF I HAD ONE OR TWO DAYS A WEEK WHERE I DIDN'T FEEL TOO BAD.

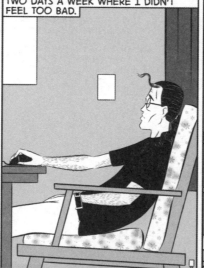

NOW, I WAS HAVING ONE OR TWO BAD DAYS A WEEK AT MOST AND THE REST OF THE TIME I EITHER FELT OKAY OR JUST MILDLY UNCOMFORTABLE.

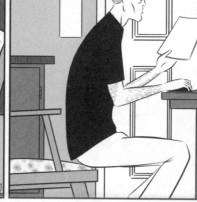

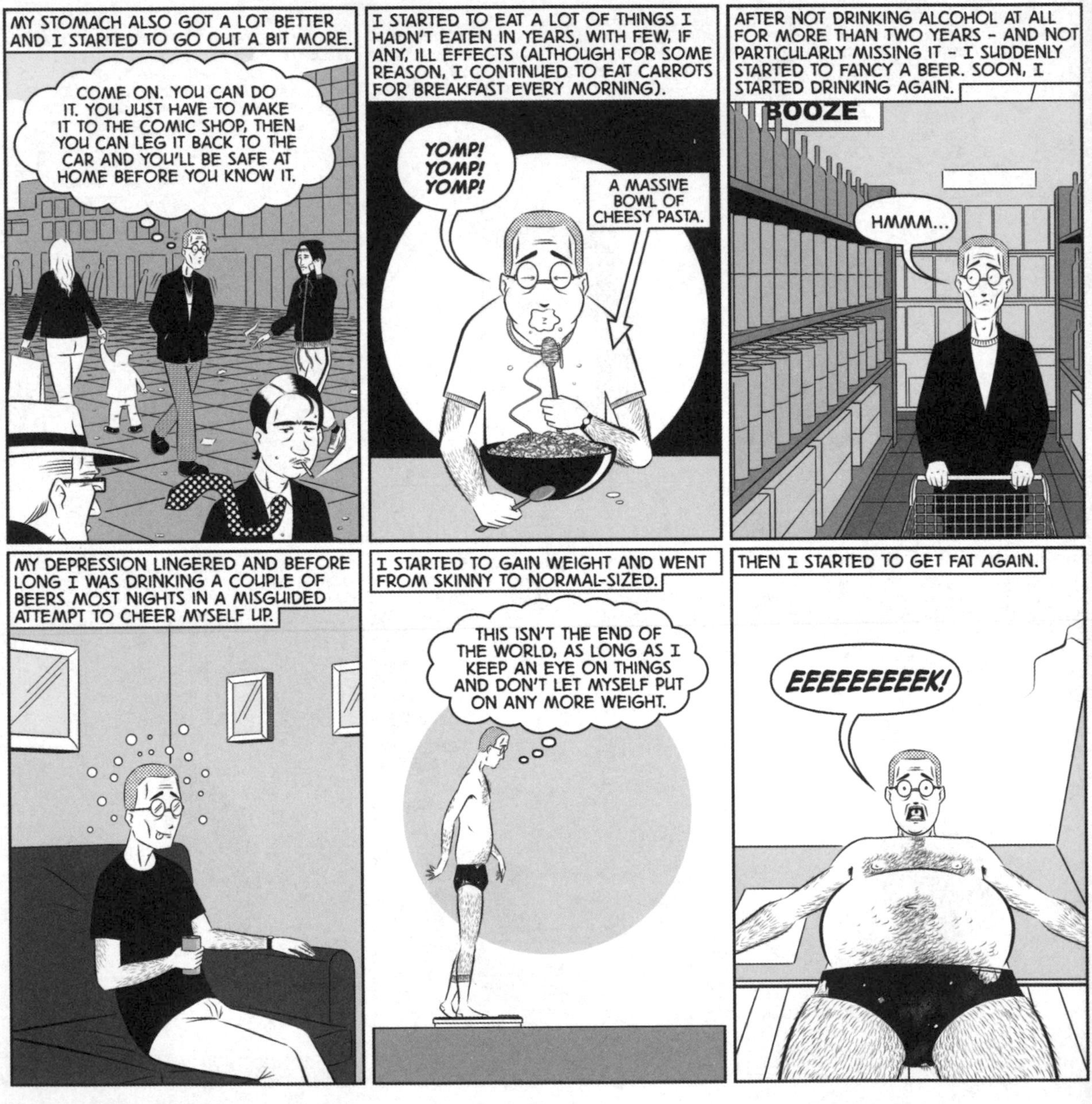
MY STOMACH ALSO GOT A LOT BETTER AND I STARTED TO GO OUT A BIT MORE.
COME ON. YOU CAN DO IT. YOU JUST HAVE TO MAKE IT TO THE COMIC SHOP, THEN YOU CAN LEG IT BACK TO THE CAR AND YOU'LL BE SAFE AT HOME BEFORE YOU KNOW IT.
I STARTED TO EAT A LOT OF THINGS I HADN'T EATEN IN YEARS, WITH FEW, IF ANY, ILL EFFECTS (ALTHOUGH FOR SOME REASON, I CONTINUED TO EAT CARROTS FOR BREAKFAST EVERY MORNING).
YOMP! YOMP! YOMP!
A MASSIVE BOWL OF CHEESY PASTA.
AFTER NOT DRINKING ALCOHOL AT ALL FOR MORE THAN TWO YEARS - AND NOT PARTICULARLY MISSING IT - I SUDDENLY STARTED TO FANCY A BEER. SOON, I STARTED DRINKING AGAIN.
BOOZE
HMMM...
MY DEPRESSION LINGERED AND BEFORE LONG I WAS DRINKING A COUPLE OF BEERS MOST NIGHTS IN A MISGUIDED ATTEMPT TO CHEER MYSELF UP.
I STARTED TO GAIN WEIGHT AND WENT FROM SKINNY TO NORMAL-SIZED.
THIS ISN'T THE END OF THE WORLD, AS LONG AS I KEEP AN EYE ON THINGS AND DON'T LET MYSELF PUT ON ANY MORE WEIGHT.
THEN I STARTED TO GET FAT AGAIN.
EEEEEEEEEK!

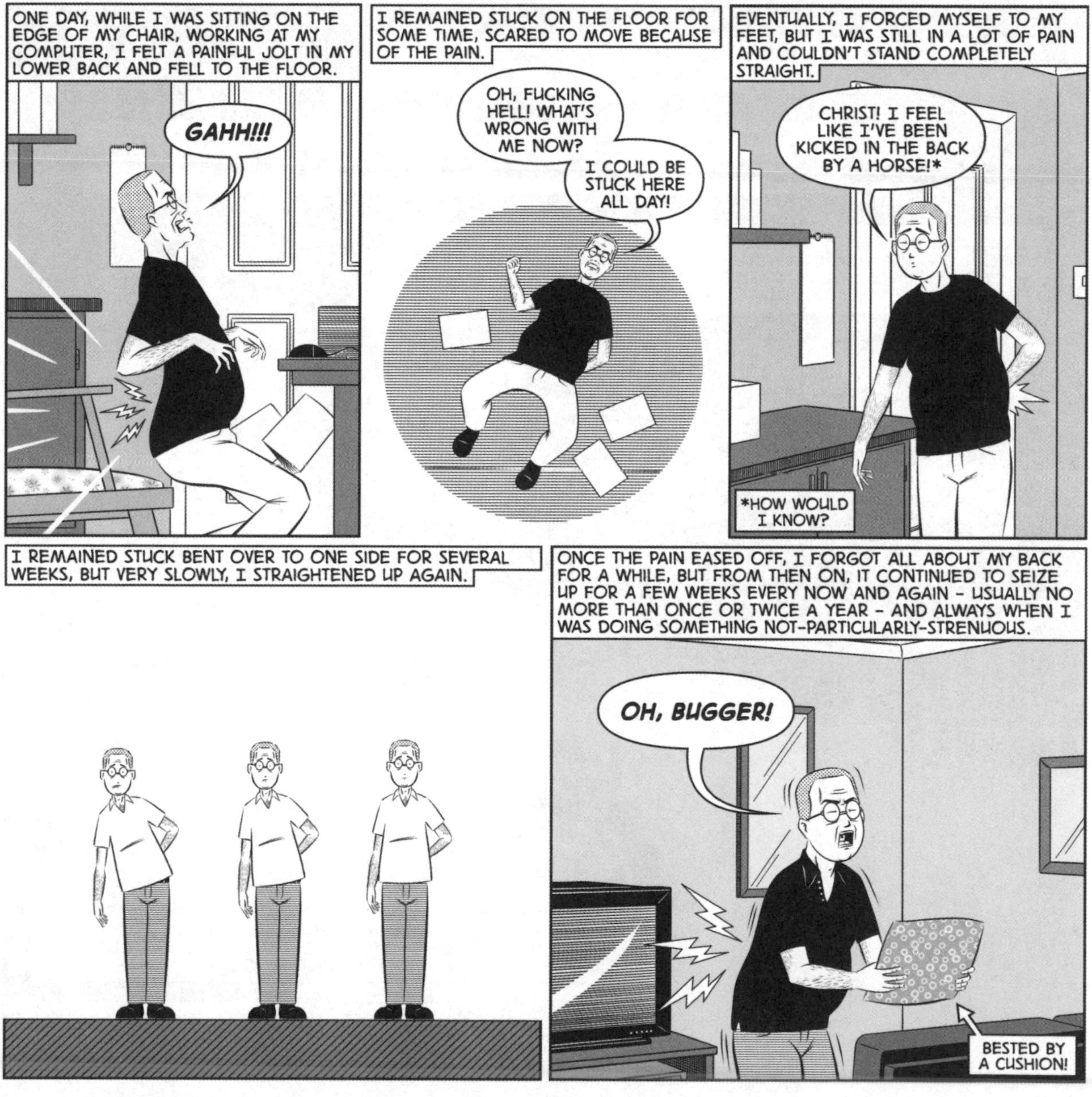
ONE DAY, WHILE I WAS SITTING ON THE EDGE OF MY CHAIR, WORKING AT MY COMPUTER, I FELT A PAINFUL JOLT IN MY LOWER BACK AND FELL TO THE FLOOR.
GAHH!!!
I REMAINED STUCK ON THE FLOOR FOR SOME TIME, SCARED TO MOVE BECAUSE OF THE PAIN.
OH, FUCKING HELL! WHAT'S WRONG WITH ME NOW?
I COULD BE STUCK HERE ALL DAY!
EVENTUALLY, I FORCED MYSELF TO MY FEET, BUT I WAS STILL IN A LOT OF PAIN AND COULDN'T STAND COMPLETELY STRAIGHT.
CHRIST! I FEEL LIKE I'VE BEEN KICKED IN THE BACK BY A HORSE!*
*HOW WOULD I KNOW?
I REMAINED STUCK BENT OVER TO ONE SIDE FOR SEVERAL WEEKS, BUT VERY SLOWLY, I STRAIGHTENED UP AGAIN.
ONCE THE PAIN EASED OFF, I FORGOT ALL ABOUT MY BACK FOR A WHILE, BUT FROM THEN ON, IT CONTINUED TO SEIZE UP FOR A FEW WEEKS EVERY NOW AND AGAIN - USUALLY NO MORE THAN ONCE OR TWICE A YEAR - AND ALWAYS WHEN I WAS DOING SOMETHING NOT-PARTICULARLY-STRENUOUS.
OH, BUGGER!
BESTED BY A CUSHION!

9. THE BRIDGES OF MAIDSTONE COUNTY

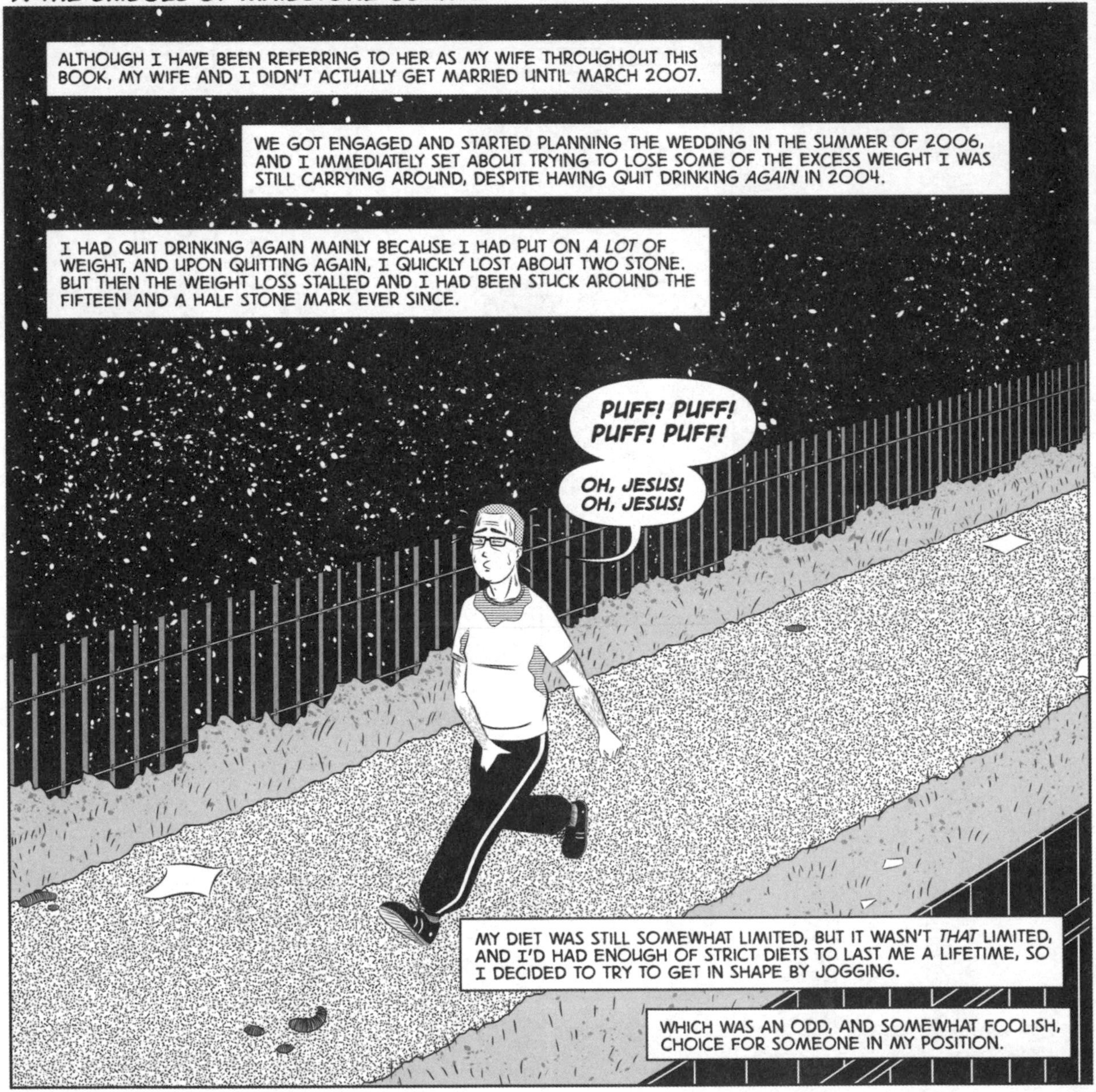
ALTHOUGH I HAVE BEEN REFERRING TO HER AS MY WIFE THROUGHOUT THIS BOOK, MY WIFE AND I DIDN'T ACTUALLY GET MARRIED UNTIL MARCH 2007.
WE GOT ENGAGED AND STARTED PLANNING THE WEDDING IN THE SUMMER OF 2006, AND I IMMEDIATELY SET ABOUT TRYING TO LOSE SOME OF THE EXCESS WEIGHT I WAS STILL CARRYING AROUND, DESPITE HAVING QUIT DRINKING *AGAIN* IN 2004.
I HAD QUIT DRINKING AGAIN MAINLY BECAUSE I HAD PUT ON *A LOT* OF WEIGHT, AND UPON QUITTING AGAIN, I QUICKLY LOST ABOUT TWO STONE. BUT THEN THE WEIGHT LOSS STALLED AND I HAD BEEN STUCK AROUND THE FIFTEEN AND A HALF STONE MARK EVER SINCE.
PUFF! PUFF! PUFF! PUFF!
OH, JESUS! OH, JESUS!
MY DIET WAS STILL SOMEWHAT LIMITED, BUT IT WASN'T *THAT* LIMITED, AND I'D HAD ENOUGH OF STRICT DIETS TO LAST ME A LIFETIME, SO I DECIDED TO TRY TO GET IN SHAPE BY JOGGING.
WHICH WAS AN ODD, AND SOMEWHAT FOOLISH, CHOICE FOR SOMEONE IN MY POSITION.

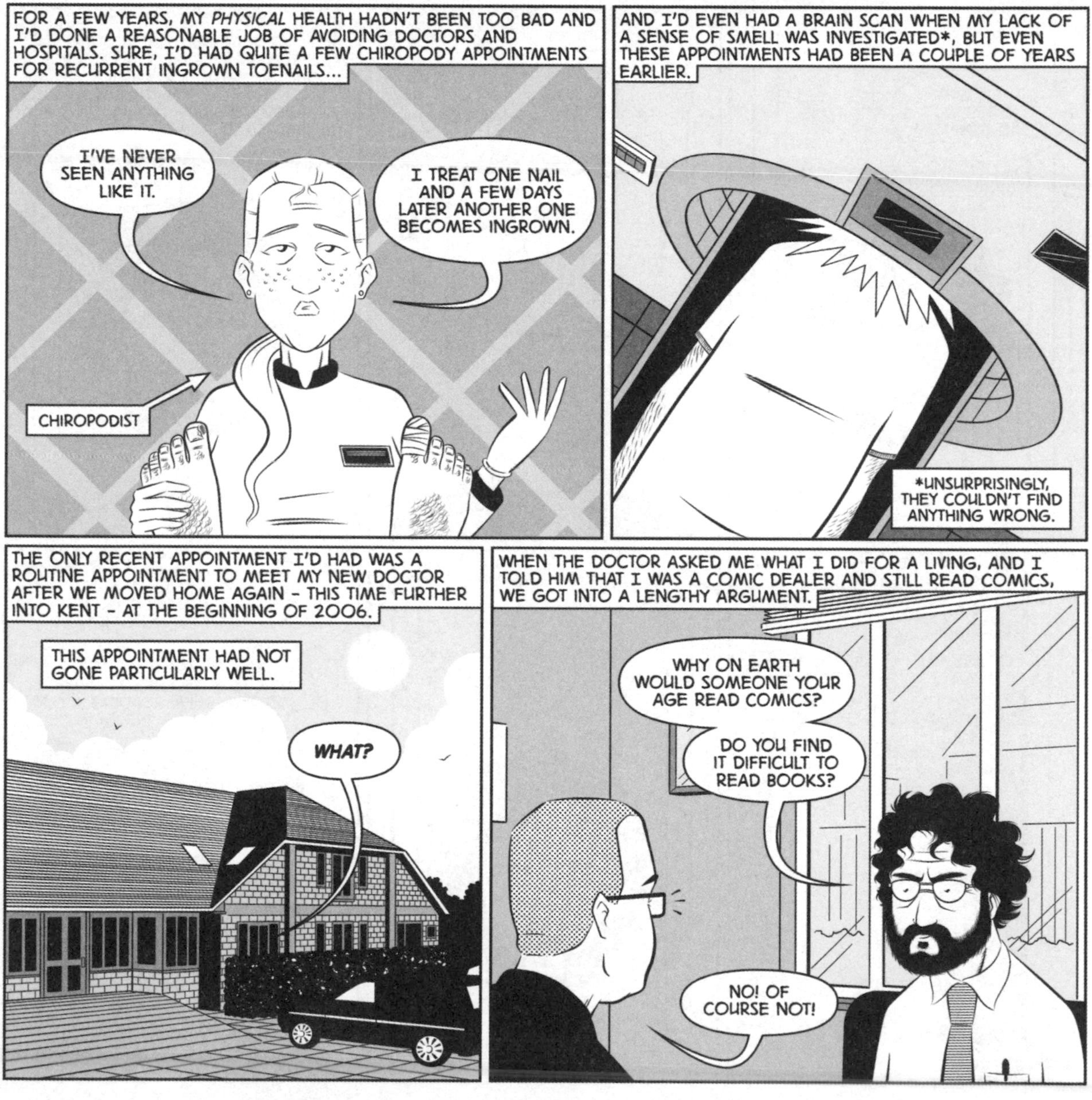
FOR A FEW YEARS, MY *PHYSICAL* HEALTH HADN'T BEEN TOO BAD AND I'D DONE A REASONABLE JOB OF AVOIDING DOCTORS AND HOSPITALS. SURE, I'D HAD QUITE A FEW CHIROPODY APPOINTMENTS FOR RECURRENT INGROWN TOENAILS...
I'VE NEVER SEEN ANYTHING LIKE IT.
I TREAT ONE NAIL AND A FEW DAYS LATER ANOTHER ONE BECOMES INGROWN.
CHIROPODIST
AND I'D EVEN HAD A BRAIN SCAN WHEN MY LACK OF A SENSE OF SMELL WAS INVESTIGATED*, BUT EVEN THESE APPOINTMENTS HAD BEEN A COUPLE OF YEARS EARLIER.
*UNSURPRISINGLY, THEY COULDN'T FIND ANYTHING WRONG.
THE ONLY RECENT APPOINTMENT I'D HAD WAS A ROUTINE APPOINTMENT TO MEET MY NEW DOCTOR AFTER WE MOVED HOME AGAIN - THIS TIME FURTHER INTO KENT - AT THE BEGINNING OF 2006.
THIS APPOINTMENT HAD NOT GONE PARTICULARLY WELL.
WHAT?
WHEN THE DOCTOR ASKED ME WHAT I DID FOR A LIVING, AND I TOLD HIM THAT I WAS A COMIC DEALER AND STILL READ COMICS, WE GOT INTO A LENGTHY ARGUMENT.
WHY ON EARTH WOULD SOMEONE YOUR AGE READ COMICS?
DO YOU FIND IT DIFFICULT TO READ BOOKS?
NO! OF COURSE NOT!

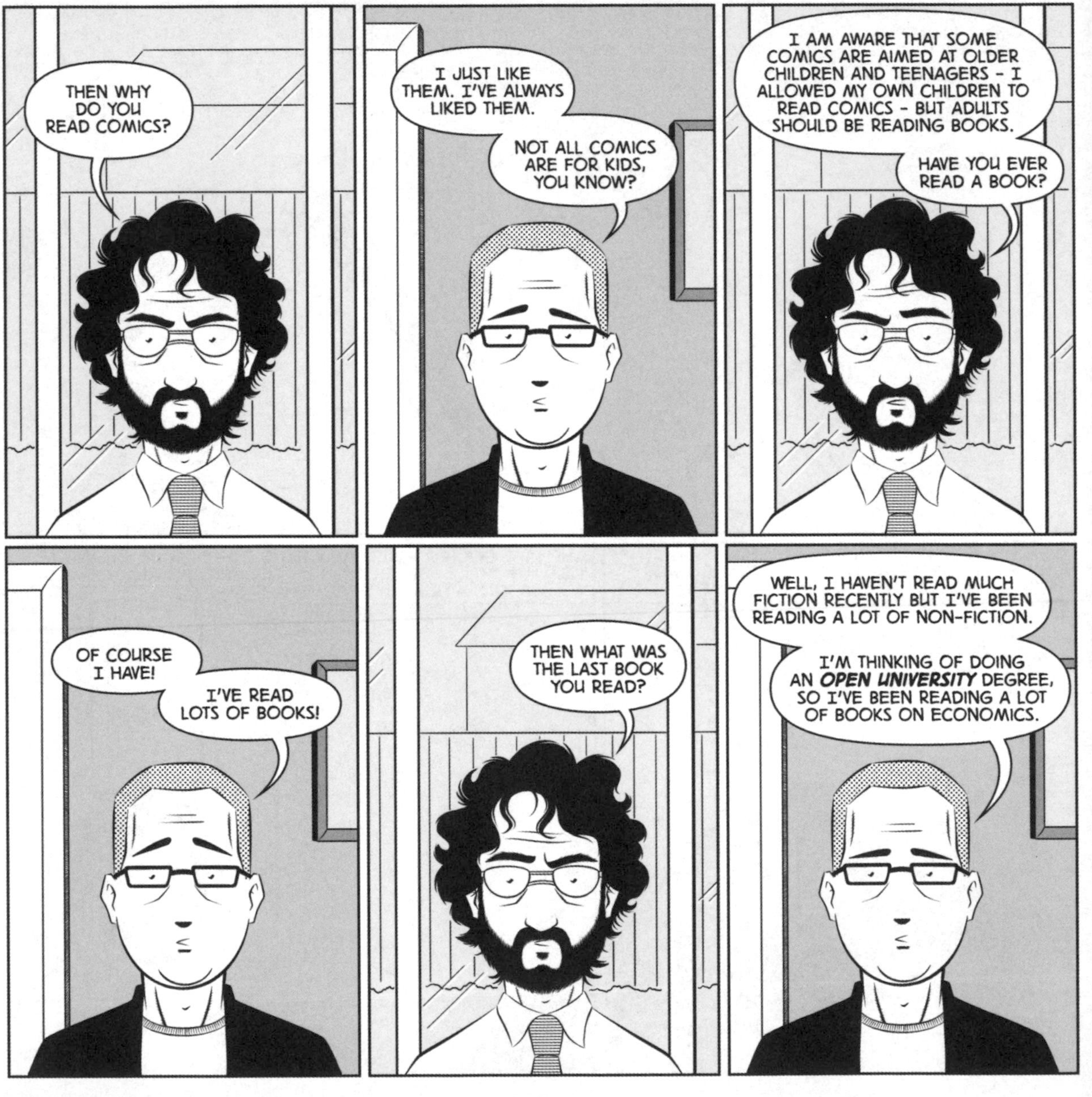
THEN WHY DO YOU READ COMICS?
I JUST LIKE THEM. I'VE ALWAYS LIKED THEM.
NOT ALL COMICS ARE FOR KIDS, YOU KNOW?
I AM AWARE THAT SOME COMICS ARE AIMED AT OLDER CHILDREN AND TEENAGERS - I ALLOWED MY OWN CHILDREN TO READ COMICS - BUT ADULTS SHOULD BE READING BOOKS.
HAVE YOU EVER READ A BOOK?
OF COURSE I HAVE!
I'VE READ LOTS OF BOOKS!
THEN WHAT WAS THE LAST BOOK YOU READ?
WELL, I HAVEN'T READ MUCH FICTION RECENTLY BUT I'VE BEEN READING A LOT OF NON-FICTION.
I'M THINKING OF DOING AN ***OPEN UNIVERSITY*** DEGREE, SO I'VE BEEN READING A LOT OF BOOKS ON ECONOMICS.

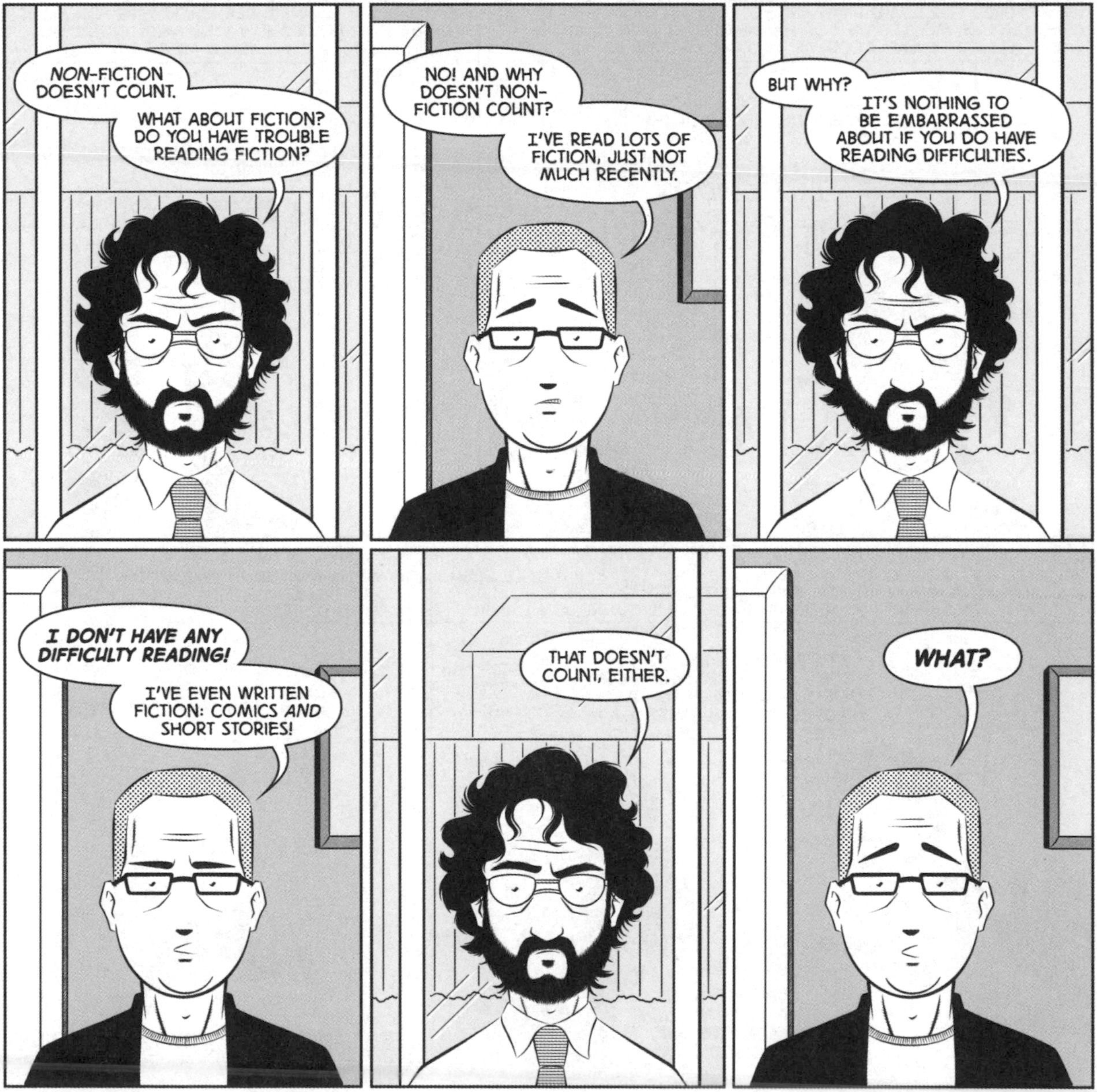
NON-FICTION DOESN'T COUNT.
WHAT ABOUT FICTION? DO YOU HAVE TROUBLE READING FICTION?
NO! AND WHY DOESN'T NON-FICTION COUNT?
I'VE READ LOTS OF FICTION, JUST NOT MUCH RECENTLY.
BUT WHY?
IT'S NOTHING TO BE EMBARRASSED ABOUT IF YOU DO HAVE READING DIFFICULTIES.
I DON'T HAVE ANY DIFFICULTY READING!
I'VE EVEN WRITTEN FICTION: COMICS AND SHORT STORIES!
THAT DOESN'T COUNT, EITHER.
WHAT?

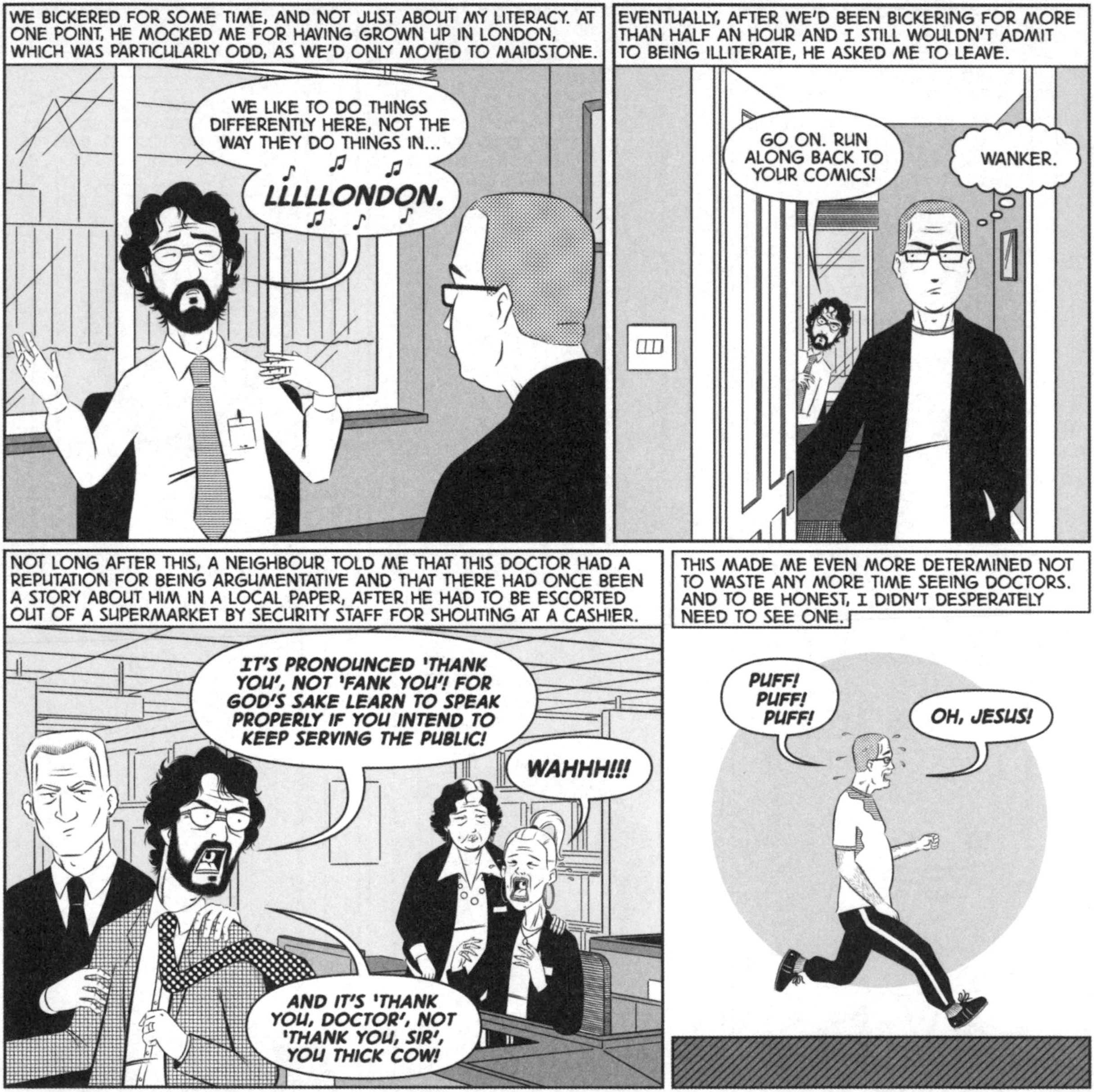
WE BICKERED FOR SOME TIME, AND NOT JUST ABOUT MY LITERACY. AT ONE POINT, HE MOCKED ME FOR HAVING GROWN UP IN LONDON, WHICH WAS PARTICULARLY ODD, AS WE'D ONLY MOVED TO MAIDSTONE.
WE LIKE TO DO THINGS DIFFERENTLY HERE, NOT THE WAY THEY DO THINGS IN...
LLLLLONDON.
EVENTUALLY, AFTER WE'D BEEN BICKERING FOR MORE THAN HALF AN HOUR AND I STILL WOULDN'T ADMIT TO BEING ILLITERATE, HE ASKED ME TO LEAVE.
GO ON. RUN ALONG BACK TO YOUR COMICS!
WANKER.
NOT LONG AFTER THIS, A NEIGHBOUR TOLD ME THAT THIS DOCTOR HAD A REPUTATION FOR BEING ARGUMENTATIVE AND THAT THERE HAD ONCE BEEN A STORY ABOUT HIM IN A LOCAL PAPER, AFTER HE HAD TO BE ESCORTED OUT OF A SUPERMARKET BY SECURITY STAFF FOR SHOUTING AT A CASHIER.
IT'S PRONOUNCED 'THANK YOU', NOT 'FANK YOU'! FOR GOD'S SAKE LEARN TO SPEAK PROPERLY IF YOU INTEND TO KEEP SERVING THE PUBLIC!
WAHHH!!!
AND IT'S 'THANK YOU, DOCTOR', NOT 'THANK YOU, SIR', YOU THICK COW!
THIS MADE ME EVEN MORE DETERMINED NOT TO WASTE ANY MORE TIME SEEING DOCTORS. AND TO BE HONEST, I DIDN'T DESPERATELY NEED TO SEE ONE.
PUFF! PUFF! PUFF!
OH, JESUS!

ALTHOUGH MY GROIN WAS STILL QUITE UNCOMFORTABLE A LOT OF THE TIME, IT WAS NOWHERE NEAR AS BAD AS IT HAD BEEN A FEW YEARS EARLIER.

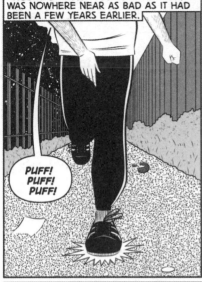

PUFF! PUFF! PUFF!

IN THE END, I THINK THOSE STEROID INJECTIONS HAD HELPED A LOT...

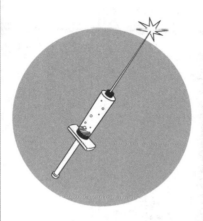

BUT I ALSO THINK I HAD BECOME USED TO THE DISCOMFORT, TO SOME DEGREE, AND HAD LEARNED TO MANAGE MY SYMPTOMS.

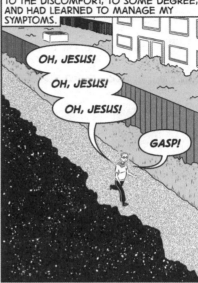

OH, JESUS!

OH, JESUS!

OH, JESUS!

GASP!

THE DISCOMFORT IN MY GROIN WOULD STILL FLARE UP BADLY EVERY NOW AND AGAIN, AND I WAS PROBABLY NEVER GOING TO BE ABLE TO RIDE A BIKE, AS I DISCOVERED WHEN MY IN-LAWS GAVE ME AN OLD MOUNTAIN BIKE TO TRY OUT...

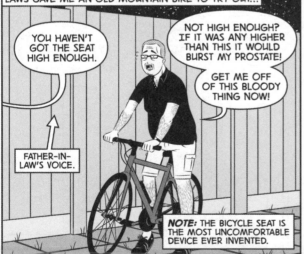

YOU HAVEN'T GOT THE SEAT HIGH ENOUGH.

NOT HIGH ENOUGH? IF IT WAS ANY HIGHER THAN THIS IT WOULD BURST MY PROSTATE!

GET ME OFF OF THIS BLOODY THING NOW!

FATHER-IN-LAW'S VOICE.

NOTE: THE BICYCLE SEAT IS THE MOST UNCOMFORTABLE DEVICE EVER INVENTED.

BUT MOST OF THE TIME, AS LONG AS I HAD A HOT BATH IN THE MORNING, I WASN'T TOO BAD.

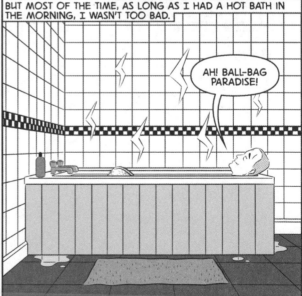

AH! BALL-BAG PARADISE!

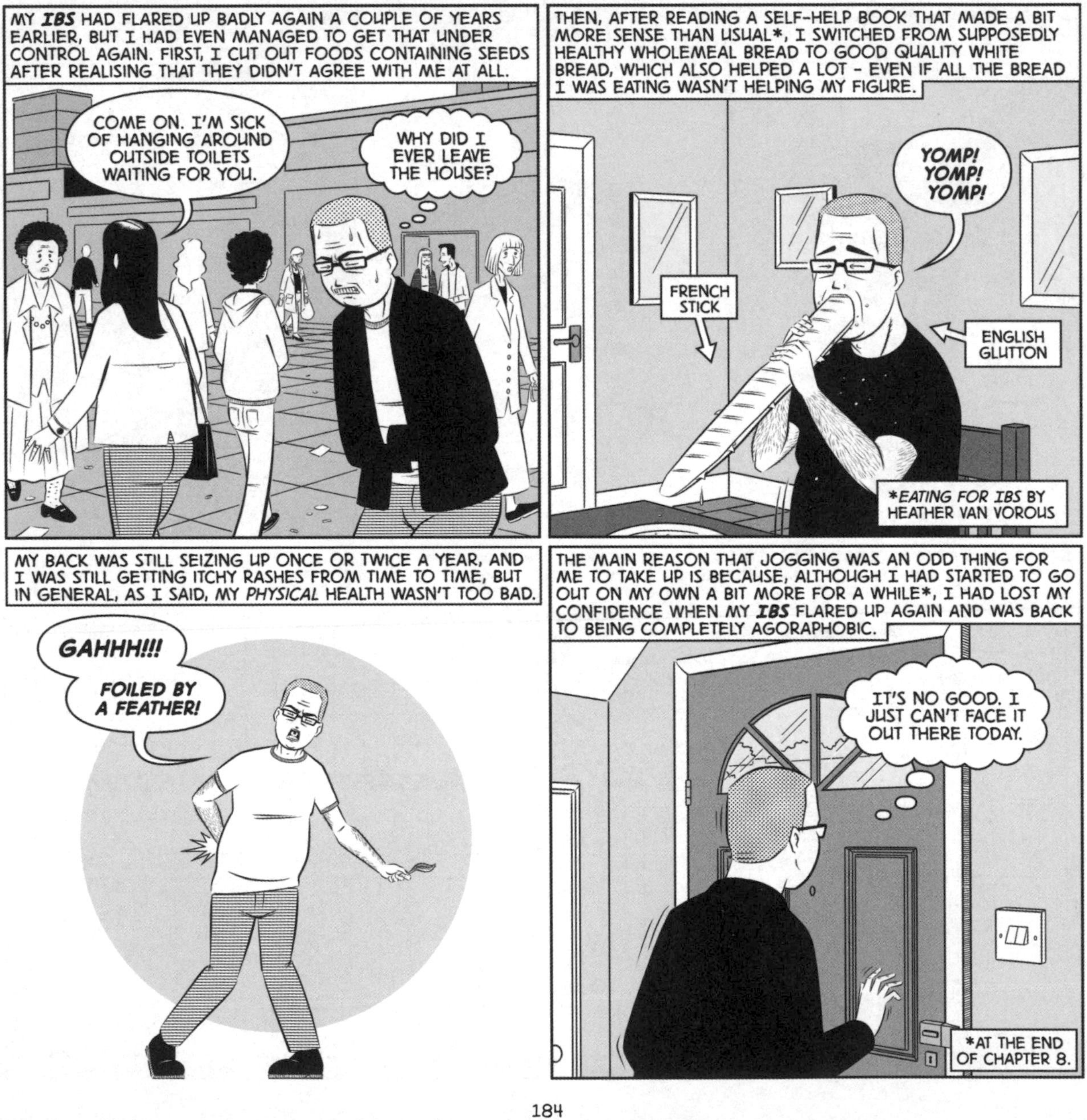
MY IBS HAD FLARED UP BADLY AGAIN A COUPLE OF YEARS EARLIER, BUT I HAD EVEN MANAGED TO GET THAT UNDER CONTROL AGAIN. FIRST, I CUT OUT FOODS CONTAINING SEEDS AFTER REALISING THAT THEY DIDN'T AGREE WITH ME AT ALL.
COME ON. I'M SICK OF HANGING AROUND OUTSIDE TOILETS WAITING FOR YOU.
WHY DID I EVER LEAVE THE HOUSE?
THEN, AFTER READING A SELF-HELP BOOK THAT MADE A BIT MORE SENSE THAN USUAL*, I SWITCHED FROM SUPPOSEDLY HEALTHY WHOLEMEAL BREAD TO GOOD QUALITY WHITE BREAD, WHICH ALSO HELPED A LOT - EVEN IF ALL THE BREAD I WAS EATING WASN'T HELPING MY FIGURE.
YOMP! YOMP! YOMP!
FRENCH STICK
ENGLISH GLUTTON
*EATING FOR IBS BY HEATHER VAN VOROUS
MY BACK WAS STILL SEIZING UP ONCE OR TWICE A YEAR, AND I WAS STILL GETTING ITCHY RASHES FROM TIME TO TIME, BUT IN GENERAL, AS I SAID, MY PHYSICAL HEALTH WASN'T TOO BAD.
GAHHH!!!
FOILED BY A FEATHER!
THE MAIN REASON THAT JOGGING WAS AN ODD THING FOR ME TO TAKE UP IS BECAUSE, ALTHOUGH I HAD STARTED TO GO OUT ON MY OWN A BIT MORE FOR A WHILE*, I HAD LOST MY CONFIDENCE WHEN MY IBS FLARED UP AGAIN AND WAS BACK TO BEING COMPLETELY AGORAPHOBIC.
IT'S NO GOOD. I JUST CAN'T FACE IT OUT THERE TODAY.
*AT THE END OF CHAPTER 8.

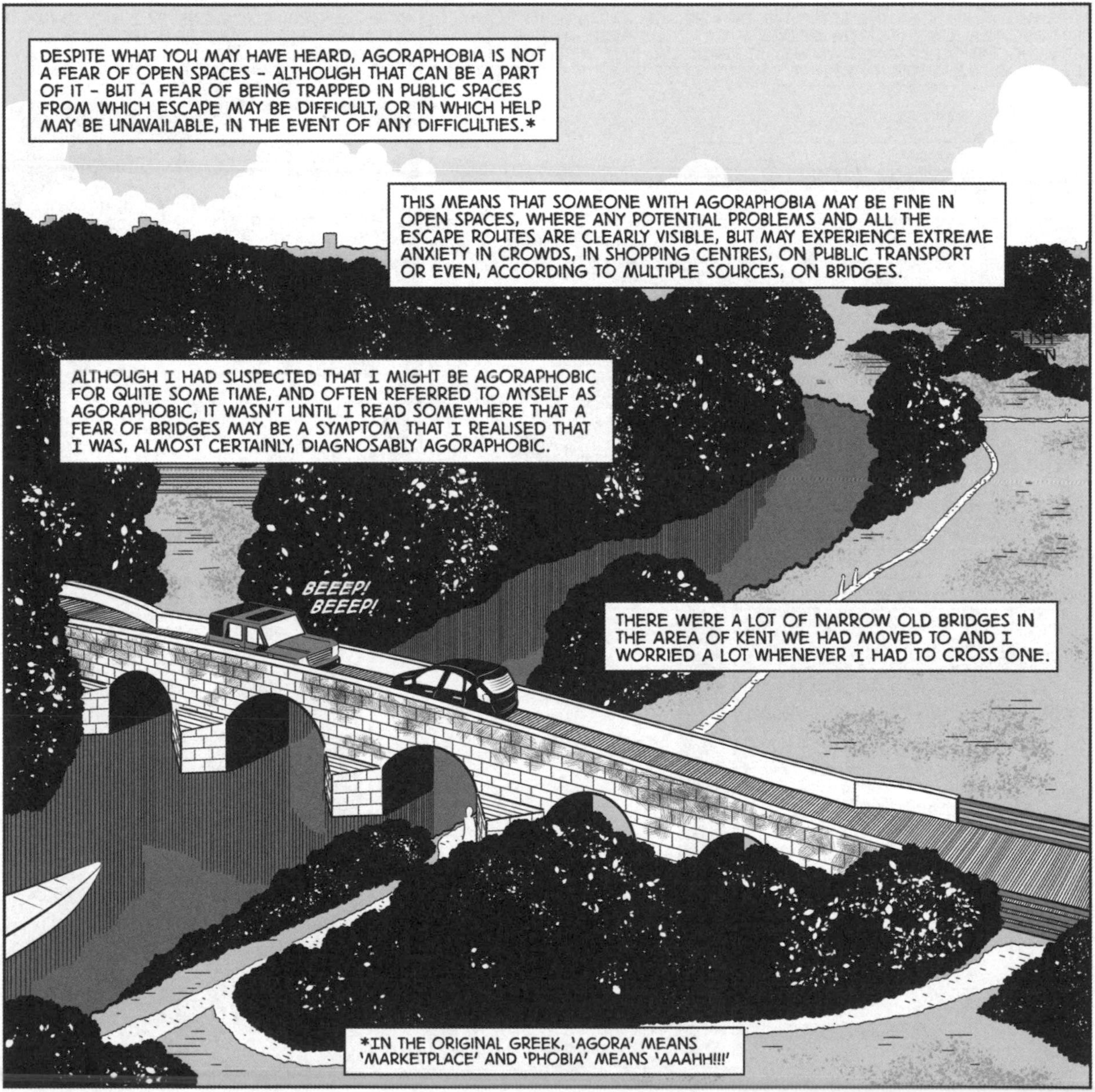

DESPITE WHAT YOU MAY HAVE HEARD, AGORAPHOBIA IS NOT A FEAR OF OPEN SPACES - ALTHOUGH THAT CAN BE A PART OF IT - BUT A FEAR OF BEING TRAPPED IN PUBLIC SPACES FROM WHICH ESCAPE MAY BE DIFFICULT, OR IN WHICH HELP MAY BE UNAVAILABLE, IN THE EVENT OF ANY DIFFICULTIES.*
THIS MEANS THAT SOMEONE WITH AGORAPHOBIA MAY BE FINE IN OPEN SPACES, WHERE ANY POTENTIAL PROBLEMS AND ALL THE ESCAPE ROUTES ARE CLEARLY VISIBLE, BUT MAY EXPERIENCE EXTREME ANXIETY IN CROWDS, IN SHOPPING CENTRES, ON PUBLIC TRANSPORT OR EVEN, ACCORDING TO MULTIPLE SOURCES, ON BRIDGES.
ALTHOUGH I HAD SUSPECTED THAT I MIGHT BE AGORAPHOBIC FOR QUITE SOME TIME, AND OFTEN REFERRED TO MYSELF AS AGORAPHOBIC, IT WASN'T UNTIL I READ SOMEWHERE THAT A FEAR OF BRIDGES MAY BE A SYMPTOM THAT I REALISED THAT I WAS, ALMOST CERTAINLY, DIAGNOSABLY AGORAPHOBIC.
BEEEP! BEEEP!
THERE WERE A LOT OF NARROW OLD BRIDGES IN THE AREA OF KENT WE HAD MOVED TO AND I WORRIED A LOT WHENEVER I HAD TO CROSS ONE.
*IN THE ORIGINAL GREEK, 'AGORA' MEANS 'MARKETPLACE' AND 'PHOBIA' MEANS 'AAAHH!!!'

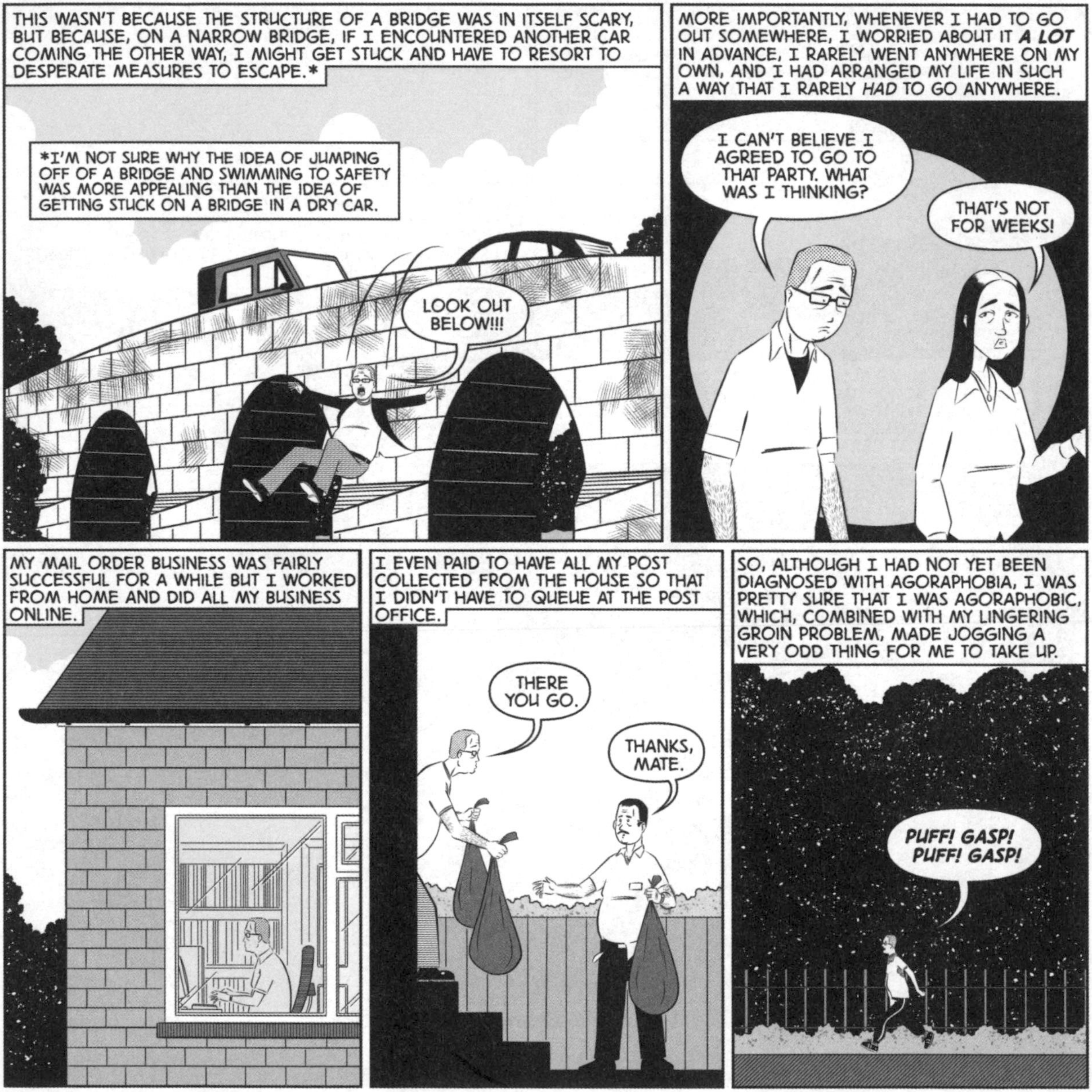
THIS WASN'T BECAUSE THE STRUCTURE OF A BRIDGE WAS IN ITSELF SCARY, BUT BECAUSE, ON A NARROW BRIDGE, IF I ENCOUNTERED ANOTHER CAR COMING THE OTHER WAY, I MIGHT GET STUCK AND HAVE TO RESORT TO DESPERATE MEASURES TO ESCAPE.*
*I'M NOT SURE WHY THE IDEA OF JUMPING OFF OF A BRIDGE AND SWIMMING TO SAFETY WAS MORE APPEALING THAN THE IDEA OF GETTING STUCK ON A BRIDGE IN A DRY CAR.
LOOK OUT BELOW!!!
MORE IMPORTANTLY, WHENEVER I HAD TO GO OUT SOMEWHERE, I WORRIED ABOUT IT ***A LOT*** IN ADVANCE, I RARELY WENT ANYWHERE ON MY OWN, AND I HAD ARRANGED MY LIFE IN SUCH A WAY THAT I RARELY *HAD* TO GO ANYWHERE.
I CAN'T BELIEVE I AGREED TO GO TO THAT PARTY. WHAT WAS I THINKING?
THAT'S NOT FOR WEEKS!
MY MAIL ORDER BUSINESS WAS FAIRLY SUCCESSFUL FOR A WHILE BUT I WORKED FROM HOME AND DID ALL MY BUSINESS ONLINE.
I EVEN PAID TO HAVE ALL MY POST COLLECTED FROM THE HOUSE SO THAT I DIDN'T HAVE TO QUEUE AT THE POST OFFICE.
THERE YOU GO.
THANKS, MATE.
SO, ALTHOUGH I HAD NOT YET BEEN DIAGNOSED WITH AGORAPHOBIA, I WAS PRETTY SURE THAT I WAS AGORAPHOBIC, WHICH, COMBINED WITH MY LINGERING GROIN PROBLEM, MADE JOGGING A VERY ODD THING FOR ME TO TAKE UP.
PUFF! GASP! PUFF! GASP!

PERHAPS I AM EXAGGERATING SLIGHTLY BY REFERRING TO WHAT I WAS DOING AS JOGGING, AS I WAS REALLY ONLY GOING FOR VERY SHORT RUNS, AND I WOULD STOP FREQUENTLY TO CATCH MY BREATH AND TO MAKE SURE MY BALLS WERE STILL WHERE THEY SHOULD BE.

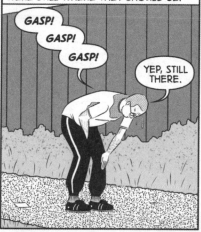

GASP!

GASP!

GASP!

YEP, STILL THERE.

I WOULD BASICALLY RUN UP A NARROW TRACK THAT WAS VERY CLOSE TO OUR HOUSE, AND WHEN I STARTED TO LOSE SIGHT OF THE HOUSE, I WOULD TURN AROUND AND RUN BACK HOME.

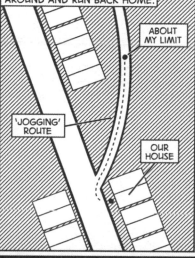

ABOUT MY LIMIT

'JOGGING' ROUTE

OUR HOUSE

I WOULD ALSO TURN AROUND AND RUN HOME IF I SAW ANY PEOPLE COMING MY WAY, BECAUSE I DIDN'T WANT ANY OF MY NEIGHBOURS TO WITNESS ME HAVING A PANIC ATTACK.*

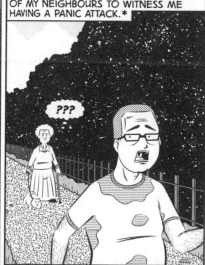

???

*THE SYMPTOMS OF A PANIC ATTACK (FOR ME) INCLUDE...

A RAPID HEARTBEAT AND FEELING LIKE I MIGHT LOSE CONTROL OF MY BODILY FUNCTIONS - PARTICULARLY MY BOWELS AND BLADDER.

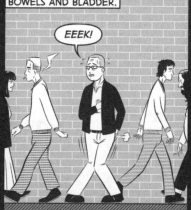

EEEK!

TUNNEL VISION: LITERALLY FEELING AS THOUGH I AM LOOKING AT THINGS THROUGH A TUNNEL, WHICH ONLY ADDS TO THE SENSE THAT I AM NO LONGER IN CONTROL OF MY BODY.

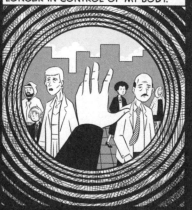

AND BLIND PANIC: AN ALMOST OVER-WHELMING DESIRE TO RUN AWAY, OR JUST CURL UP IN A BALL AND SCREAM.

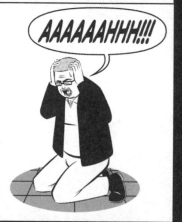

AAAAAAHHH!!!

I CARRIED ON 'JOGGING' LIKE THIS, SEVERAL TIMES A WEEK, FOR AT LEAST A COUPLE OF MONTHS.

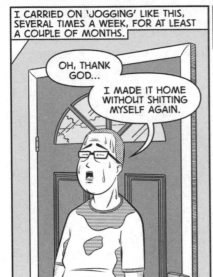

OH, THANK GOD...

I MADE IT HOME WITHOUT SHITTING MYSELF AGAIN.

MY BACK BECAME VERY PAINFUL DURING THIS PERIOD AND SOON HURT MOST OF THE TIME - APART FROM WHEN I WAS ACTUALLY JOGGING, FOR SOME REASON.

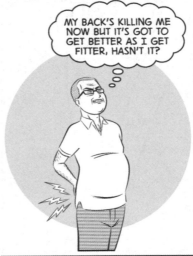

MY BACK'S KILLING ME NOW BUT IT'S GOT TO GET BETTER AS I GET FITTER, HASN'T IT?

CONVERSELY, MY GROIN WOULD GET VERY TIGHT AND UNCOMFORTABLE WHILE I WAS JOGGING BUT WOULD ALWAYS EASE OFF AGAIN DURING A POST-JOG BATH.

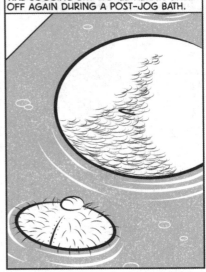

EXCEPT, OF COURSE, FOR THE TIME THAT IT DIDN'T.

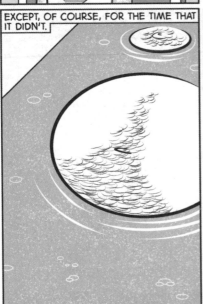

THE LAST TIME I WENT FOR A RUN, I PUSHED MYSELF HARDER THAN USUAL, AND MANAGED TO RUN ALL THE WAY UP THE TRACK AND BACK AGAIN WITHOUT STOPPING ONCE.

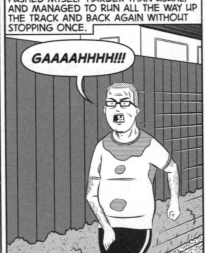

GAAAAHHHH!!!

MY GROIN GOT VERY UNCOMFORTABLE, AS USUAL, ONLY THIS TIME IT DIDN'T GET ANY BETTER IN THE BATH.

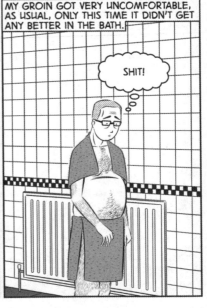

SHIT!

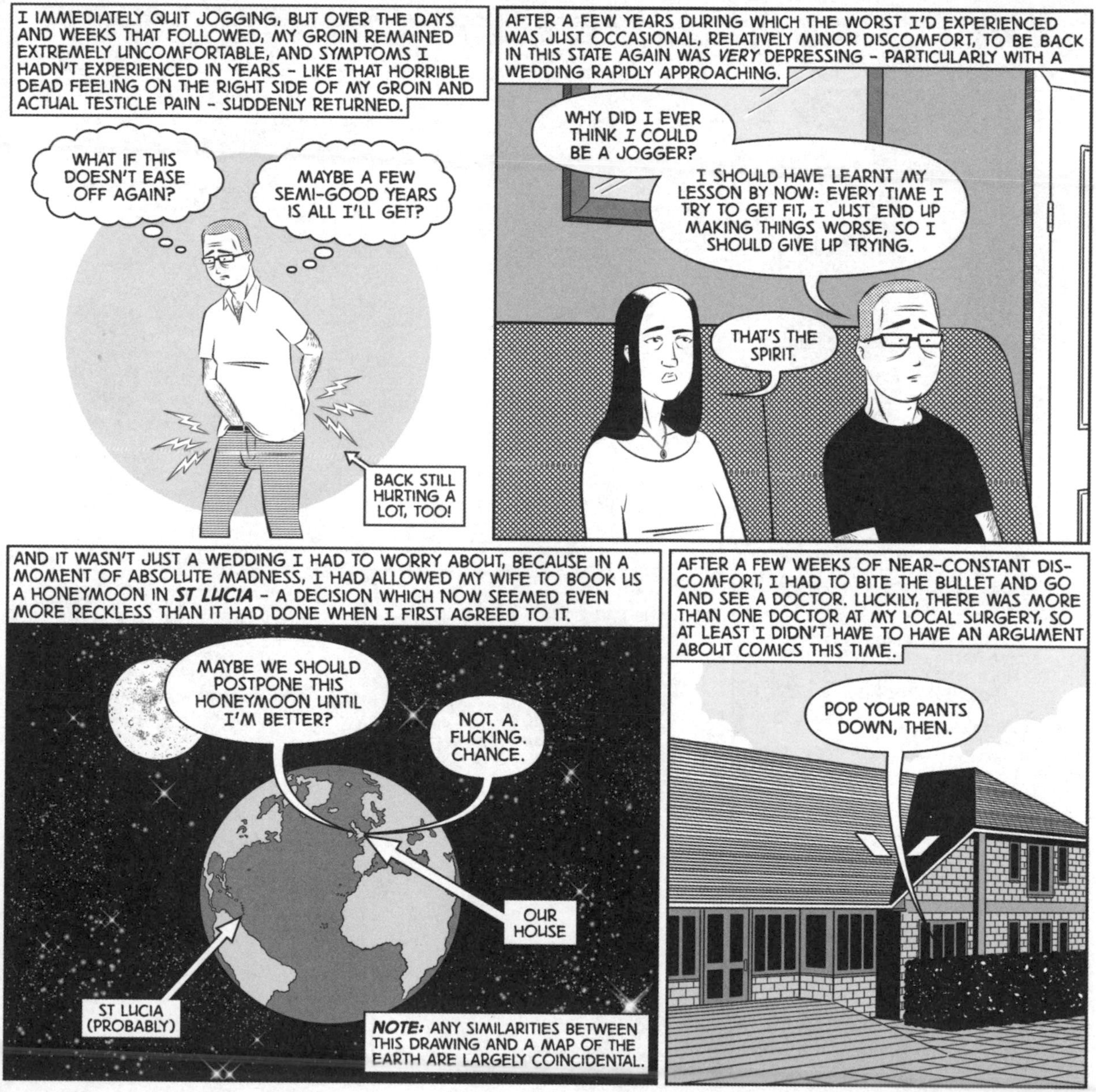
I IMMEDIATELY QUIT JOGGING, BUT OVER THE DAYS AND WEEKS THAT FOLLOWED, MY GROIN REMAINED EXTREMELY UNCOMFORTABLE, AND SYMPTOMS I HADN'T EXPERIENCED IN YEARS - LIKE THAT HORRIBLE DEAD FEELING ON THE RIGHT SIDE OF MY GROIN AND ACTUAL TESTICLE PAIN - SUDDENLY RETURNED.
WHAT IF THIS DOESN'T EASE OFF AGAIN?
MAYBE A FEW SEMI-GOOD YEARS IS ALL I'LL GET?
BACK STILL HURTING A LOT, TOO!
AFTER A FEW YEARS DURING WHICH THE WORST I'D EXPERIENCED WAS JUST OCCASIONAL, RELATIVELY MINOR DISCOMFORT, TO BE BACK IN THIS STATE AGAIN WAS *VERY* DEPRESSING - PARTICULARLY WITH A WEDDING RAPIDLY APPROACHING.
WHY DID I EVER THINK *I* COULD BE A JOGGER?
I SHOULD HAVE LEARNT MY LESSON BY NOW: EVERY TIME I TRY TO GET FIT, I JUST END UP MAKING THINGS WORSE, SO I SHOULD GIVE UP TRYING.
THAT'S THE SPIRIT.
AND IT WASN'T JUST A WEDDING I HAD TO WORRY ABOUT, BECAUSE IN A MOMENT OF ABSOLUTE MADNESS, I HAD ALLOWED MY WIFE TO BOOK US A HONEYMOON IN ***ST LUCIA*** - A DECISION WHICH NOW SEEMED EVEN MORE RECKLESS THAN IT HAD DONE WHEN I FIRST AGREED TO IT.
MAYBE WE SHOULD POSTPONE THIS HONEYMOON UNTIL I'M BETTER?
NOT. A. FUCKING. CHANCE.
OUR HOUSE
ST LUCIA (PROBABLY)
NOTE: ANY SIMILARITIES BETWEEN THIS DRAWING AND A MAP OF THE EARTH ARE LARGELY COINCIDENTAL.
AFTER A FEW WEEKS OF NEAR-CONSTANT DISCOMFORT, I HAD TO BITE THE BULLET AND GO AND SEE A DOCTOR. LUCKILY, THERE WAS MORE THAN ONE DOCTOR AT MY LOCAL SURGERY, SO AT LEAST I DIDN'T HAVE TO HAVE AN ARGUMENT ABOUT COMICS THIS TIME.
POP YOUR PANTS DOWN, THEN.

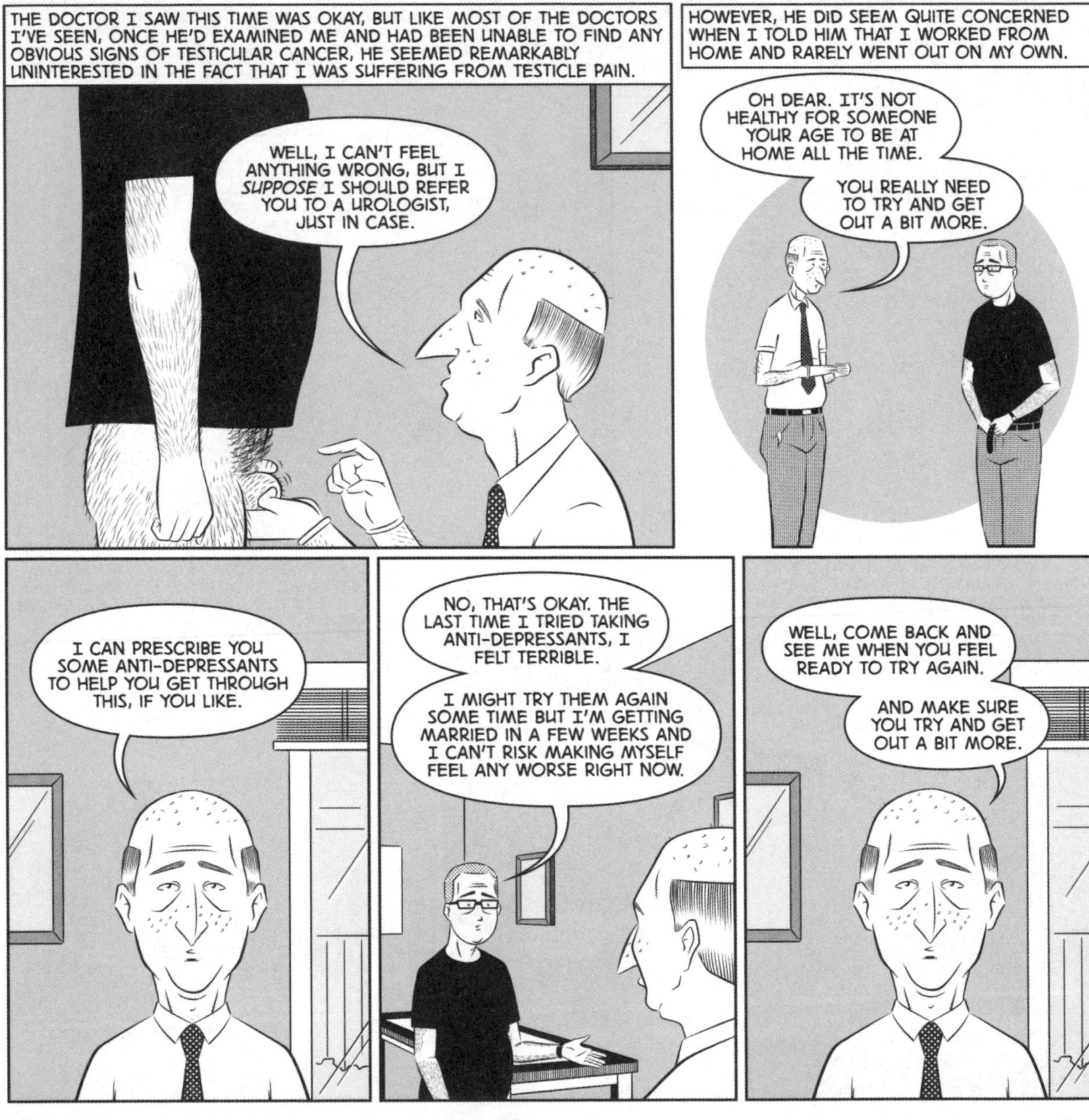

THE DOCTOR I SAW THIS TIME WAS OKAY, BUT LIKE MOST OF THE DOCTORS I'VE SEEN, ONCE HE'D EXAMINED ME AND HAD BEEN UNABLE TO FIND ANY OBVIOUS SIGNS OF TESTICULAR CANCER, HE SEEMED REMARKABLY UNINTERESTED IN THE FACT THAT I WAS SUFFERING FROM TESTICLE PAIN.
WELL, I CAN'T FEEL ANYTHING WRONG, BUT I *SUPPOSE* I SHOULD REFER YOU TO A UROLOGIST, JUST IN CASE.
HOWEVER, HE DID SEEM QUITE CONCERNED WHEN I TOLD HIM THAT I WORKED FROM HOME AND RARELY WENT OUT ON MY OWN.
OH DEAR. IT'S NOT HEALTHY FOR SOMEONE YOUR AGE TO BE AT HOME ALL THE TIME.
YOU REALLY NEED TO TRY AND GET OUT A BIT MORE.
I CAN PRESCRIBE YOU SOME ANTI-DEPRESSANTS TO HELP YOU GET THROUGH THIS, IF YOU LIKE.
NO, THAT'S OKAY. THE LAST TIME I TRIED TAKING ANTI-DEPRESSANTS, I FELT TERRIBLE.
I MIGHT TRY THEM AGAIN SOME TIME BUT I'M GETTING MARRIED IN A FEW WEEKS AND I CAN'T RISK MAKING MYSELF FEEL ANY WORSE RIGHT NOW.
WELL, COME BACK AND SEE ME WHEN YOU FEEL READY TO TRY AGAIN.
AND MAKE SURE YOU TRY AND GET OUT A BIT MORE.

I ASKED MY DOCTOR TO REFER ME TO SEE A UROLOGIST PRIVATELY, AS AN **NHS** APPOINTMENT WOULDN'T HAVE COME THROUGH UNTIL AFTER THE WEDDING, AND A WEEK OR SO LATER, I PAID £100, OR THEREABOUTS, TO SEE A UROLOGIST AT A NEARBY PRIVATE HOSPITAL.

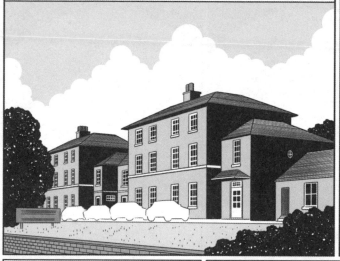

HE SEEMED VERY GOOD BUT COULDN'T FIND ANYTHING WRONG WHEN HE EXAMINED ME AND RECOMMENDED AN **MRI** SCAN.

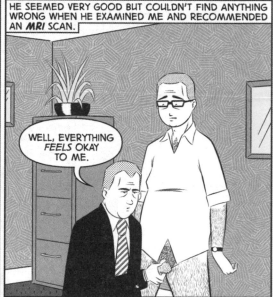

WELL, EVERYTHING *FEELS* OKAY TO ME.

THIS **MRI** TOOK PLACE IN THE BACK OF A VAN IN THE HOSPITAL CAR PARK, USING AN **MRI** SCANNER LESS POWERFUL THAN THE ONES MOST **NHS** HOSPITALS USE*, AND THIS COST ME ANOTHER £600.

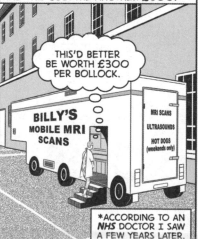

THIS'D BETTER BE WORTH £300 PER BOLLOCK.

BILLY'S MOBILE MRI SCANS

MRI SCANS
ULTRASOUNDS
HOT DOGS (weekends only)

*ACCORDING TO AN **NHS** DOCTOR I SAW A FEW YEARS LATER.

THE UROLOGIST THEN PRESCRIBED ME SOME POWERFUL ANTI-INFLAMMATORY DRUGS, SOME PROSTATE-RELAXING DRUGS AND AMITRIPTYLINE* TO TIDE ME OVER WHILE I WAITED FOR THE RESULTS OF THE **MRI**.

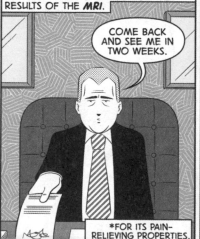

COME BACK AND SEE ME IN TWO WEEKS.

*FOR ITS PAIN-RELIEVING PROPERTIES.

BECAUSE THE PRESCRIPTION HAD BEEN WRITTEN BY A DOCTOR I'D SEEN PRIVATELY, I HAD TO PAY THE FULL PRICE FOR THE DRUGS WHEN I COLLECTED THEM FROM A PHARMACIST, AND THIS WAS NEARLY £90.

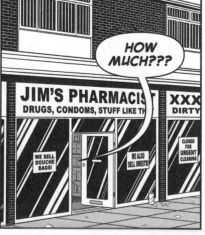

HOW MUCH???

JIM'S PHARMACIST
DRUGS, CONDOMS, STUFF LIKE TH

XXX DIRTY

WE SELL DOUCHE BAGS!

WE ALSO SELL SHEETS!

CLOSED FOR URGENT CLEANING

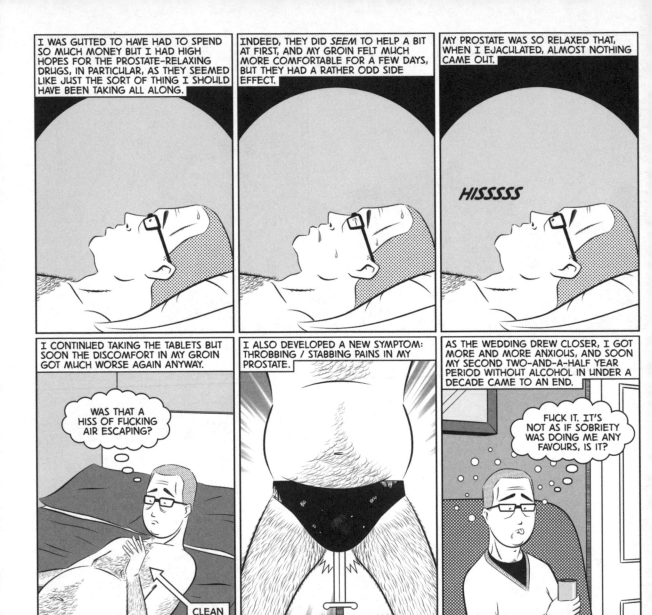

I WAS GUTTED TO HAVE HAD TO SPEND SO MUCH MONEY BUT I HAD HIGH HOPES FOR THE PROSTATE-RELAXING DRUGS, IN PARTICULAR, AS THEY SEEMED LIKE JUST THE SORT OF THING I SHOULD HAVE BEEN TAKING ALL ALONG.

INDEED, THEY DID *SEEM* TO HELP A BIT AT FIRST, AND MY GROIN FELT MUCH MORE COMFORTABLE FOR A FEW DAYS, BUT THEY HAD A RATHER ODD SIDE EFFECT.

MY PROSTATE WAS SO RELAXED THAT, WHEN I EJACULATED, ALMOST NOTHING CAME OUT.

HISSSSS

I CONTINUED TAKING THE TABLETS BUT SOON THE DISCOMFORT IN MY GROIN GOT MUCH WORSE AGAIN ANYWAY.

WAS THAT A HISS OF FUCKING AIR ESCAPING?

CLEAN HAND!

I ALSO DEVELOPED A NEW SYMPTOM: THROBBING / STABBING PAINS IN MY PROSTATE.

AS THE WEDDING DREW CLOSER, I GOT MORE AND MORE ANXIOUS, AND SOON MY SECOND TWO-AND-A-HALF YEAR PERIOD WITHOUT ALCOHOL IN UNDER A DECADE CAME TO AN END.

FUCK IT. IT'S NOT AS IF SOBRIETY WAS DOING ME ANY FAVOURS, IS IT?

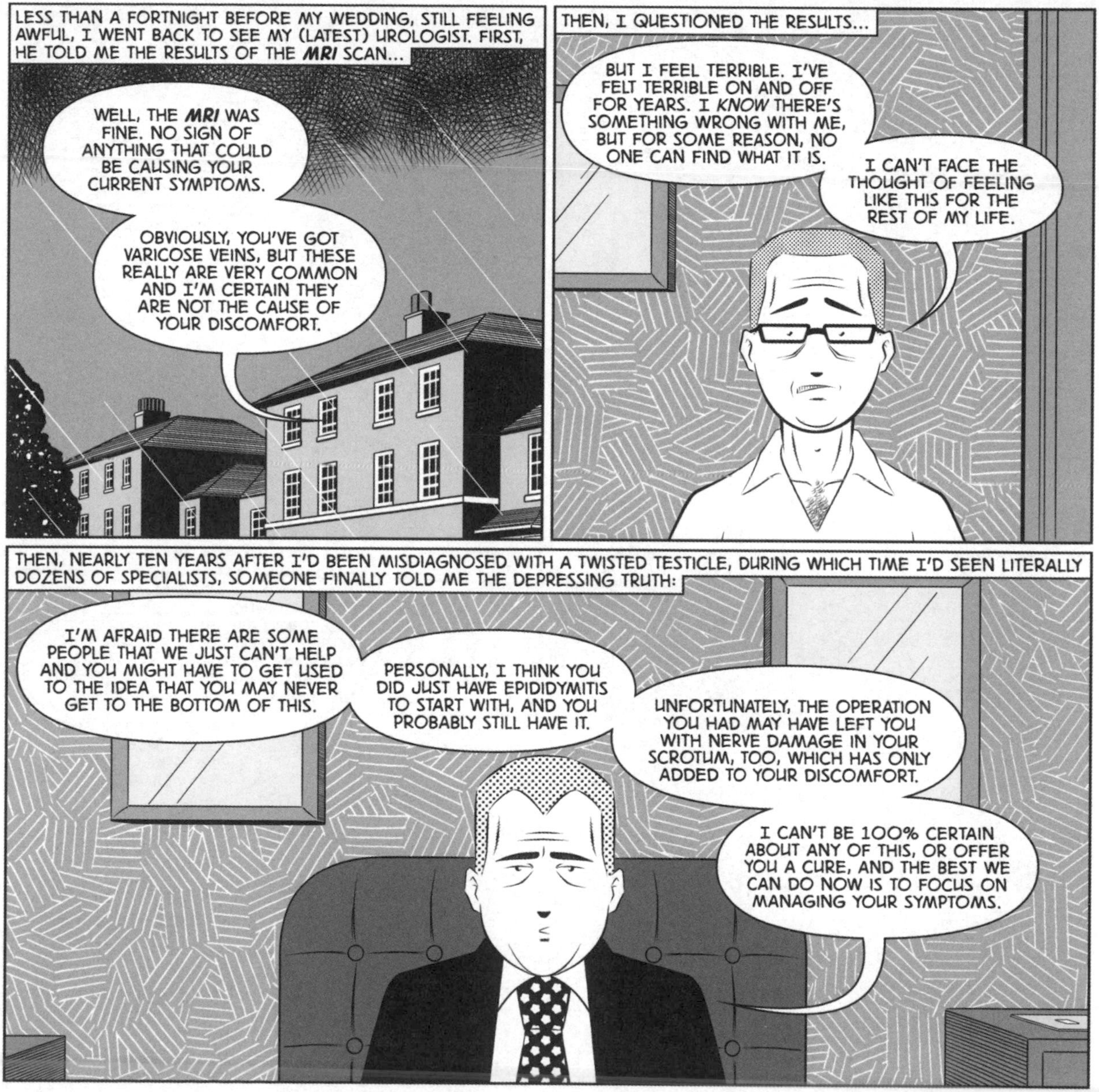
LESS THAN A FORTNIGHT BEFORE MY WEDDING, STILL FEELING AWFUL, I WENT BACK TO SEE MY (LATEST) UROLOGIST. FIRST, HE TOLD ME THE RESULTS OF THE MRI SCAN...
WELL, THE MRI WAS FINE. NO SIGN OF ANYTHING THAT COULD BE CAUSING YOUR CURRENT SYMPTOMS.
OBVIOUSLY, YOU'VE GOT VARICOSE VEINS, BUT THESE REALLY ARE VERY COMMON AND I'M CERTAIN THEY ARE NOT THE CAUSE OF YOUR DISCOMFORT.
THEN, I QUESTIONED THE RESULTS...
BUT I FEEL TERRIBLE. I'VE FELT TERRIBLE ON AND OFF FOR YEARS. I KNOW THERE'S SOMETHING WRONG WITH ME, BUT FOR SOME REASON, NO ONE CAN FIND WHAT IT IS.
I CAN'T FACE THE THOUGHT OF FEELING LIKE THIS FOR THE REST OF MY LIFE.
THEN, NEARLY TEN YEARS AFTER I'D BEEN MISDIAGNOSED WITH A TWISTED TESTICLE, DURING WHICH TIME I'D SEEN LITERALLY DOZENS OF SPECIALISTS, SOMEONE FINALLY TOLD ME THE DEPRESSING TRUTH:
I'M AFRAID THERE ARE SOME PEOPLE THAT WE JUST CAN'T HELP AND YOU MIGHT HAVE TO GET USED TO THE IDEA THAT YOU MAY NEVER GET TO THE BOTTOM OF THIS.
PERSONALLY, I THINK YOU DID JUST HAVE EPIDIDYMITIS TO START WITH, AND YOU PROBABLY STILL HAVE IT.
UNFORTUNATELY, THE OPERATION YOU HAD MAY HAVE LEFT YOU WITH NERVE DAMAGE IN YOUR SCROTUM, TOO, WHICH HAS ONLY ADDED TO YOUR DISCOMFORT.
I CAN'T BE 100% CERTAIN ABOUT ANY OF THIS, OR OFFER YOU A CURE, AND THE BEST WE CAN DO NOW IS TO FOCUS ON MANAGING YOUR SYMPTOMS.

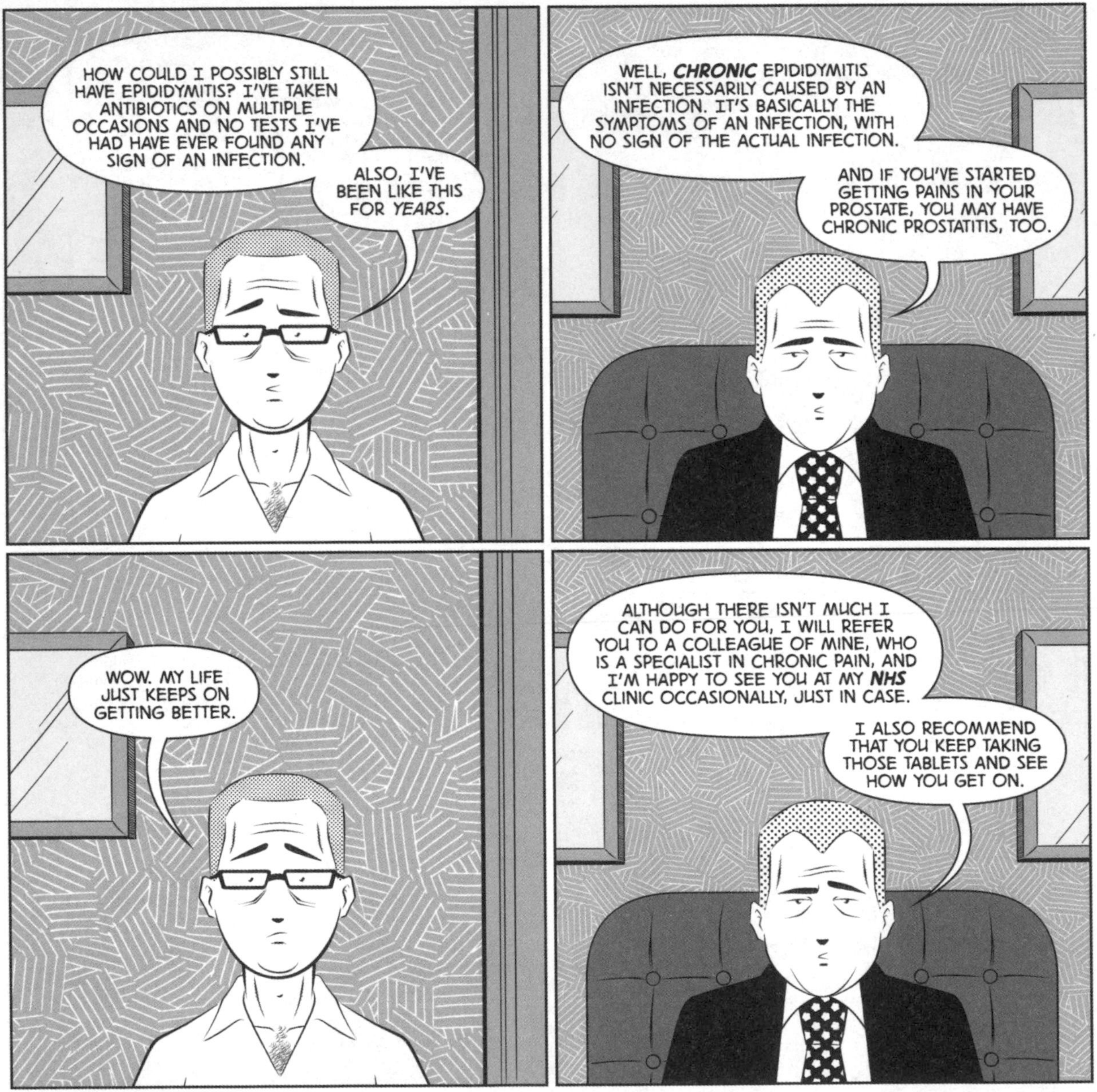
HOW COULD I POSSIBLY STILL HAVE EPIDIDYMITIS? I'VE TAKEN ANTIBIOTICS ON MULTIPLE OCCASIONS AND NO TESTS I'VE HAD HAVE EVER FOUND ANY SIGN OF AN INFECTION.
ALSO, I'VE BEEN LIKE THIS FOR *YEARS*.
WELL, ***CHRONIC*** EPIDIDYMITIS ISN'T NECESSARILY CAUSED BY AN INFECTION. IT'S BASICALLY THE SYMPTOMS OF AN INFECTION, WITH NO SIGN OF THE ACTUAL INFECTION.
AND IF YOU'VE STARTED GETTING PAINS IN YOUR PROSTATE, YOU MAY HAVE CHRONIC PROSTATITIS, TOO.
WOW. MY LIFE JUST KEEPS ON GETTING BETTER.
ALTHOUGH THERE ISN'T MUCH I CAN DO FOR YOU, I WILL REFER YOU TO A COLLEAGUE OF MINE, WHO IS A SPECIALIST IN CHRONIC PAIN, AND I'M HAPPY TO SEE YOU AT MY ***NHS*** CLINIC OCCASIONALLY, JUST IN CASE.
I ALSO RECOMMEND THAT YOU KEEP TAKING THOSE TABLETS AND SEE HOW YOU GET ON.

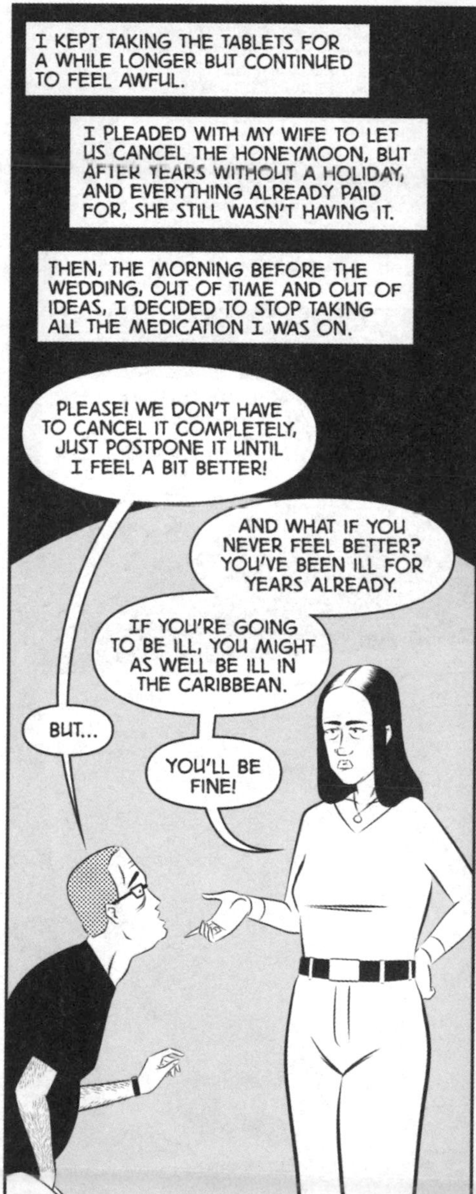
I KEPT TAKING THE TABLETS FOR A WHILE LONGER BUT CONTINUED TO FEEL AWFUL.
I PLEADED WITH MY WIFE TO LET US CANCEL THE HONEYMOON, BUT AFTER YEARS WITHOUT A HOLIDAY, AND EVERYTHING ALREADY PAID FOR, SHE STILL WASN'T HAVING IT.
THEN, THE MORNING BEFORE THE WEDDING, OUT OF TIME AND OUT OF IDEAS, I DECIDED TO STOP TAKING ALL THE MEDICATION I WAS ON.
PLEASE! WE DON'T HAVE TO CANCEL IT COMPLETELY, JUST POSTPONE IT UNTIL I FEEL A BIT BETTER!
AND WHAT IF YOU NEVER FEEL BETTER? YOU'VE BEEN ILL FOR YEARS ALREADY.
IF YOU'RE GOING TO BE ILL, YOU MIGHT AS WELL BE ILL IN THE CARIBBEAN.
BUT...
YOU'LL BE FINE!

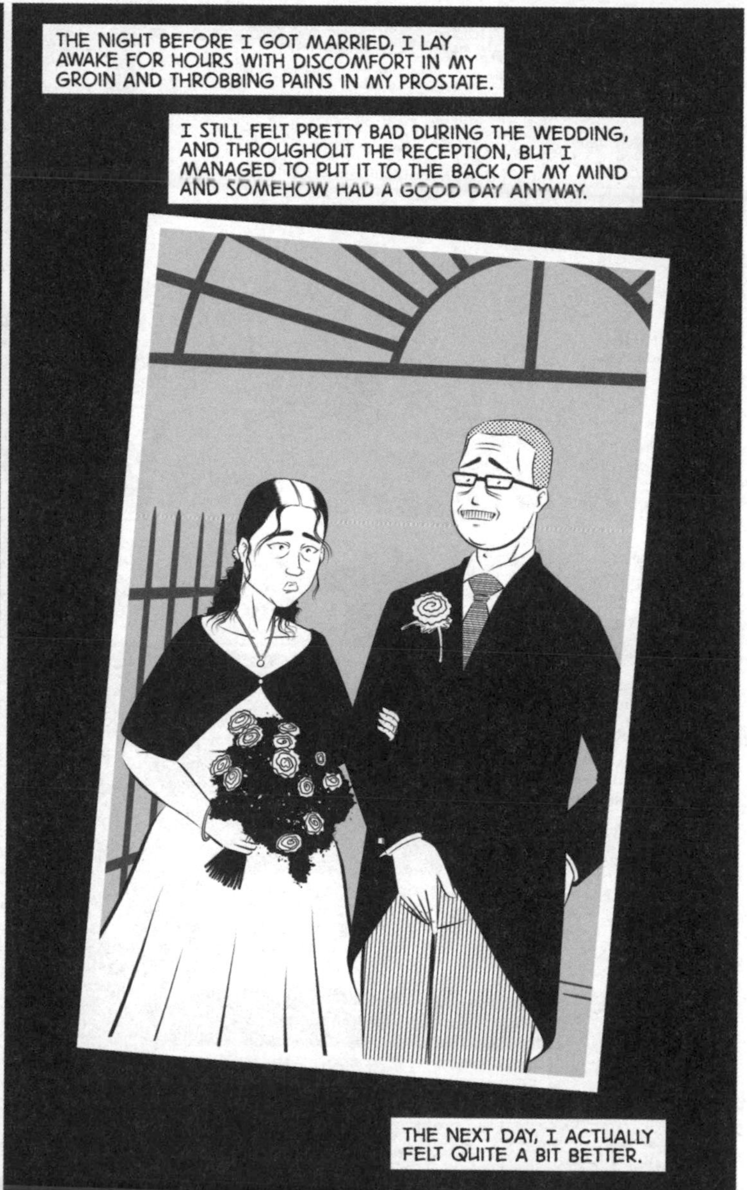
THE NIGHT BEFORE I GOT MARRIED, I LAY AWAKE FOR HOURS WITH DISCOMFORT IN MY GROIN AND THROBBING PAINS IN MY PROSTATE.
I STILL FELT PRETTY BAD DURING THE WEDDING, AND THROUGHOUT THE RECEPTION, BUT I MANAGED TO PUT IT TO THE BACK OF MY MIND AND SOMEHOW HAD A GOOD DAY ANYWAY.
THE NEXT DAY, I ACTUALLY FELT QUITE A BIT BETTER.

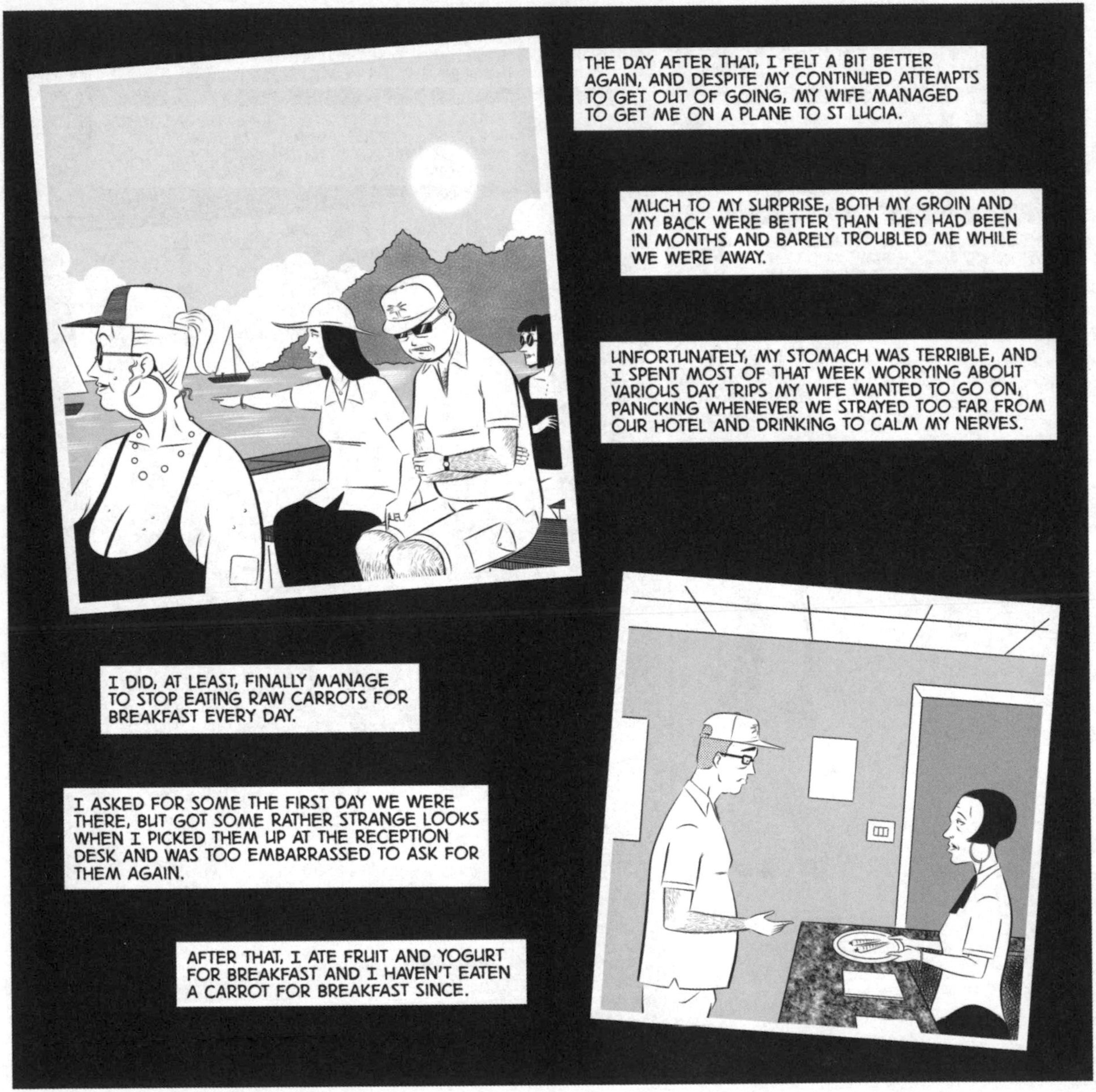
THE DAY AFTER THAT, I FELT A BIT BETTER AGAIN, AND DESPITE MY CONTINUED ATTEMPTS TO GET OUT OF GOING, MY WIFE MANAGED TO GET ME ON A PLANE TO ST LUCIA.
MUCH TO MY SURPRISE, BOTH MY GROIN AND MY BACK WERE BETTER THAN THEY HAD BEEN IN MONTHS AND BARELY TROUBLED ME WHILE WE WERE AWAY.
UNFORTUNATELY, MY STOMACH WAS TERRIBLE, AND I SPENT MOST OF THAT WEEK WORRYING ABOUT VARIOUS DAY TRIPS MY WIFE WANTED TO GO ON, PANICKING WHENEVER WE STRAYED TOO FAR FROM OUR HOTEL AND DRINKING TO CALM MY NERVES.
I DID, AT LEAST, FINALLY MANAGE TO STOP EATING RAW CARROTS FOR BREAKFAST EVERY DAY.
I ASKED FOR SOME THE FIRST DAY WE WERE THERE, BUT GOT SOME RATHER STRANGE LOOKS WHEN I PICKED THEM UP AT THE RECEPTION DESK AND WAS TOO EMBARRASSED TO ASK FOR THEM AGAIN.
AFTER THAT, I ATE FRUIT AND YOGURT FOR BREAKFAST AND I HAVEN'T EATEN A CARROT FOR BREAKFAST SINCE.

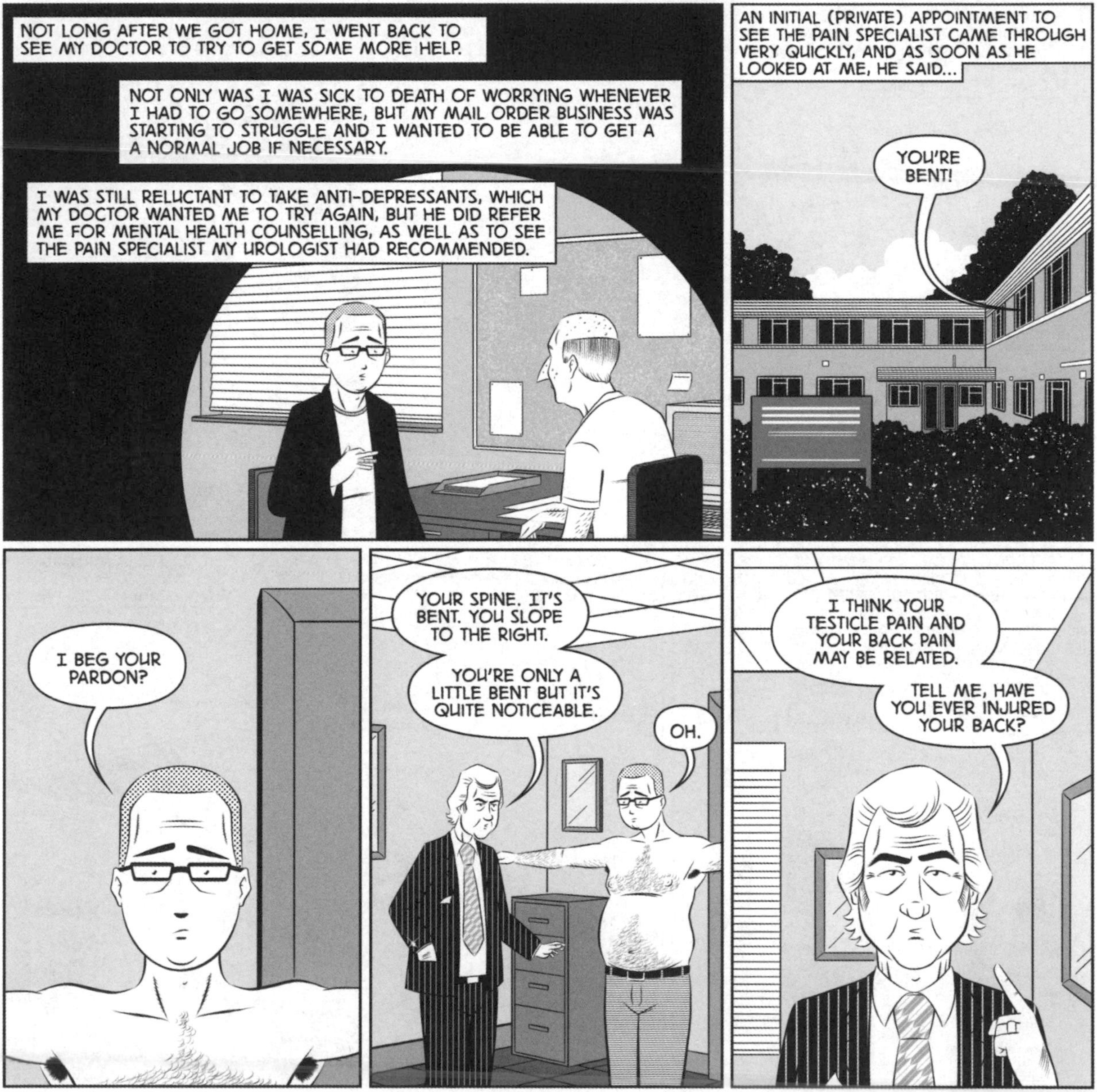
NOT LONG AFTER WE GOT HOME, I WENT BACK TO SEE MY DOCTOR TO TRY TO GET SOME MORE HELP.
NOT ONLY WAS I WAS SICK TO DEATH OF WORRYING WHENEVER I HAD TO GO SOMEWHERE, BUT MY MAIL ORDER BUSINESS WAS STARTING TO STRUGGLE AND I WANTED TO BE ABLE TO GET A A NORMAL JOB IF NECESSARY.
I WAS STILL RELUCTANT TO TAKE ANTI-DEPRESSANTS, WHICH MY DOCTOR WANTED ME TO TRY AGAIN, BUT HE DID REFER ME FOR MENTAL HEALTH COUNSELLING, AS WELL AS TO SEE THE PAIN SPECIALIST MY UROLOGIST HAD RECOMMENDED.
AN INITIAL (PRIVATE) APPOINTMENT TO SEE THE PAIN SPECIALIST CAME THROUGH VERY QUICKLY, AND AS SOON AS HE LOOKED AT ME, HE SAID...
YOU'RE BENT!
I BEG YOUR PARDON?
YOUR SPINE. IT'S BENT. YOU SLOPE TO THE RIGHT.
YOU'RE ONLY A LITTLE BENT BUT IT'S QUITE NOTICEABLE.
OH.
I THINK YOUR TESTICLE PAIN AND YOUR BACK PAIN MAY BE RELATED.
TELL ME, HAVE YOU EVER INJURED YOUR BACK?

I TOLD HIM ABOUT THE TIME I HURT MY BACK WEIGHT-LIFTING WHEN I WAS IN MY EARLY-20S, WHICH WAS ALSO THE FIRST TIME I EXPERIENCED PAIN AND DISCOMFORT IN MY GROIN.

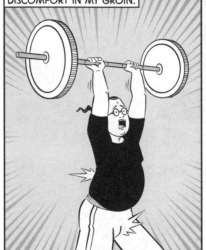

THEN HE TOLD ME HOW THE NERVES IN THE TESTICLES ORIGINATE IN THE SPINE, SO A BACK PROBLEM COULD LEAD TO SO-CALLED REFERRED PAIN IN THE TESTICLES.

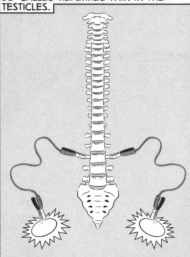

HE RECOMMENDED THAT I HAVE SOME STEROID INJECTIONS IN MY SPINE, WHICH WOULD AT LEAST HELP DETERMINE IF MY TESTICLE PAIN WAS CAUSED BY A BACK PROBLEM.

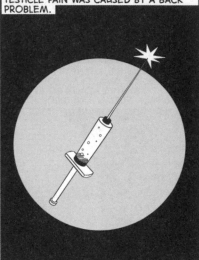

I COULDN'T AFFORD TO HAVE THIS DONE PRIVATELY — I COULD BARELY AFFORD THIS FIRST APPOINTMENT — BUT HE AGREED TO CONTINUE SEEING ME AT HIS **NHS** CLINIC, AND I WENT HOME THAT DAY FEELING LIKE I WAS *FINALLY* GETTING SOMEWHERE.

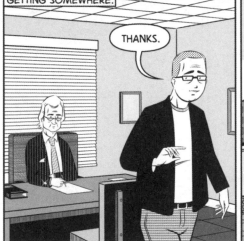

THANKS.

NOT LONG AFTER THIS, MY FIRST (**NHS**) APPOINTMENT TO SEE A MENTAL HEALTH COUNCILLOR CAME THROUGH. I GOT ON VERY WELL WITH THE COUNCILLOR I SAW, AND AFTER WE'D CHATTED FOR AN HOUR OR SO, HE CONFIRMED WHAT I'D LONG SUSPECTED:

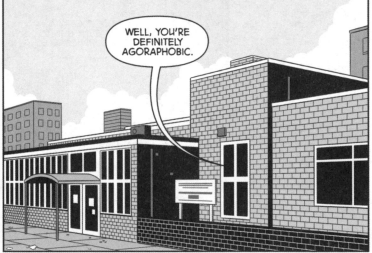

WELL, YOU'RE DEFINITELY AGORAPHOBIC.

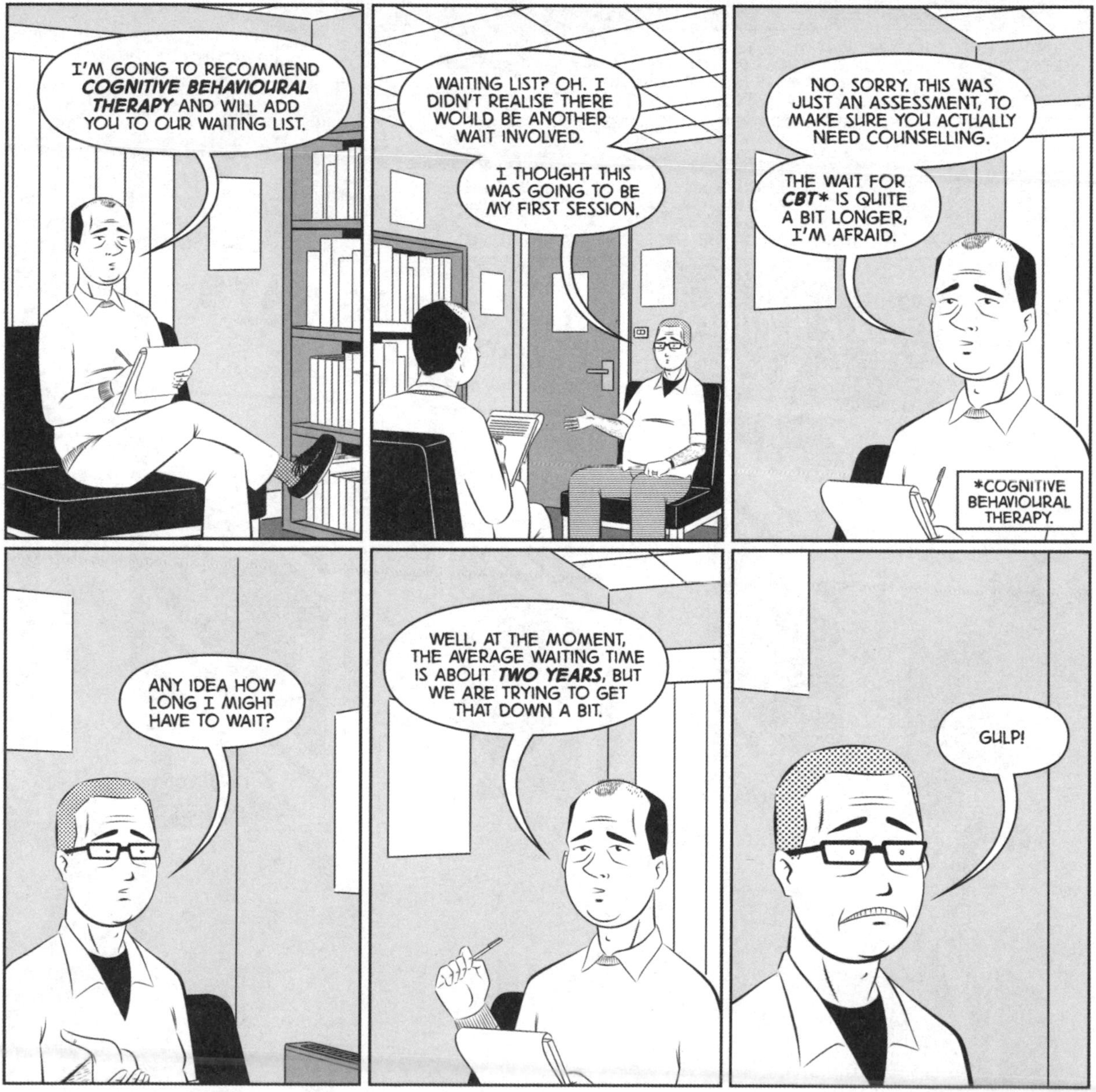
I'M GOING TO RECOMMEND **COGNITIVE BEHAVIOURAL THERAPY** AND WILL ADD YOU TO OUR WAITING LIST.
WAITING LIST? OH. I DIDN'T REALISE THERE WOULD BE ANOTHER WAIT INVOLVED.
I THOUGHT THIS WAS GOING TO BE MY FIRST SESSION.
NO. SORRY. THIS WAS JUST AN ASSESSMENT, TO MAKE SURE YOU ACTUALLY NEED COUNSELLING.
THE WAIT FOR **CBT*** IS QUITE A BIT LONGER, I'M AFRAID.
*COGNITIVE BEHAVIOURAL THERAPY.
ANY IDEA HOW LONG I MIGHT HAVE TO WAIT?
WELL, AT THE MOMENT, THE AVERAGE WAITING TIME IS ABOUT **TWO YEARS**, BUT WE ARE TRYING TO GET THAT DOWN A BIT.
GULP!

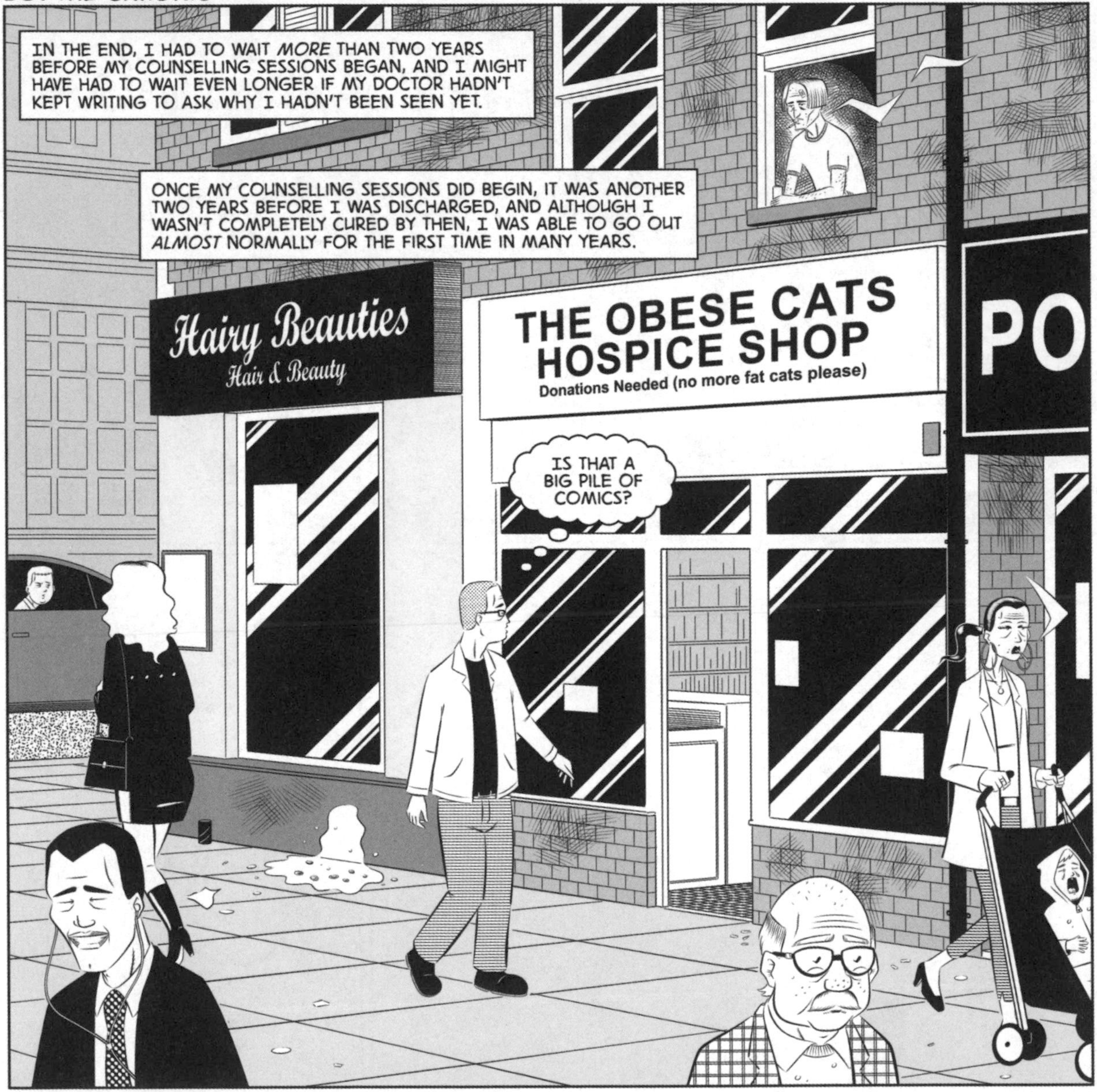
IN THE END, I HAD TO WAIT *MORE* THAN TWO YEARS BEFORE MY COUNSELLING SESSIONS BEGAN, AND I MIGHT HAVE HAD TO WAIT EVEN LONGER IF MY DOCTOR HADN'T KEPT WRITING TO ASK WHY I HADN'T BEEN SEEN YET.
ONCE MY COUNSELLING SESSIONS DID BEGIN, IT WAS ANOTHER TWO YEARS BEFORE I WAS DISCHARGED, AND ALTHOUGH I WASN'T COMPLETELY CURED BY THEN, I WAS ABLE TO GO OUT *ALMOST* NORMALLY FOR THE FIRST TIME IN MANY YEARS.
Hairy Beauties
Hair & Beauty
THE OBESE CATS HOSPICE SHOP
Donations Needed (no more fat cats please)
PO
IS THAT A BIG PILE OF COMICS?

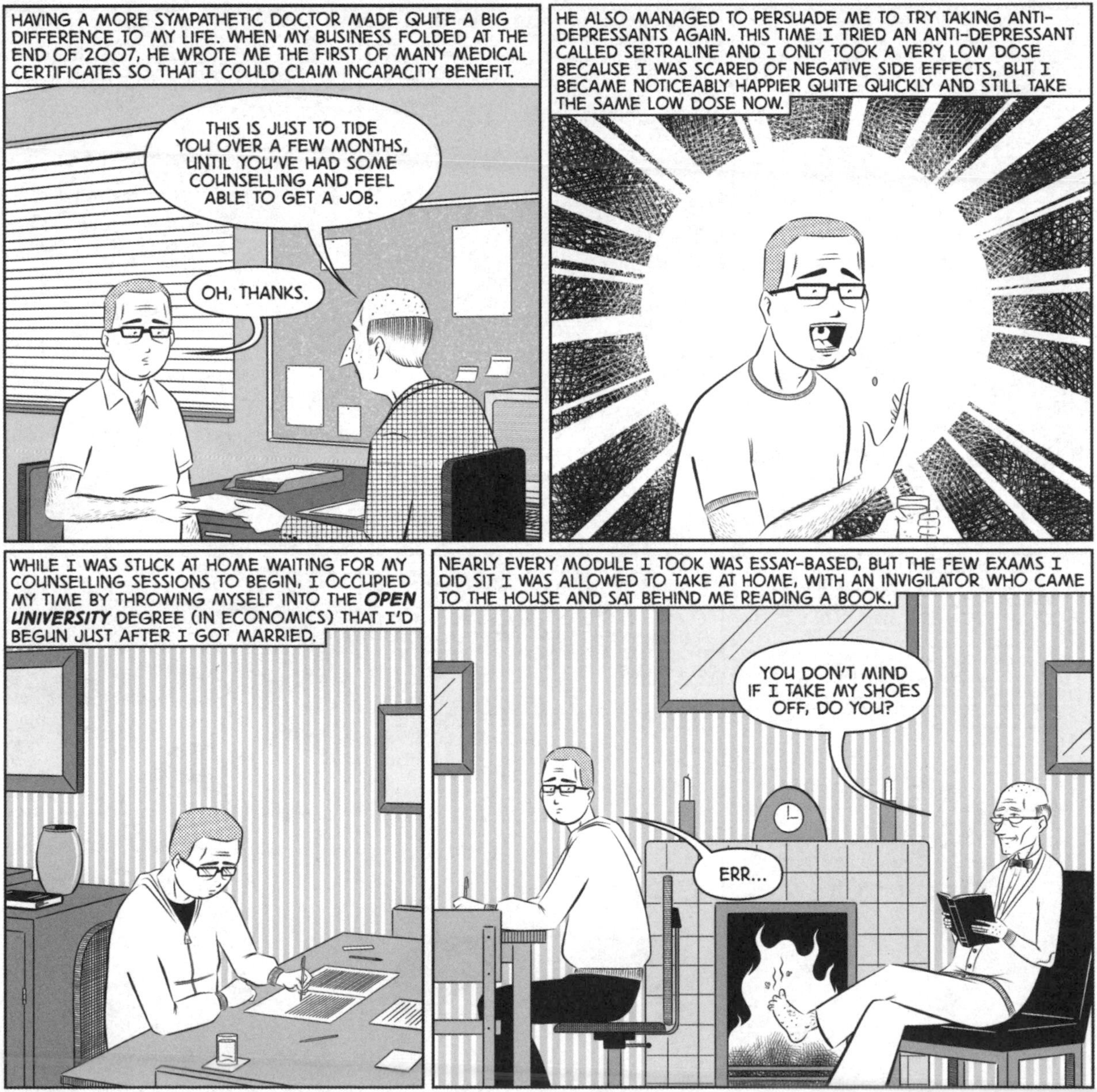
HAVING A MORE SYMPATHETIC DOCTOR MADE QUITE A BIG DIFFERENCE TO MY LIFE. WHEN MY BUSINESS FOLDED AT THE END OF 2007, HE WROTE ME THE FIRST OF MANY MEDICAL CERTIFICATES SO THAT I COULD CLAIM INCAPACITY BENEFIT.
THIS IS JUST TO TIDE YOU OVER A FEW MONTHS, UNTIL YOU'VE HAD SOME COUNSELLING AND FEEL ABLE TO GET A JOB.
OH, THANKS.
HE ALSO MANAGED TO PERSUADE ME TO TRY TAKING ANTI-DEPRESSANTS AGAIN. THIS TIME I TRIED AN ANTI-DEPRESSANT CALLED SERTRALINE AND I ONLY TOOK A VERY LOW DOSE BECAUSE I WAS SCARED OF NEGATIVE SIDE EFFECTS, BUT I BECAME NOTICEABLY HAPPIER QUITE QUICKLY AND STILL TAKE THE SAME LOW DOSE NOW.
WHILE I WAS STUCK AT HOME WAITING FOR MY COUNSELLING SESSIONS TO BEGIN, I OCCUPIED MY TIME BY THROWING MYSELF INTO THE ***OPEN UNIVERSITY*** DEGREE (IN ECONOMICS) THAT I'D BEGUN JUST AFTER I GOT MARRIED.
NEARLY EVERY MODULE I TOOK WAS ESSAY-BASED, BUT THE FEW EXAMS I DID SIT I WAS ALLOWED TO TAKE AT HOME, WITH AN INVIGILATOR WHO CAME TO THE HOUSE AND SAT BEHIND ME READING A BOOK.
YOU DON'T MIND IF I TAKE MY SHOES OFF, DO YOU?
ERR...

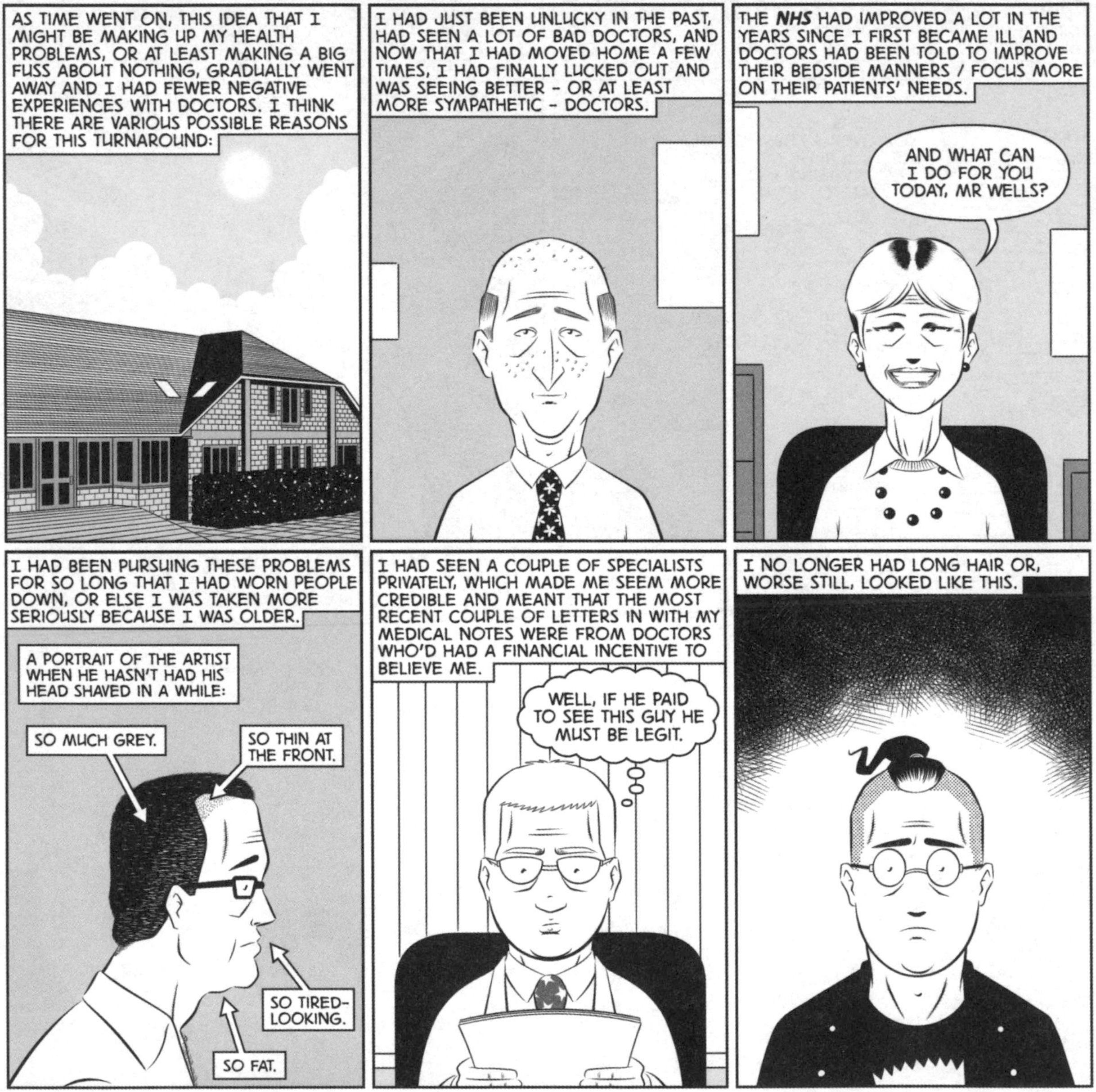
AS TIME WENT ON, THIS IDEA THAT I MIGHT BE MAKING UP MY HEALTH PROBLEMS, OR AT LEAST MAKING A BIG FUSS ABOUT NOTHING, GRADUALLY WENT AWAY AND I HAD FEWER NEGATIVE EXPERIENCES WITH DOCTORS. I THINK THERE ARE VARIOUS POSSIBLE REASONS FOR THIS TURNAROUND:
I HAD JUST BEEN UNLUCKY IN THE PAST, HAD SEEN A LOT OF BAD DOCTORS, AND NOW THAT I HAD MOVED HOME A FEW TIMES, I HAD FINALLY LUCKED OUT AND WAS SEEING BETTER - OR AT LEAST MORE SYMPATHETIC - DOCTORS.
THE **NHS** HAD IMPROVED A LOT IN THE YEARS SINCE I FIRST BECAME ILL AND DOCTORS HAD BEEN TOLD TO IMPROVE THEIR BEDSIDE MANNERS / FOCUS MORE ON THEIR PATIENTS' NEEDS.
AND WHAT CAN I DO FOR YOU TODAY, MR WELLS?
I HAD BEEN PURSUING THESE PROBLEMS FOR SO LONG THAT I HAD WORN PEOPLE DOWN, OR ELSE I WAS TAKEN MORE SERIOUSLY BECAUSE I WAS OLDER.
A PORTRAIT OF THE ARTIST WHEN HE HASN'T HAD HIS HEAD SHAVED IN A WHILE:
SO MUCH GREY.
SO THIN AT THE FRONT.
SO TIRED-LOOKING.
SO FAT.
I HAD SEEN A COUPLE OF SPECIALISTS PRIVATELY, WHICH MADE ME SEEM MORE CREDIBLE AND MEANT THAT THE MOST RECENT COUPLE OF LETTERS IN WITH MY MEDICAL NOTES WERE FROM DOCTORS WHO'D HAD A FINANCIAL INCENTIVE TO BELIEVE ME.
WELL, IF HE PAID TO SEE THIS GUY HE MUST BE LEGIT.
I NO LONGER HAD LONG HAIR OR, WORSE STILL, LOOKED LIKE THIS.

WHATEVER THE REASON, I HAD FEWER NEGATIVE EXPERIENCES WITH DOCTORS, BUT THEY DID STILL OCCUR FROM TIME TO TIME.

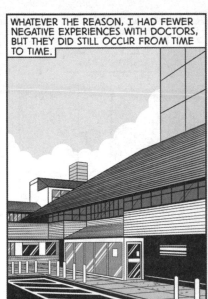

AFTER MY WEDDING, I CONTINUED TO SEE THE UROLOGIST I'D SEEN PRIVATELY JUST BEFORE THE WEDDING ON THE **NHS**, BUT THIS PROVED TO BE A WASTE OF TIME, AS THERE WAS LITTLE HE COULD DO FOR ME AND HE QUICKLY LOST INTEREST.

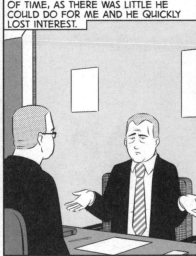

THE LAST TIME I WENT TO HIS CLINIC, I WAS SEEN BY ANOTHER MEMBER OF HIS TEAM INSTEAD, AND THIS UROLOGIST WAS LESS THAN SYMPATHETIC.

YOU PEOPLE...

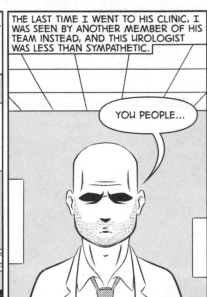

YOU DON'T KNOW *REAL* SUFFERING.

IN MY COUNTRY, I SAW THINGS YOU WOULDN'T BELIEVE. *TERRIBLE* THINGS.

AND YOU COMPLAIN ABOUT SOMETHING LIKE THIS? THIS IS *NOTHING*. YOU DON'T KNOW HOW LUCKY YOU ARE.

JUST FORGET ABOUT THIS AND LIVE YOUR LIFE!

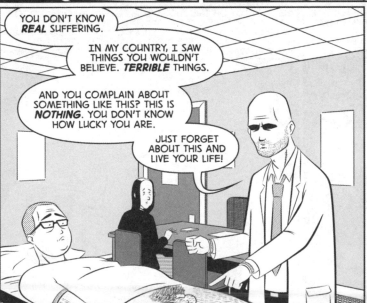

HE HAD A POINT. I MEAN, COMPARED TO THINGS LIKE WAR AND ETHNIC CLEANSING, MY YEARS OF TESTICLE PAIN WERE UTTERLY TRIVIAL, BUT THAT'S NOT REALLY WHAT YOU WANT TO HEAR FROM YOUR UROLOGIST.

OH, THE HORROR...

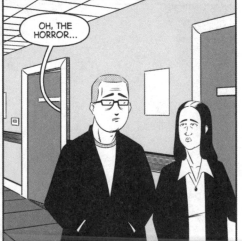

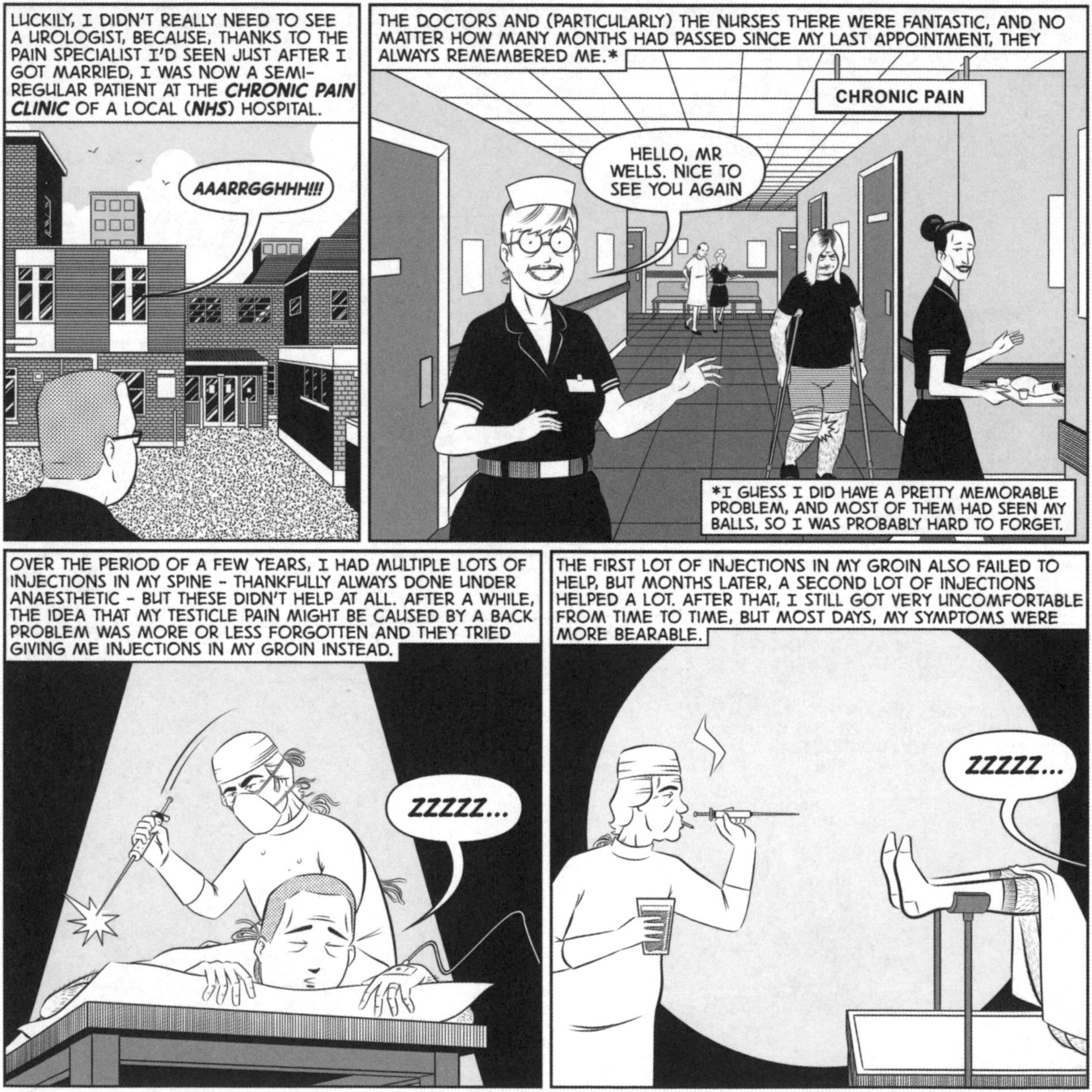
LUCKILY, I DIDN'T REALLY NEED TO SEE A UROLOGIST, BECAUSE, THANKS TO THE PAIN SPECIALIST I'D SEEN JUST AFTER I GOT MARRIED, I WAS NOW A SEMI-REGULAR PATIENT AT THE ***CHRONIC PAIN CLINIC*** OF A LOCAL (***NHS***) HOSPITAL.
AAARRGGHHH!!!
THE DOCTORS AND (PARTICULARLY) THE NURSES THERE WERE FANTASTIC, AND NO MATTER HOW MANY MONTHS HAD PASSED SINCE MY LAST APPOINTMENT, THEY ALWAYS REMEMBERED ME.*
CHRONIC PAIN
HELLO, MR WELLS. NICE TO SEE YOU AGAIN
*I GUESS I DID HAVE A PRETTY MEMORABLE PROBLEM, AND MOST OF THEM HAD SEEN MY BALLS, SO I WAS PROBABLY HARD TO FORGET.
OVER THE PERIOD OF A FEW YEARS, I HAD MULTIPLE LOTS OF INJECTIONS IN MY SPINE - THANKFULLY ALWAYS DONE UNDER ANAESTHETIC - BUT THESE DIDN'T HELP AT ALL. AFTER A WHILE, THE IDEA THAT MY TESTICLE PAIN MIGHT BE CAUSED BY A BACK PROBLEM WAS MORE OR LESS FORGOTTEN AND THEY TRIED GIVING ME INJECTIONS IN MY GROIN INSTEAD.
ZZZZZ...
THE FIRST LOT OF INJECTIONS IN MY GROIN ALSO FAILED TO HELP, BUT MONTHS LATER, A SECOND LOT OF INJECTIONS HELPED A LOT. AFTER THAT, I STILL GOT VERY UNCOMFORTABLE FROM TIME TO TIME, BUT MOST DAYS, MY SYMPTOMS WERE MORE BEARABLE.
ZZZZZ...

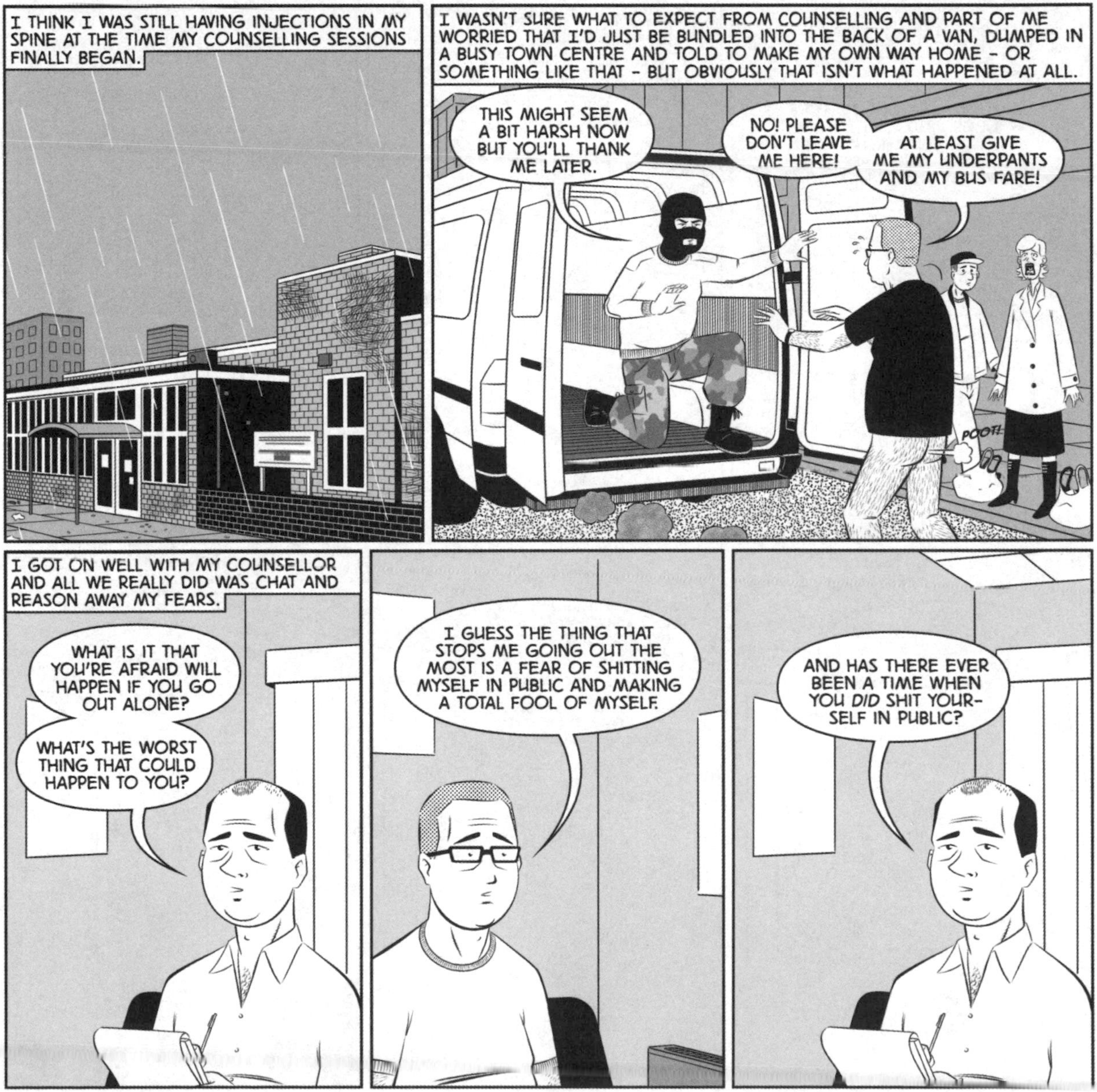
I THINK I WAS STILL HAVING INJECTIONS IN MY SPINE AT THE TIME MY COUNSELLING SESSIONS FINALLY BEGAN.
I WASN'T SURE WHAT TO EXPECT FROM COUNSELLING AND PART OF ME WORRIED THAT I'D JUST BE BUNDLED INTO THE BACK OF A VAN, DUMPED IN A BUSY TOWN CENTRE AND TOLD TO MAKE MY OWN WAY HOME - OR SOMETHING LIKE THAT - BUT OBVIOUSLY THAT ISN'T WHAT HAPPENED AT ALL.
THIS MIGHT SEEM A BIT HARSH NOW BUT YOU'LL THANK ME LATER.
NO! PLEASE DON'T LEAVE ME HERE!
AT LEAST GIVE ME MY UNDERPANTS AND MY BUS FARE!
POOT!
I GOT ON WELL WITH MY COUNSELLOR AND ALL WE REALLY DID WAS CHAT AND REASON AWAY MY FEARS.
WHAT IS IT THAT YOU'RE AFRAID WILL HAPPEN IF YOU GO OUT ALONE?
WHAT'S THE WORST THING THAT COULD HAPPEN TO YOU?
I GUESS THE THING THAT STOPS ME GOING OUT THE MOST IS A FEAR OF SHITTING MYSELF IN PUBLIC AND MAKING A TOTAL FOOL OF MYSELF.
AND HAS THERE EVER BEEN A TIME WHEN YOU *DID* SHIT YOURSELF IN PUBLIC?

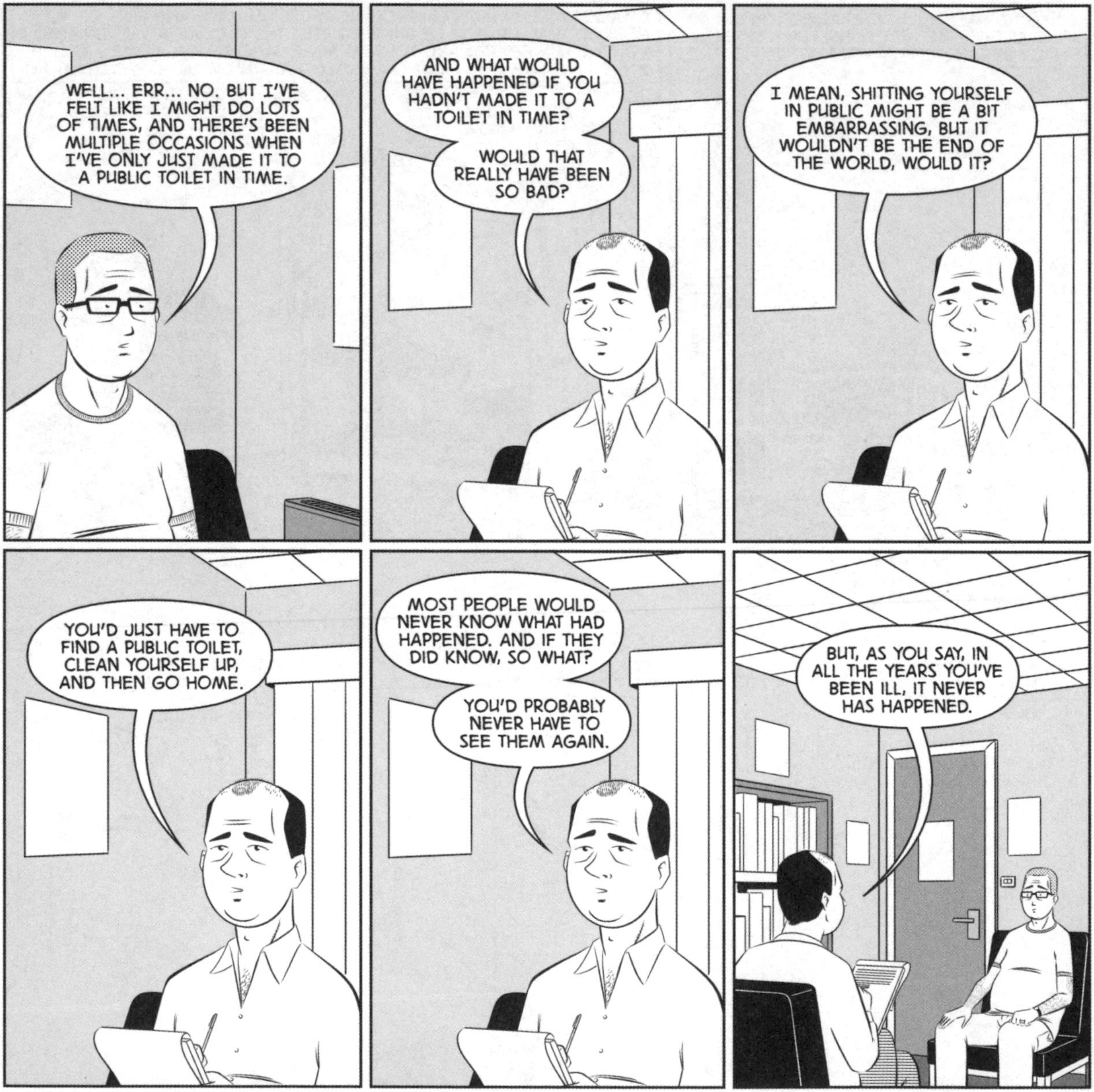
WELL... ERR... NO. BUT I'VE FELT LIKE I MIGHT DO LOTS OF TIMES, AND THERE'S BEEN MULTIPLE OCCASIONS WHEN I'VE ONLY JUST MADE IT TO A PUBLIC TOILET IN TIME.
AND WHAT WOULD HAVE HAPPENED IF YOU HADN'T MADE IT TO A TOILET IN TIME?
WOULD THAT REALLY HAVE BEEN SO BAD?
I MEAN, SHITTING YOURSELF IN PUBLIC MIGHT BE A BIT EMBARRASSING, BUT IT WOULDN'T BE THE END OF THE WORLD, WOULD IT?
YOU'D JUST HAVE TO FIND A PUBLIC TOILET, CLEAN YOURSELF UP, AND THEN GO HOME.
MOST PEOPLE WOULD NEVER KNOW WHAT HAD HAPPENED. AND IF THEY DID KNOW, SO WHAT?
YOU'D PROBABLY NEVER HAVE TO SEE THEM AGAIN.
BUT, AS YOU SAY, IN ALL THE YEARS YOU'VE BEEN ILL, IT NEVER HAS HAPPENED.

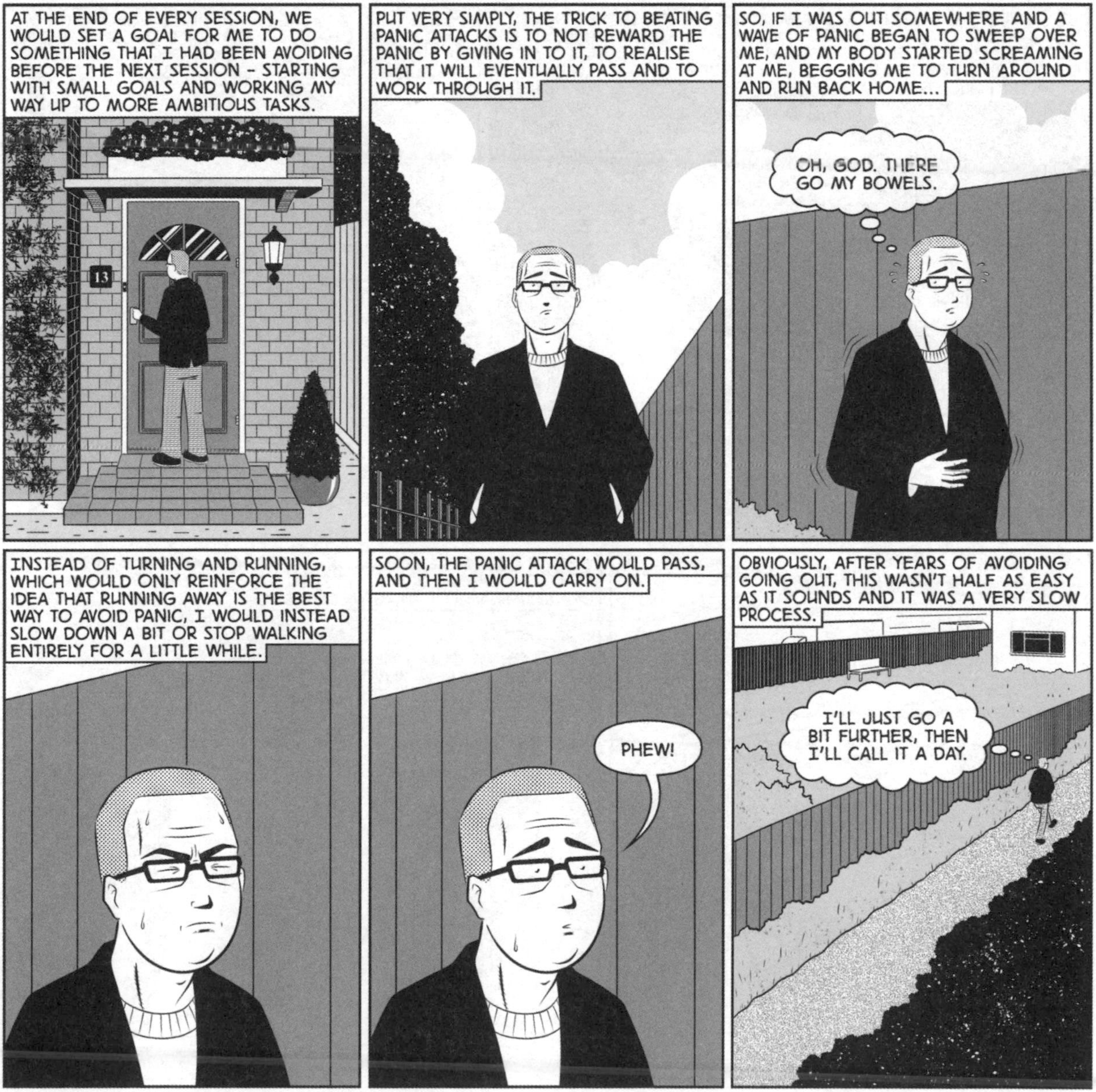
AT THE END OF EVERY SESSION, WE WOULD SET A GOAL FOR ME TO DO SOMETHING THAT I HAD BEEN AVOIDING BEFORE THE NEXT SESSION - STARTING WITH SMALL GOALS AND WORKING MY WAY UP TO MORE AMBITIOUS TASKS.
13
PUT VERY SIMPLY, THE TRICK TO BEATING PANIC ATTACKS IS TO NOT REWARD THE PANIC BY GIVING IN TO IT, TO REALISE THAT IT WILL EVENTUALLY PASS AND TO WORK THROUGH IT.
SO, IF I WAS OUT SOMEWHERE AND A WAVE OF PANIC BEGAN TO SWEEP OVER ME, AND MY BODY STARTED SCREAMING AT ME, BEGGING ME TO TURN AROUND AND RUN BACK HOME...
OH, GOD. THERE GO MY BOWELS.
INSTEAD OF TURNING AND RUNNING, WHICH WOULD ONLY REINFORCE THE IDEA THAT RUNNING AWAY IS THE BEST WAY TO AVOID PANIC, I WOULD INSTEAD SLOW DOWN A BIT OR STOP WALKING ENTIRELY FOR A LITTLE WHILE.
SOON, THE PANIC ATTACK WOULD PASS, AND THEN I WOULD CARRY ON.
PHEW!
OBVIOUSLY, AFTER YEARS OF AVOIDING GOING OUT, THIS WASN'T HALF AS EASY AS IT SOUNDS AND IT WAS A VERY SLOW PROCESS.
I'LL JUST GO A BIT FURTHER, THEN I'LL CALL IT A DAY.

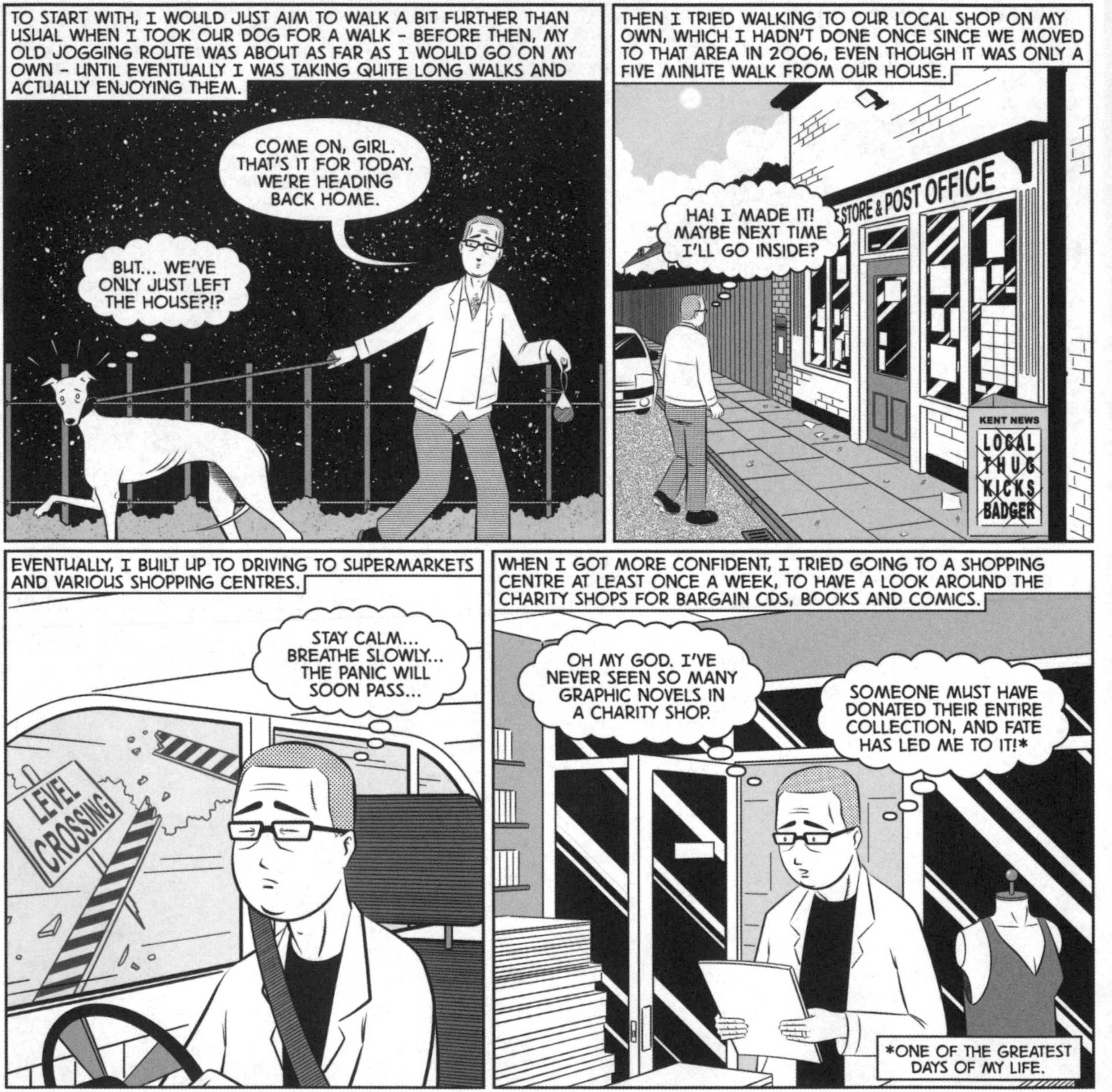

TO START WITH, I WOULD JUST AIM TO WALK A BIT FURTHER THAN USUAL WHEN I TOOK OUR DOG FOR A WALK - BEFORE THEN, MY OLD JOGGING ROUTE WAS ABOUT AS FAR AS I WOULD GO ON MY OWN - UNTIL EVENTUALLY I WAS TAKING QUITE LONG WALKS AND ACTUALLY ENJOYING THEM.
COME ON, GIRL. THAT'S IT FOR TODAY. WE'RE HEADING BACK HOME.
BUT... WE'VE ONLY JUST LEFT THE HOUSE?!?
THEN I TRIED WALKING TO OUR LOCAL SHOP ON MY OWN, WHICH I HADN'T DONE ONCE SINCE WE MOVED TO THAT AREA IN 2006, EVEN THOUGH IT WAS ONLY A FIVE MINUTE WALK FROM OUR HOUSE.
STORE & POST OFFICE
HA! I MADE IT! MAYBE NEXT TIME I'LL GO INSIDE?
KENT NEWS
LOCAL THUG KICKS BADGER
EVENTUALLY, I BUILT UP TO DRIVING TO SUPERMARKETS AND VARIOUS SHOPPING CENTRES.
STAY CALM... BREATHE SLOWLY... THE PANIC WILL SOON PASS...
LEVEL CROSSING
WHEN I GOT MORE CONFIDENT, I TRIED GOING TO A SHOPPING CENTRE AT LEAST ONCE A WEEK, TO HAVE A LOOK AROUND THE CHARITY SHOPS FOR BARGAIN CDS, BOOKS AND COMICS.
OH MY GOD. I'VE NEVER SEEN SO MANY GRAPHIC NOVELS IN A CHARITY SHOP.
SOMEONE MUST HAVE DONATED THEIR ENTIRE COLLECTION, AND FATE HAS LED ME TO IT!*
*ONE OF THE GREATEST DAYS OF MY LIFE.

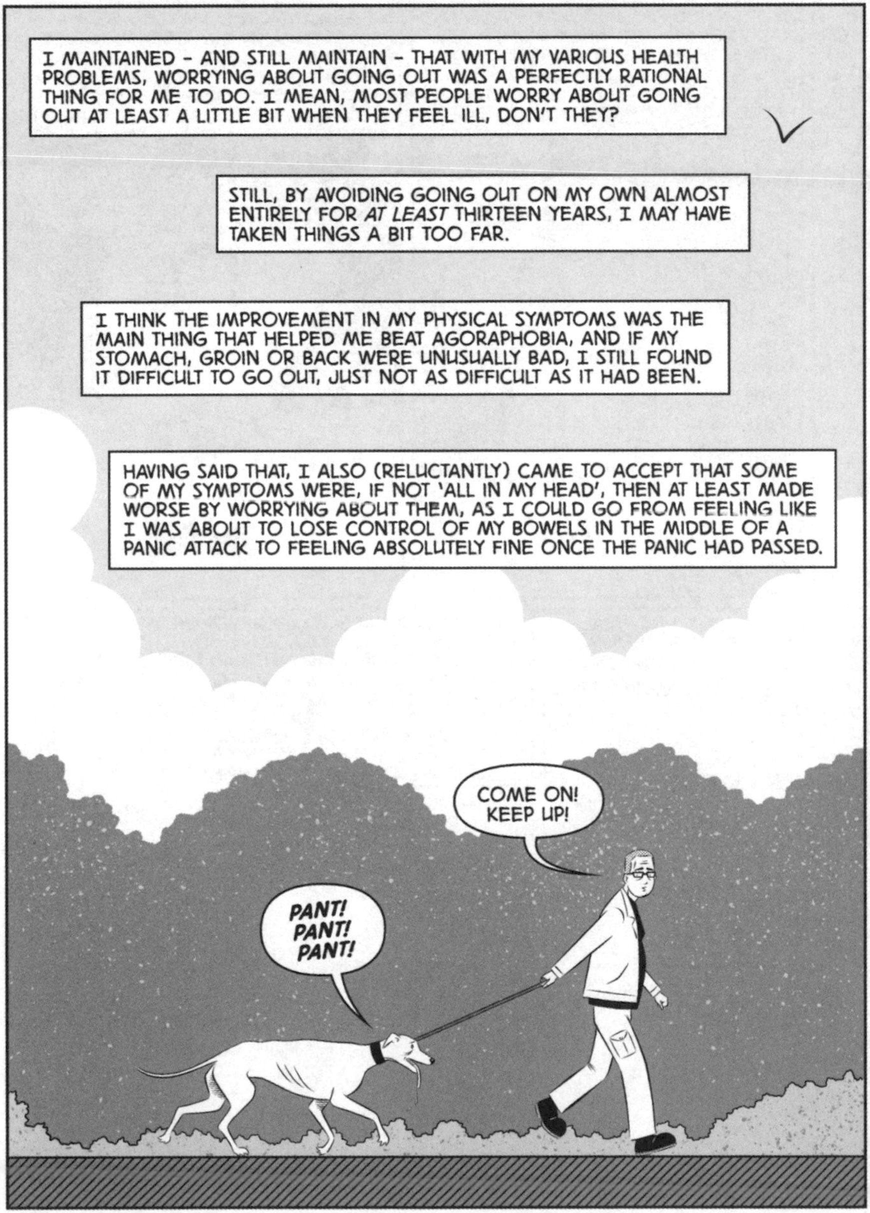
I MAINTAINED - AND STILL MAINTAIN - THAT WITH MY VARIOUS HEALTH PROBLEMS, WORRYING ABOUT GOING OUT WAS A PERFECTLY RATIONAL THING FOR ME TO DO. I MEAN, MOST PEOPLE WORRY ABOUT GOING OUT AT LEAST A LITTLE BIT WHEN THEY FEEL ILL, DON'T THEY?
STILL, BY AVOIDING GOING OUT ON MY OWN ALMOST ENTIRELY FOR *AT LEAST* THIRTEEN YEARS, I MAY HAVE TAKEN THINGS A BIT TOO FAR.
I THINK THE IMPROVEMENT IN MY PHYSICAL SYMPTOMS WAS THE MAIN THING THAT HELPED ME BEAT AGORAPHOBIA, AND IF MY STOMACH, GROIN OR BACK WERE UNUSUALLY BAD, I STILL FOUND IT DIFFICULT TO GO OUT, JUST NOT AS DIFFICULT AS IT HAD BEEN.
HAVING SAID THAT, I ALSO (RELUCTANTLY) CAME TO ACCEPT THAT SOME OF MY SYMPTOMS WERE, IF NOT 'ALL IN MY HEAD', THEN AT LEAST MADE WORSE BY WORRYING ABOUT THEM, AS I COULD GO FROM FEELING LIKE I WAS ABOUT TO LOSE CONTROL OF MY BOWELS IN THE MIDDLE OF A PANIC ATTACK TO FEELING ABSOLUTELY FINE ONCE THE PANIC HAD PASSED.
COME ON! KEEP UP!
PANT! PANT! PANT!

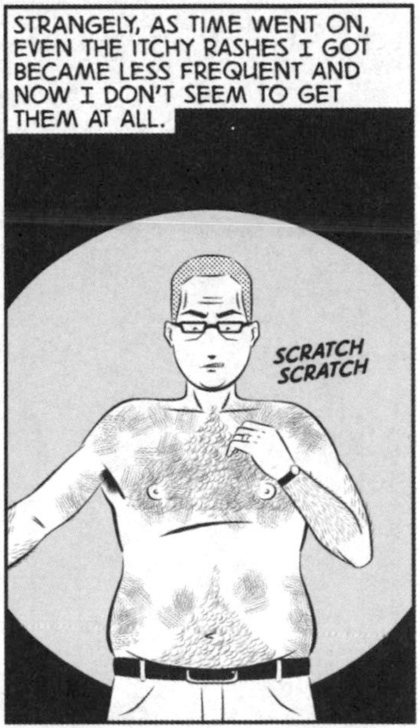
STRANGELY, AS TIME WENT ON, EVEN THE ITCHY RASHES I GOT BECAME LESS FREQUENT AND NOW I DON'T SEEM TO GET THEM AT ALL.
SCRATCH SCRATCH

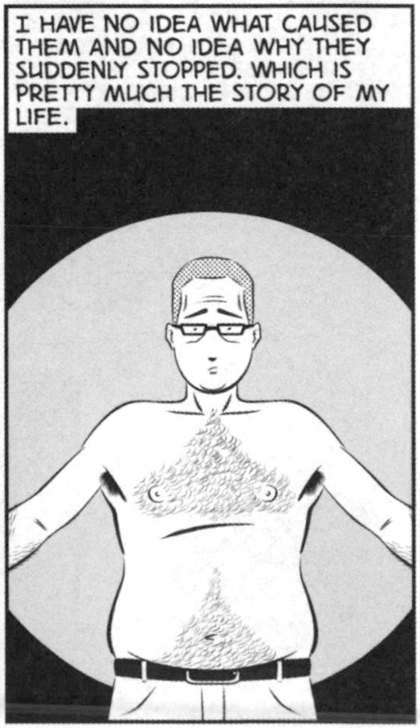
I HAVE NO IDEA WHAT CAUSED THEM AND NO IDEA WHY THEY SUDDENLY STOPPED. WHICH IS PRETTY MUCH THE STORY OF MY LIFE.

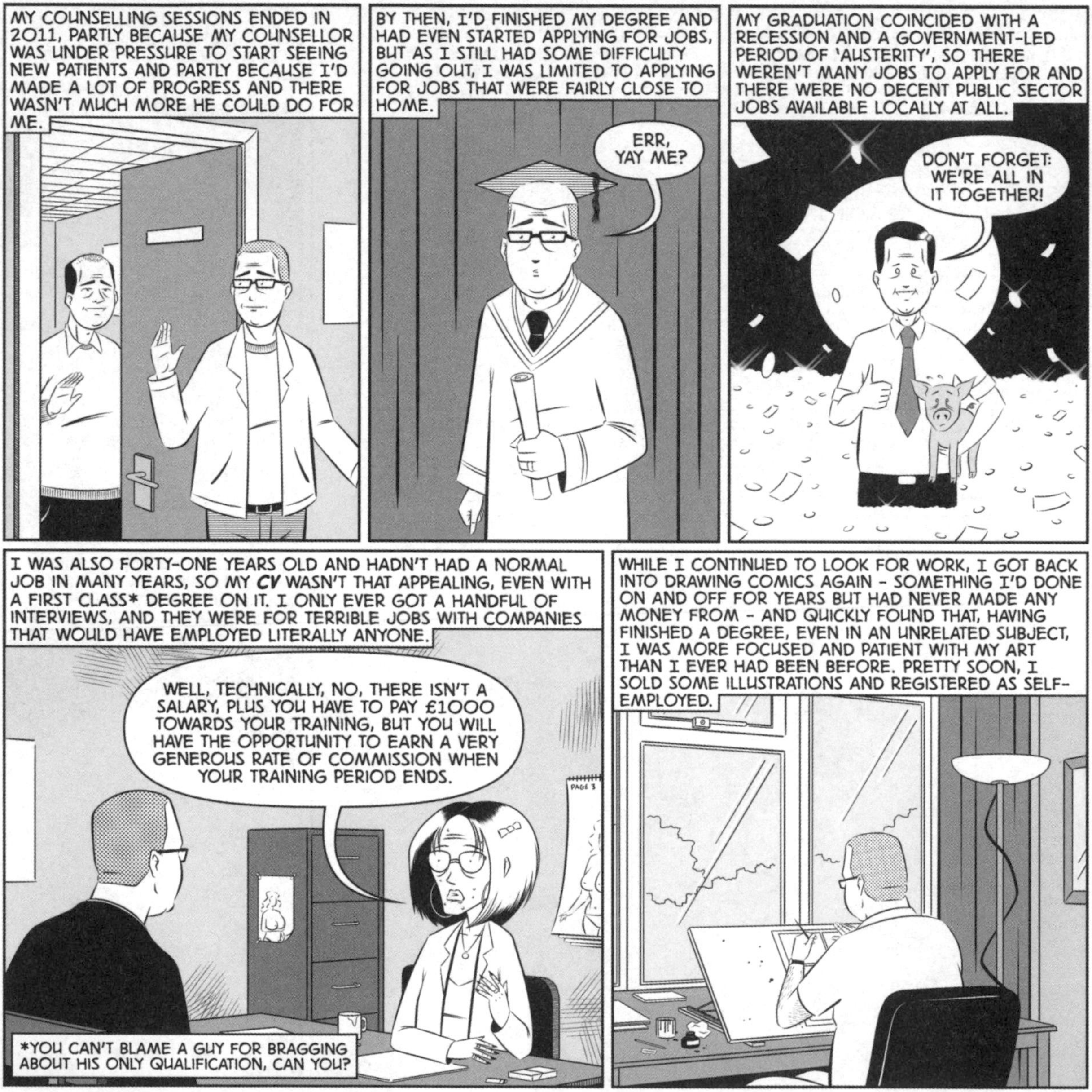
MY COUNSELLING SESSIONS ENDED IN 2011, PARTLY BECAUSE MY COUNSELLOR WAS UNDER PRESSURE TO START SEEING NEW PATIENTS AND PARTLY BECAUSE I'D MADE A LOT OF PROGRESS AND THERE WASN'T MUCH MORE HE COULD DO FOR ME.
BY THEN, I'D FINISHED MY DEGREE AND HAD EVEN STARTED APPLYING FOR JOBS, BUT AS I STILL HAD SOME DIFFICULTY GOING OUT, I WAS LIMITED TO APPLYING FOR JOBS THAT WERE FAIRLY CLOSE TO HOME.
ERR, YAY ME?
MY GRADUATION COINCIDED WITH A RECESSION AND A GOVERNMENT-LED PERIOD OF 'AUSTERITY', SO THERE WEREN'T MANY JOBS TO APPLY FOR AND THERE WERE NO DECENT PUBLIC SECTOR JOBS AVAILABLE LOCALLY AT ALL.
DON'T FORGET: WE'RE ALL IN IT TOGETHER!
I WAS ALSO FORTY-ONE YEARS OLD AND HADN'T HAD A NORMAL JOB IN MANY YEARS, SO MY ***CV*** WASN'T THAT APPEALING, EVEN WITH A FIRST CLASS* DEGREE ON IT. I ONLY EVER GOT A HANDFUL OF INTERVIEWS, AND THEY WERE FOR TERRIBLE JOBS WITH COMPANIES THAT WOULD HAVE EMPLOYED LITERALLY ANYONE.
WELL, TECHNICALLY, NO, THERE ISN'T A SALARY, PLUS YOU HAVE TO PAY £1000 TOWARDS YOUR TRAINING, BUT YOU WILL HAVE THE OPPORTUNITY TO EARN A VERY GENEROUS RATE OF COMMISSION WHEN YOUR TRAINING PERIOD ENDS.
PAGE 3
*YOU CAN'T BLAME A GUY FOR BRAGGING ABOUT HIS ONLY QUALIFICATION, CAN YOU?
WHILE I CONTINUED TO LOOK FOR WORK, I GOT BACK INTO DRAWING COMICS AGAIN - SOMETHING I'D DONE ON AND OFF FOR YEARS BUT HAD NEVER MADE ANY MONEY FROM - AND QUICKLY FOUND THAT, HAVING FINISHED A DEGREE, EVEN IN AN UNRELATED SUBJECT, I WAS MORE FOCUSED AND PATIENT WITH MY ART THAN I EVER HAD BEEN BEFORE. PRETTY SOON, I SOLD SOME ILLUSTRATIONS AND REGISTERED AS SELF-EMPLOYED.

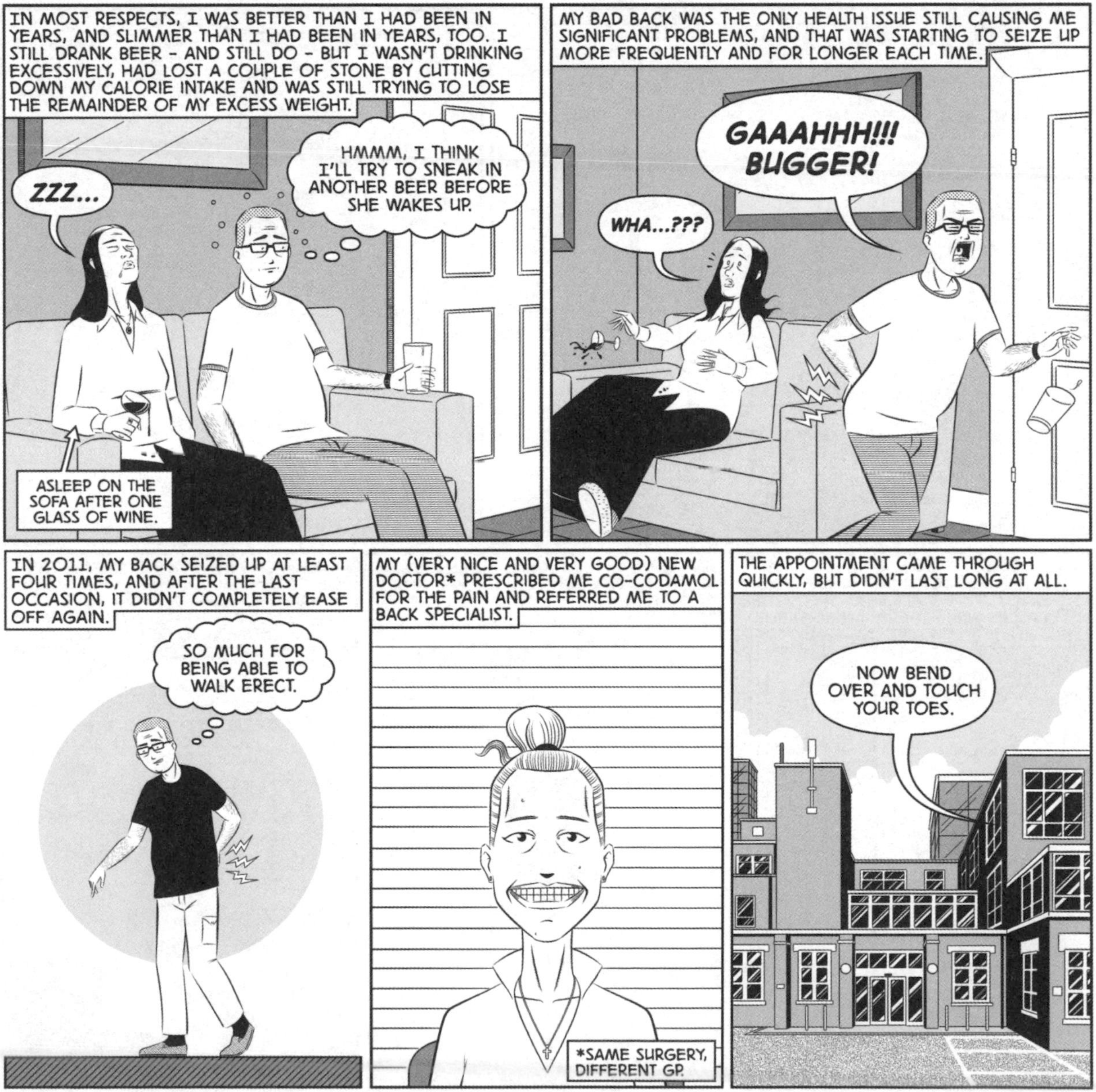
IN MOST RESPECTS, I WAS BETTER THAN I HAD BEEN IN YEARS, AND SLIMMER THAN I HAD BEEN IN YEARS, TOO. I STILL DRANK BEER - AND STILL DO - BUT I WASN'T DRINKING EXCESSIVELY, HAD LOST A COUPLE OF STONE BY CUTTING DOWN MY CALORIE INTAKE AND WAS STILL TRYING TO LOSE THE REMAINDER OF MY EXCESS WEIGHT.
ZZZ...
HMMM, I THINK I'LL TRY TO SNEAK IN ANOTHER BEER BEFORE SHE WAKES UP.
ASLEEP ON THE SOFA AFTER ONE GLASS OF WINE.
MY BAD BACK WAS THE ONLY HEALTH ISSUE STILL CAUSING ME SIGNIFICANT PROBLEMS, AND THAT WAS STARTING TO SEIZE UP MORE FREQUENTLY AND FOR LONGER EACH TIME.
GAAAHHH!!! BUGGER!
WHA...???
IN 2011, MY BACK SEIZED UP AT LEAST FOUR TIMES, AND AFTER THE LAST OCCASION, IT DIDN'T COMPLETELY EASE OFF AGAIN.
SO MUCH FOR BEING ABLE TO WALK ERECT.
MY (VERY NICE AND VERY GOOD) NEW DOCTOR* PRESCRIBED ME CO-CODAMOL FOR THE PAIN AND REFERRED ME TO A BACK SPECIALIST.
*SAME SURGERY, DIFFERENT GP.
THE APPOINTMENT CAME THROUGH QUICKLY, BUT DIDN'T LAST LONG AT ALL.
NOW BEND OVER AND TOUCH YOUR TOES.

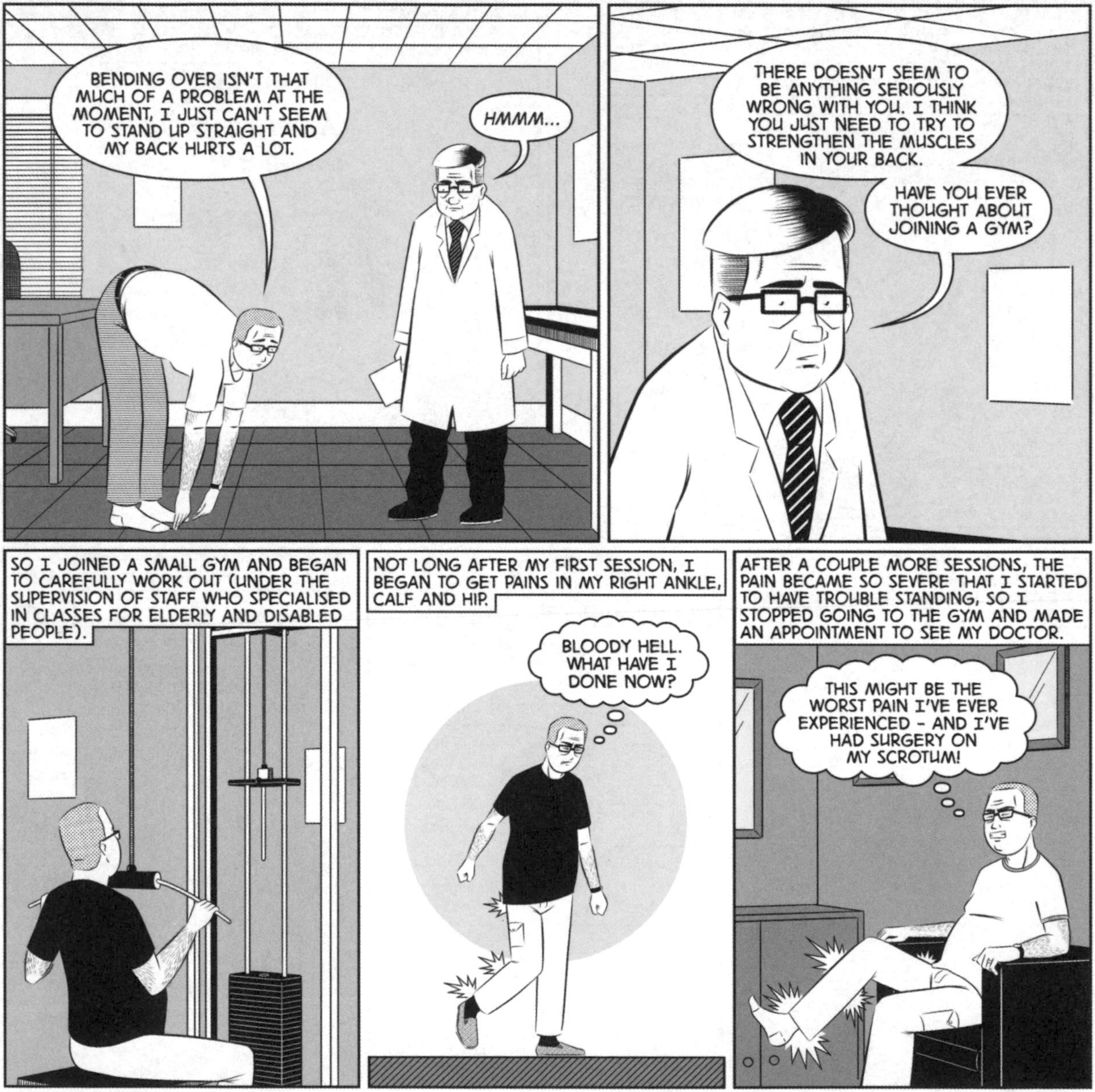
BENDING OVER ISN'T THAT MUCH OF A PROBLEM AT THE MOMENT, I JUST CAN'T SEEM TO STAND UP STRAIGHT AND MY BACK HURTS A LOT.
HMMM...
THERE DOESN'T SEEM TO BE ANYTHING SERIOUSLY WRONG WITH YOU. I THINK YOU JUST NEED TO TRY TO STRENGTHEN THE MUSCLES IN YOUR BACK.
HAVE YOU EVER THOUGHT ABOUT JOINING A GYM?
SO I JOINED A SMALL GYM AND BEGAN TO CAREFULLY WORK OUT (UNDER THE SUPERVISION OF STAFF WHO SPECIALISED IN CLASSES FOR ELDERLY AND DISABLED PEOPLE).
NOT LONG AFTER MY FIRST SESSION, I BEGAN TO GET PAINS IN MY RIGHT ANKLE, CALF AND HIP.
BLOODY HELL. WHAT HAVE I DONE NOW?
AFTER A COUPLE MORE SESSIONS, THE PAIN BECAME SO SEVERE THAT I STARTED TO HAVE TROUBLE STANDING, SO I STOPPED GOING TO THE GYM AND MADE AN APPOINTMENT TO SEE MY DOCTOR.
THIS MIGHT BE THE WORST PAIN I'VE EVER EXPERIENCED - AND I'VE HAD SURGERY ON MY SCROTUM!

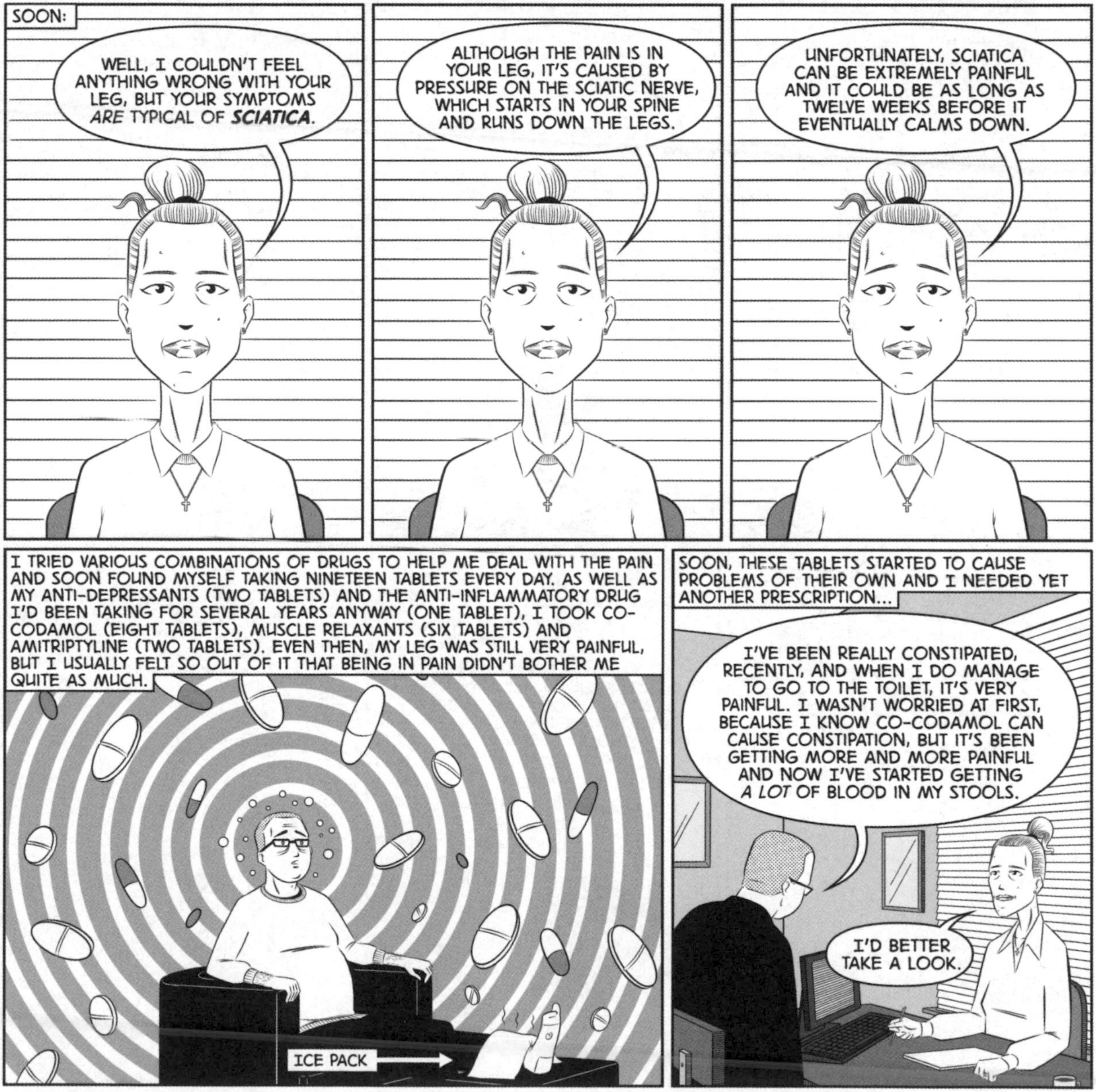
SOON:
WELL, I COULDN'T FEEL ANYTHING WRONG WITH YOUR LEG, BUT YOUR SYMPTOMS *ARE* TYPICAL OF ***SCIATICA***.
ALTHOUGH THE PAIN IS IN YOUR LEG, IT'S CAUSED BY PRESSURE ON THE SCIATIC NERVE, WHICH STARTS IN YOUR SPINE AND RUNS DOWN THE LEGS.
UNFORTUNATELY, SCIATICA CAN BE EXTREMELY PAINFUL AND IT COULD BE AS LONG AS TWELVE WEEKS BEFORE IT EVENTUALLY CALMS DOWN.
I TRIED VARIOUS COMBINATIONS OF DRUGS TO HELP ME DEAL WITH THE PAIN AND SOON FOUND MYSELF TAKING NINETEEN TABLETS EVERY DAY. AS WELL AS MY ANTI-DEPRESSANTS (TWO TABLETS) AND THE ANTI-INFLAMMATORY DRUG I'D BEEN TAKING FOR SEVERAL YEARS ANYWAY (ONE TABLET), I TOOK CO-CODAMOL (EIGHT TABLETS), MUSCLE RELAXANTS (SIX TABLETS) AND AMITRIPTYLINE (TWO TABLETS). EVEN THEN, MY LEG WAS STILL VERY PAINFUL, BUT I USUALLY FELT SO OUT OF IT THAT BEING IN PAIN DIDN'T BOTHER ME QUITE AS MUCH.
ICE PACK
SOON, THESE TABLETS STARTED TO CAUSE PROBLEMS OF THEIR OWN AND I NEEDED YET ANOTHER PRESCRIPTION...
I'VE BEEN REALLY CONSTIPATED, RECENTLY, AND WHEN I DO MANAGE TO GO TO THE TOILET, IT'S VERY PAINFUL. I WASN'T WORRIED AT FIRST, BECAUSE I KNOW CO-CODAMOL CAN CAUSE CONSTIPATION, BUT IT'S BEEN GETTING MORE AND MORE PAINFUL AND NOW I'VE STARTED GETTING *A LOT* OF BLOOD IN MY STOOLS.
I'D BETTER TAKE A LOOK.

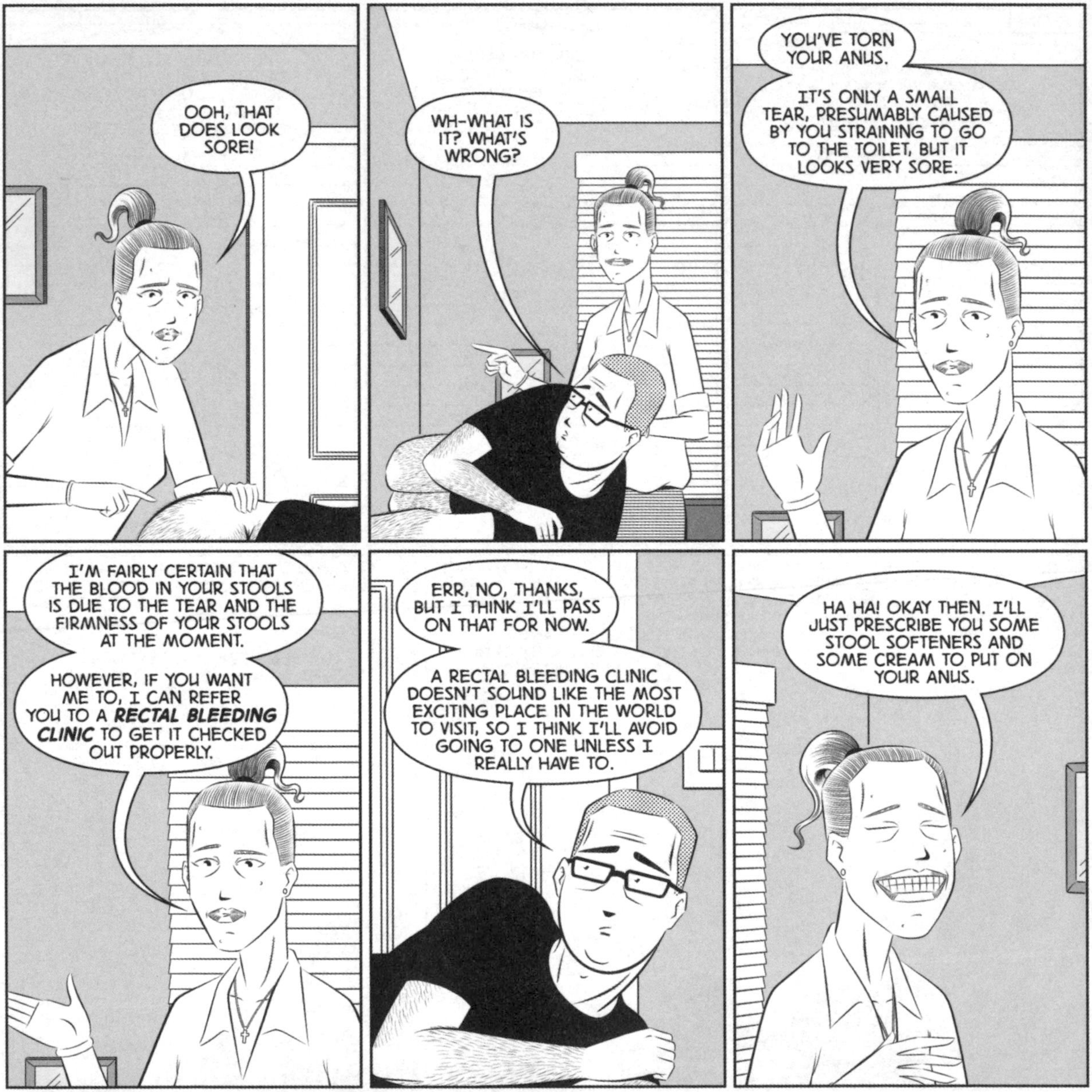
OOH, THAT DOES LOOK SORE!
WH-WHAT IS IT? WHAT'S WRONG?
YOU'VE TORN YOUR ANUS.
IT'S ONLY A SMALL TEAR, PRESUMABLY CAUSED BY YOU STRAINING TO GO TO THE TOILET, BUT IT LOOKS VERY SORE.
I'M FAIRLY CERTAIN THAT THE BLOOD IN YOUR STOOLS IS DUE TO THE TEAR AND THE FIRMNESS OF YOUR STOOLS AT THE MOMENT.
HOWEVER, IF YOU WANT ME TO, I CAN REFER YOU TO A ***RECTAL BLEEDING CLINIC*** TO GET IT CHECKED OUT PROPERLY.
ERR, NO, THANKS, BUT I THINK I'LL PASS ON THAT FOR NOW.
A RECTAL BLEEDING CLINIC DOESN'T SOUND LIKE THE MOST EXCITING PLACE IN THE WORLD TO VISIT, SO I THINK I'LL AVOID GOING TO ONE UNLESS I REALLY HAVE TO.
HA HA! OKAY THEN. I'LL JUST PRESCRIBE YOU SOME STOOL SOFTENERS AND SOME CREAM TO PUT ON YOUR ANUS.

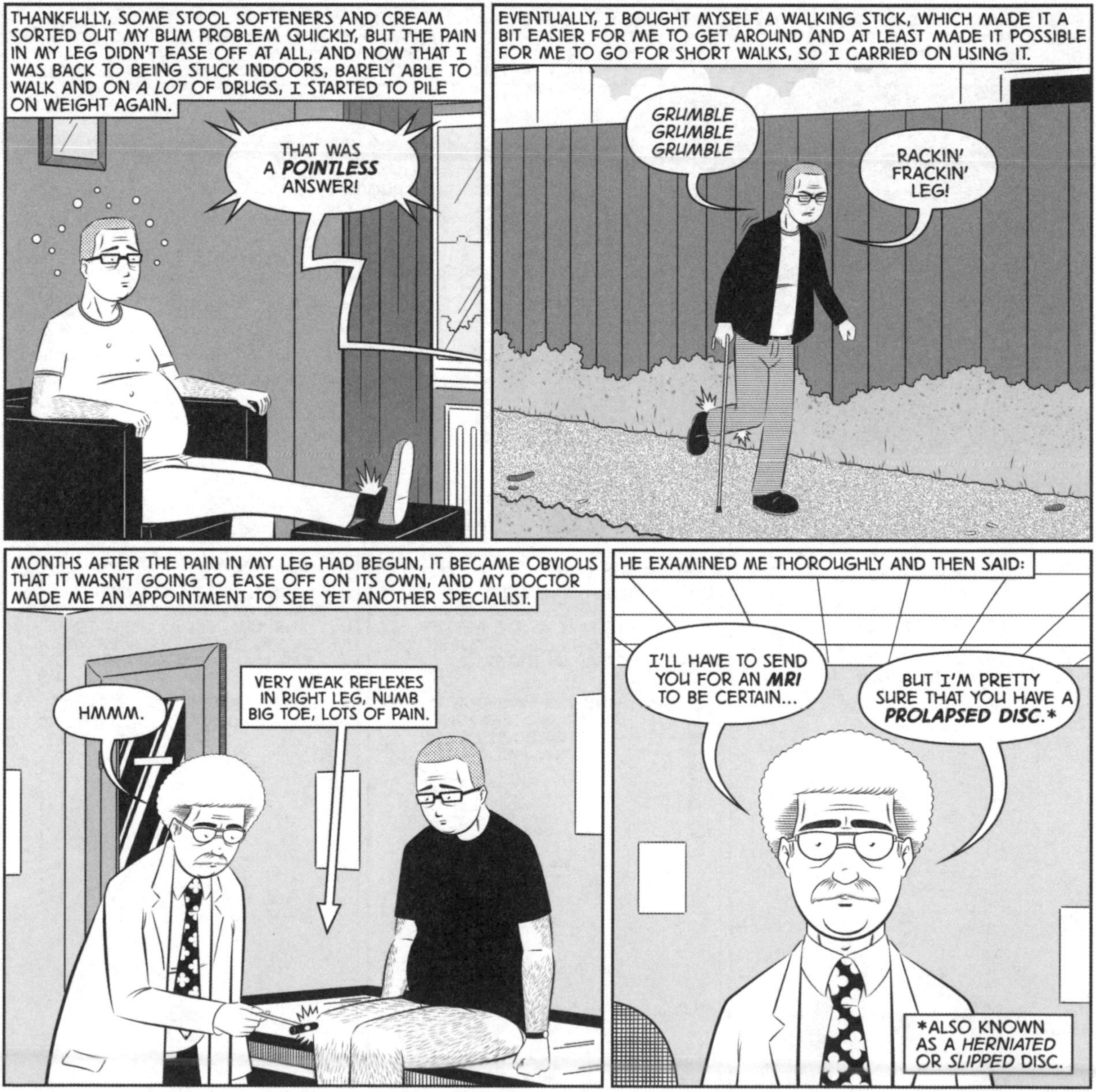
THANKFULLY, SOME STOOL SOFTENERS AND CREAM SORTED OUT MY BUM PROBLEM QUICKLY, BUT THE PAIN IN MY LEG DIDN'T EASE OFF AT ALL, AND NOW THAT I WAS BACK TO BEING STUCK INDOORS, BARELY ABLE TO WALK AND ON *A LOT* OF DRUGS, I STARTED TO PILE ON WEIGHT AGAIN.
THAT WAS A ***POINTLESS*** ANSWER!
EVENTUALLY, I BOUGHT MYSELF A WALKING STICK, WHICH MADE IT A BIT EASIER FOR ME TO GET AROUND AND AT LEAST MADE IT POSSIBLE FOR ME TO GO FOR SHORT WALKS, SO I CARRIED ON USING IT.
GRUMBLE GRUMBLE GRUMBLE
RACKIN' FRACKIN' LEG!
MONTHS AFTER THE PAIN IN MY LEG HAD BEGUN, IT BECAME OBVIOUS THAT IT WASN'T GOING TO EASE OFF ON ITS OWN, AND MY DOCTOR MADE ME AN APPOINTMENT TO SEE YET ANOTHER SPECIALIST.
HMMM.
VERY WEAK REFLEXES IN RIGHT LEG, NUMB BIG TOE, LOTS OF PAIN.
HE EXAMINED ME THOROUGHLY AND THEN SAID:
I'LL HAVE TO SEND YOU FOR AN ***MRI*** TO BE CERTAIN...
BUT I'M PRETTY SURE THAT YOU HAVE A ***PROLAPSED DISC***.*
*ALSO KNOWN AS A *HERNIATED* OR *SLIPPED* DISC.

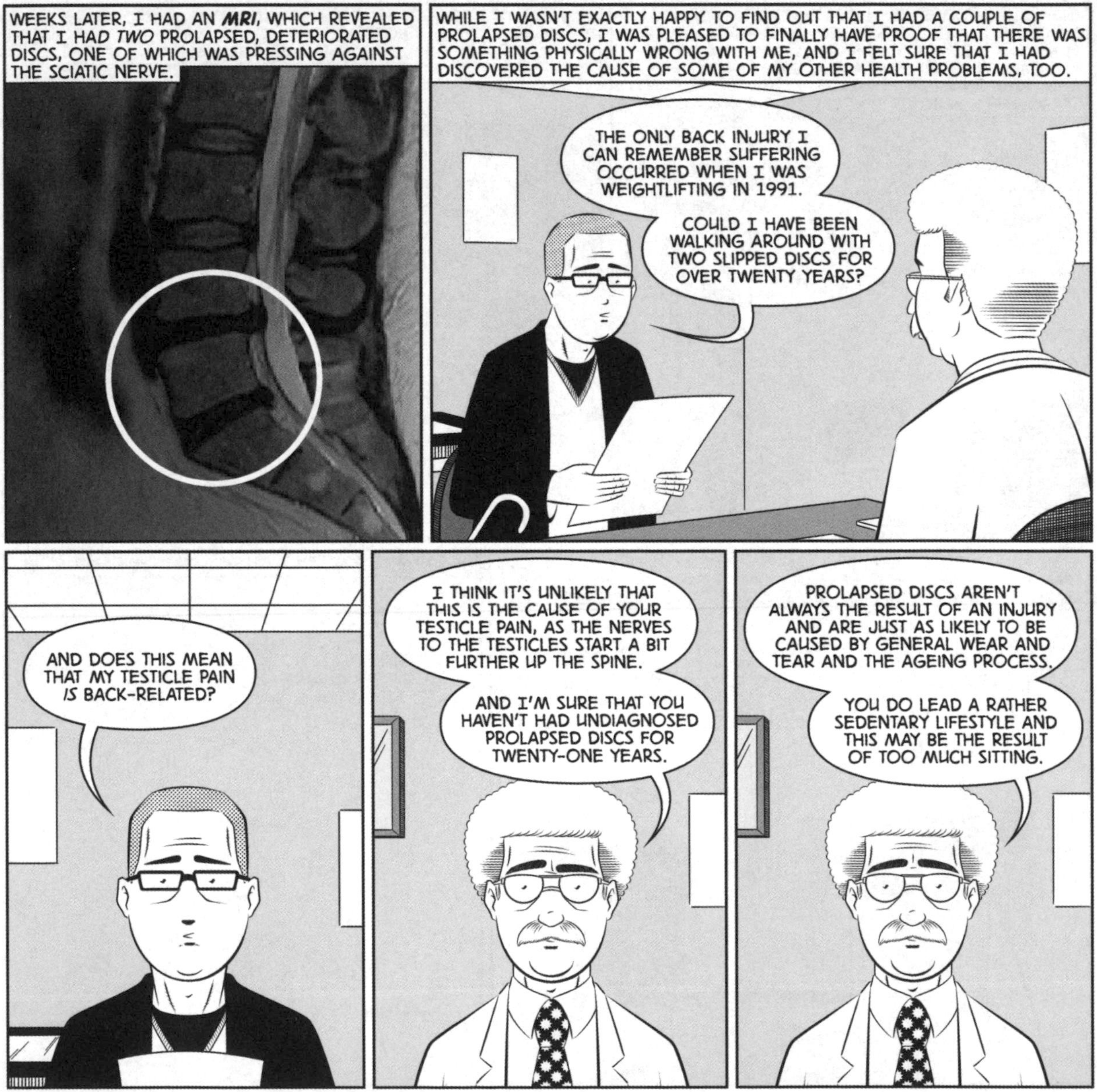
WEEKS LATER, I HAD AN *MRI*, WHICH REVEALED THAT I HAD *TWO* PROLAPSED, DETERIORATED DISCS, ONE OF WHICH WAS PRESSING AGAINST THE SCIATIC NERVE.
WHILE I WASN'T EXACTLY HAPPY TO FIND OUT THAT I HAD A COUPLE OF PROLAPSED DISCS, I WAS PLEASED TO FINALLY HAVE PROOF THAT THERE WAS SOMETHING PHYSICALLY WRONG WITH ME, AND I FELT SURE THAT I HAD DISCOVERED THE CAUSE OF SOME OF MY OTHER HEALTH PROBLEMS, TOO.
THE ONLY BACK INJURY I CAN REMEMBER SUFFERING OCCURRED WHEN I WAS WEIGHTLIFTING IN 1991.
COULD I HAVE BEEN WALKING AROUND WITH TWO SLIPPED DISCS FOR OVER TWENTY YEARS?
AND DOES THIS MEAN THAT MY TESTICLE PAIN *IS* BACK-RELATED?
I THINK IT'S UNLIKELY THAT THIS IS THE CAUSE OF YOUR TESTICLE PAIN, AS THE NERVES TO THE TESTICLES START A BIT FURTHER UP THE SPINE.
AND I'M SURE THAT YOU HAVEN'T HAD UNDIAGNOSED PROLAPSED DISCS FOR TWENTY-ONE YEARS.
PROLAPSED DISCS AREN'T ALWAYS THE RESULT OF AN INJURY AND ARE JUST AS LIKELY TO BE CAUSED BY GENERAL WEAR AND TEAR AND THE AGEING PROCESS.
YOU DO LEAD A RATHER SEDENTARY LIFESTYLE AND THIS MAY BE THE RESULT OF TOO MUCH SITTING.

I WAS PUT ON A WAITING LIST FOR SPINAL SURGERY, TO HAVE PART OF THE BULGING PROLAPSED DISCS CUT AWAY AND SOME OF THE BONE AROUND THE DISCS REMOVED TO TAKE THE PRESSURE OFF OF THEM. I WAS ALSO SENT BACK TO MY LOCAL PAIN CLINIC FOR EVEN MORE INJECTIONS INTO MY SPINE, WHICH HELPED REDUCE THE PAIN TO A MORE MANAGEABLE LEVEL.

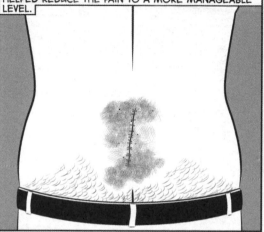

ALTHOUGH I STILL NEEDED TO USE A WALKING STICK, I CONTINUED TO TRY TO GET OUT AND ABOUT, WITH NO RETURN OF MY PANIC ATTACKS, WHILE I WAITED FOR A DATE FOR THE OPERATION TO COME THROUGH.

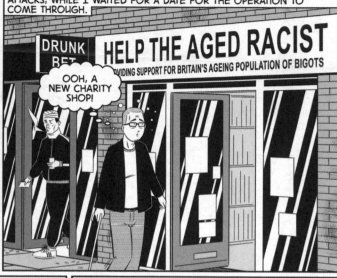

DRUNK BET

HELP THE AGED RACIST
...VIDING SUPPORT FOR BRITAIN'S AGEING POPULATION OF BIGOTS

OOH, A NEW CHARITY SHOP!

I EVENTUALLY HAD THE OPERATION IN MAY 2013. BECAUSE I HAD BEEN WAITING A LONG TIME AND BECAUSE THE HOSPITAL I WAS ATTENDING WAS UNDER PRESSURE TO CLEAR ITS LONG WAITING LISTS, I WAS OFFERED THE OPPORTUNITY TO HAVE IT DONE IN A POSH PRIVATE HOSPITAL IN CENTRAL LONDON, FULLY PAID FOR BY THE *NHS*.

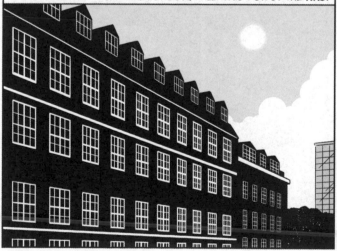

THAT SUITED ME FINE, AS I HAD A PRIVATE ROOM, AN EN-SUITE BATHROOM AND A TV WITH MOVIES ON DEMAND. IT WAS LIKE BEING IN A HOTEL.

THERE'S LOADS OF FILMS I HAVEN'T SEEN YET ON HERE. WITH ANY LUCK, THEY'LL NEED TO KEEP ME IN FOR AN EXTRA COUPLE OF DAYS.

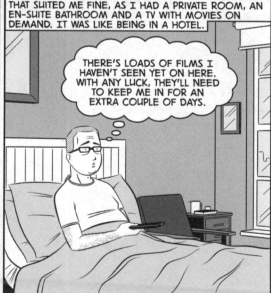

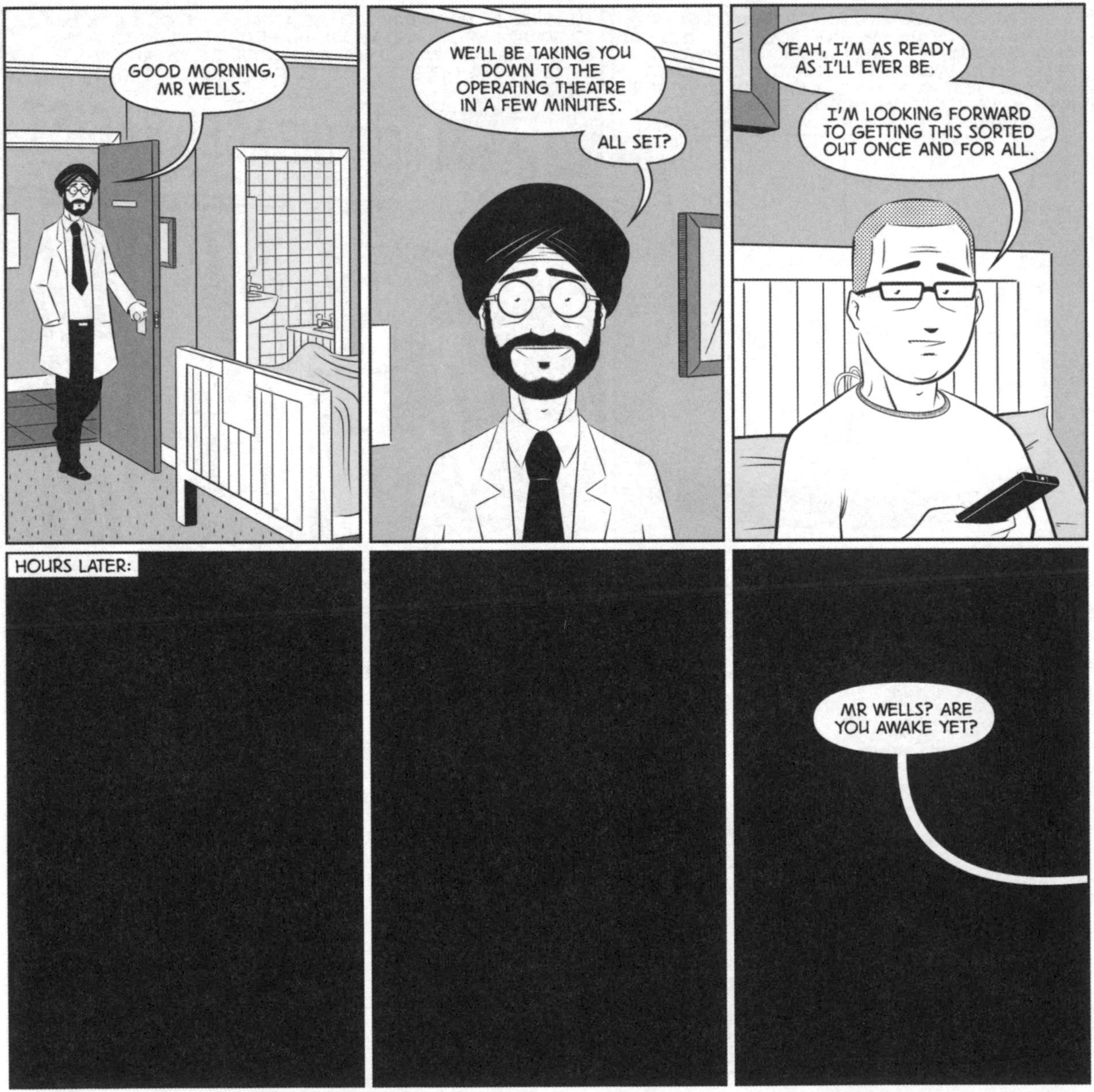
GOOD MORNING, MR WELLS.
WE'LL BE TAKING YOU DOWN TO THE OPERATING THEATRE IN A FEW MINUTES.
ALL SET?
YEAH, I'M AS READY AS I'LL EVER BE.
I'M LOOKING FORWARD TO GETTING THIS SORTED OUT ONCE AND FOR ALL.
HOURS LATER:
MR WELLS? ARE YOU AWAKE YET?

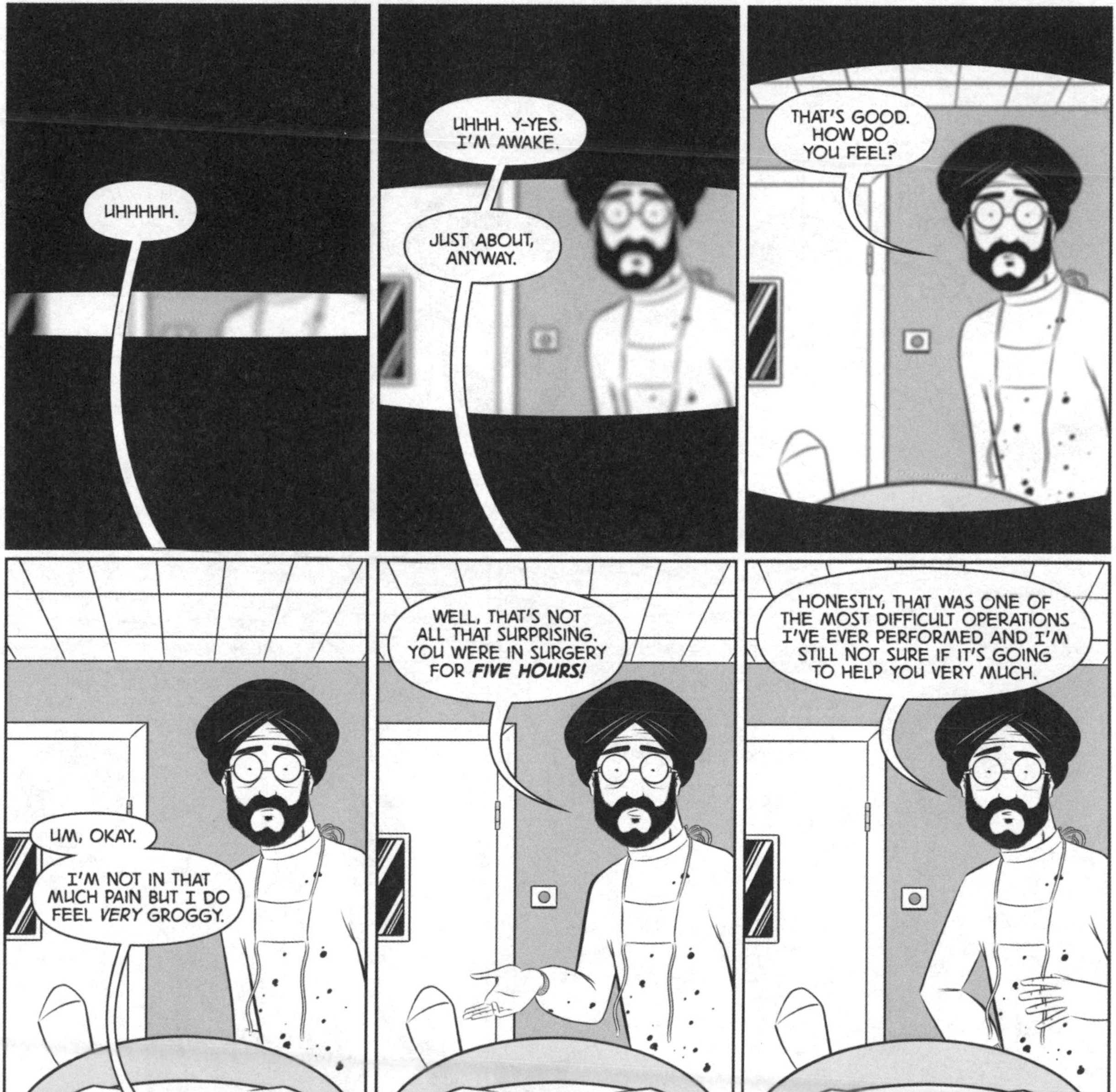
UHHHHH.
UHHH. Y-YES. I'M AWAKE.
JUST ABOUT, ANYWAY.
THAT'S GOOD. HOW DO YOU FEEL?
UM, OKAY.
I'M NOT IN THAT MUCH PAIN BUT I DO FEEL *VERY* GROGGY.
WELL, THAT'S NOT ALL THAT SURPRISING. YOU WERE IN SURGERY FOR ***FIVE HOURS!***
HONESTLY, THAT WAS ONE OF THE MOST DIFFICULT OPERATIONS I'VE EVER PERFORMED AND I'M STILL NOT SURE IF IT'S GOING TO HELP YOU VERY MUCH.

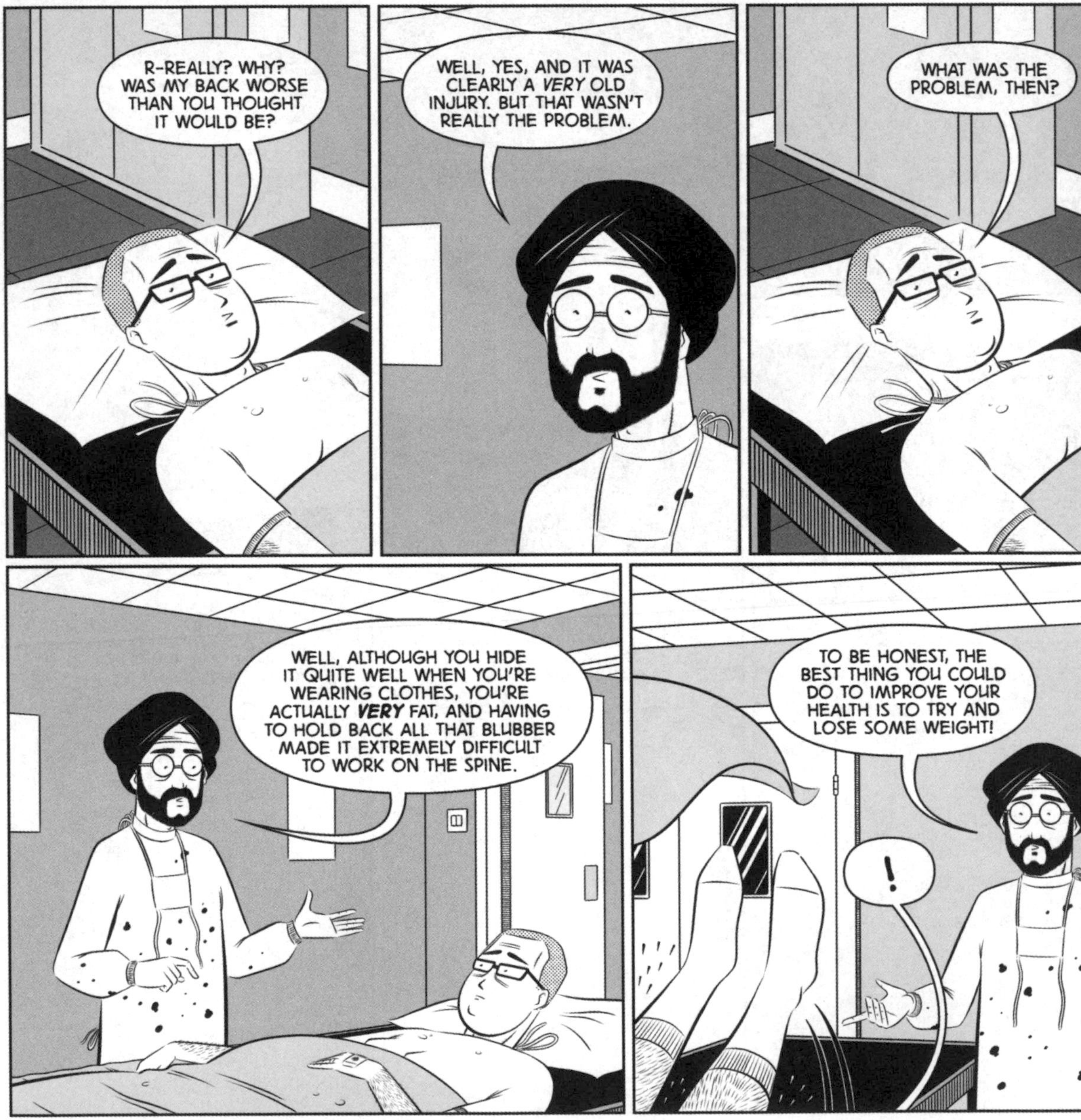
R-REALLY? WHY? WAS MY BACK WORSE THAN YOU THOUGHT IT WOULD BE?
WELL, YES, AND IT WAS CLEARLY A *VERY* OLD INJURY. BUT THAT WASN'T REALLY THE PROBLEM.
WHAT WAS THE PROBLEM, THEN?
WELL, ALTHOUGH YOU HIDE IT QUITE WELL WHEN YOU'RE WEARING CLOTHES, YOU'RE ACTUALLY **VERY** FAT, AND HAVING TO HOLD BACK ALL THAT BLUBBER MADE IT EXTREMELY DIFFICULT TO WORK ON THE SPINE.
TO BE HONEST, THE BEST THING YOU COULD DO TO IMPROVE YOUR HEALTH IS TO TRY AND LOSE SOME WEIGHT!
!

CONCLUSION:

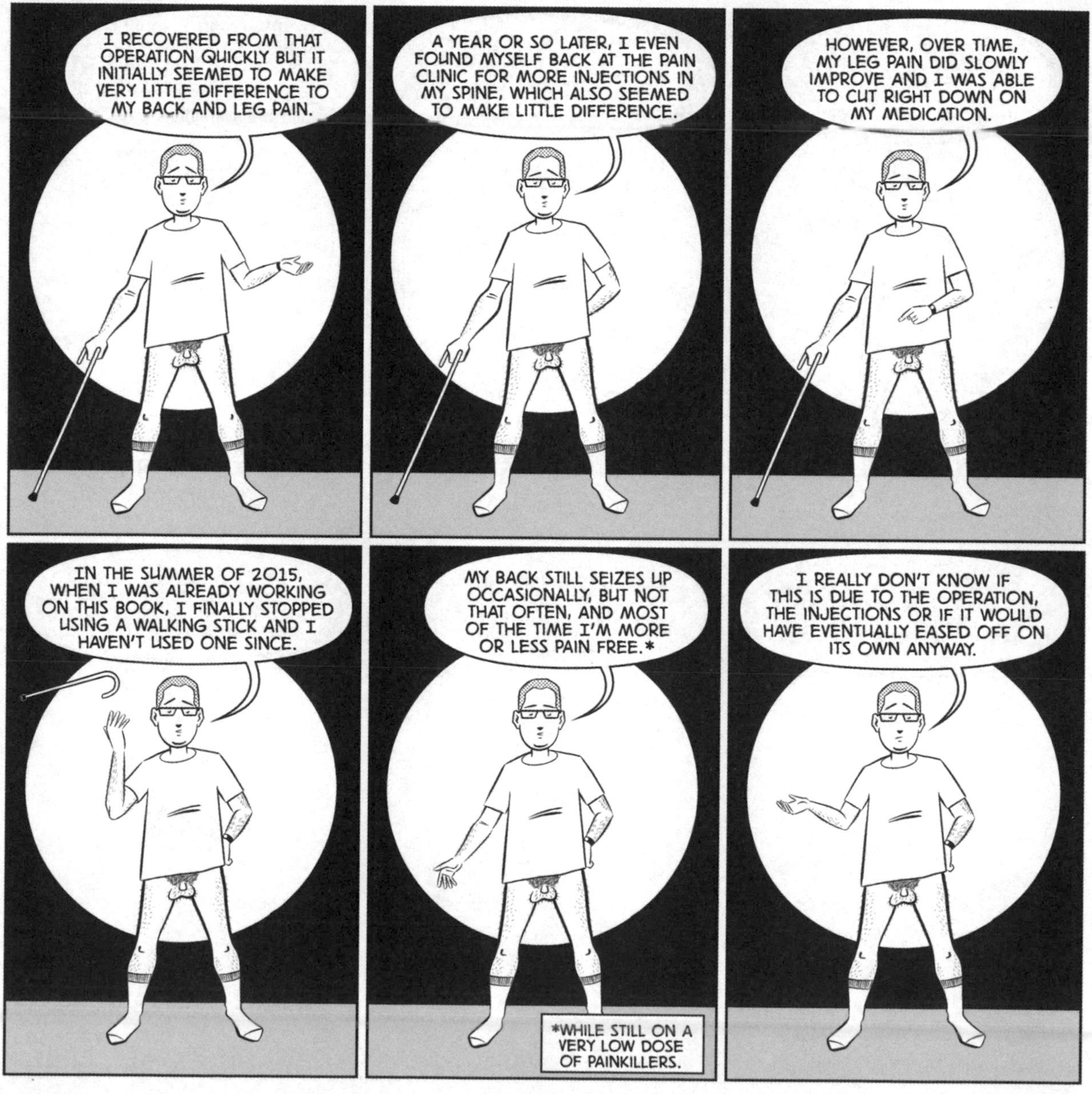
I RECOVERED FROM THAT OPERATION QUICKLY BUT IT INITIALLY SEEMED TO MAKE VERY LITTLE DIFFERENCE TO MY BACK AND LEG PAIN.
A YEAR OR SO LATER, I EVEN FOUND MYSELF BACK AT THE PAIN CLINIC FOR MORE INJECTIONS IN MY SPINE, WHICH ALSO SEEMED TO MAKE LITTLE DIFFERENCE.
HOWEVER, OVER TIME, MY LEG PAIN DID SLOWLY IMPROVE AND I WAS ABLE TO CUT RIGHT DOWN ON MY MEDICATION.
IN THE SUMMER OF 2015, WHEN I WAS ALREADY WORKING ON THIS BOOK, I FINALLY STOPPED USING A WALKING STICK AND I HAVEN'T USED ONE SINCE.
MY BACK STILL SEIZES UP OCCASIONALLY, BUT NOT THAT OFTEN, AND MOST OF THE TIME I'M MORE OR LESS PAIN FREE.*
*WHILE STILL ON A VERY LOW DOSE OF PAINKILLERS.
I REALLY DON'T KNOW IF THIS IS DUE TO THE OPERATION, THE INJECTIONS OR IF IT WOULD HAVE EVENTUALLY EASED OFF ON ITS OWN ANYWAY.

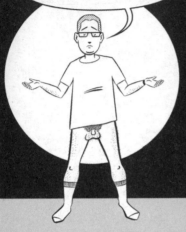

AS WITH MY OTHER HEALTH PROBLEMS, IT WAS PROBABLY A COMBINATION OF THINGS, AND I'M AFRAID I DON'T HAVE ANY CLEAR ANSWERS.

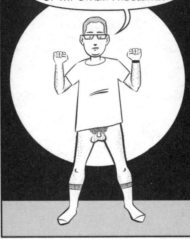

AT LEAST I HAVE A PRETTY GOOD IDEA WHAT *CAUSED* MY BACK PROBLEM, AS I HAVE NO IDEA WHAT CAUSED MOST OF MY OTHER PROBLEMS.

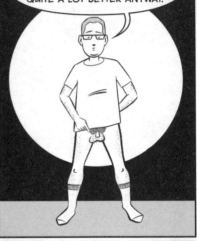

I STILL DON'T EVEN KNOW IF MY BACK AND GROIN PROBLEMS WERE RELATED. I MEAN, MY GROIN DIDN'T IMPROVE AFTER THAT BACK OPERATION, BUT BY THEN IT WAS QUITE A LOT BETTER ANYWAY.

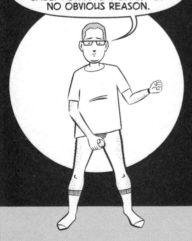

I STILL GET UNCOMFORTABLE 'DOWN THERE' QUITE OFTEN, AND EVERY NOW AND AGAIN MY OLD SYMPTOMS WILL FLARE UP BADLY FOR A FEW DAYS, FOR NO OBVIOUS REASON.

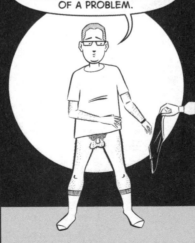

MOST OF THE TIME, THOUGH, AS LONG AS I HAVE REGULAR HOT BATHS AND DON'T OVERDO THINGS, IT ISN'T THAT MUCH OF A PROBLEM.

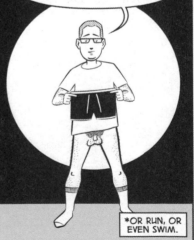

I STILL COULDN'T SIT ON A BICYCLE SEAT*, BUT AT LEAST I DON'T HAVE TROUBLE BUYING NEW UNDERWEAR ANYMORE.

*OR RUN, OR EVEN SWIM.

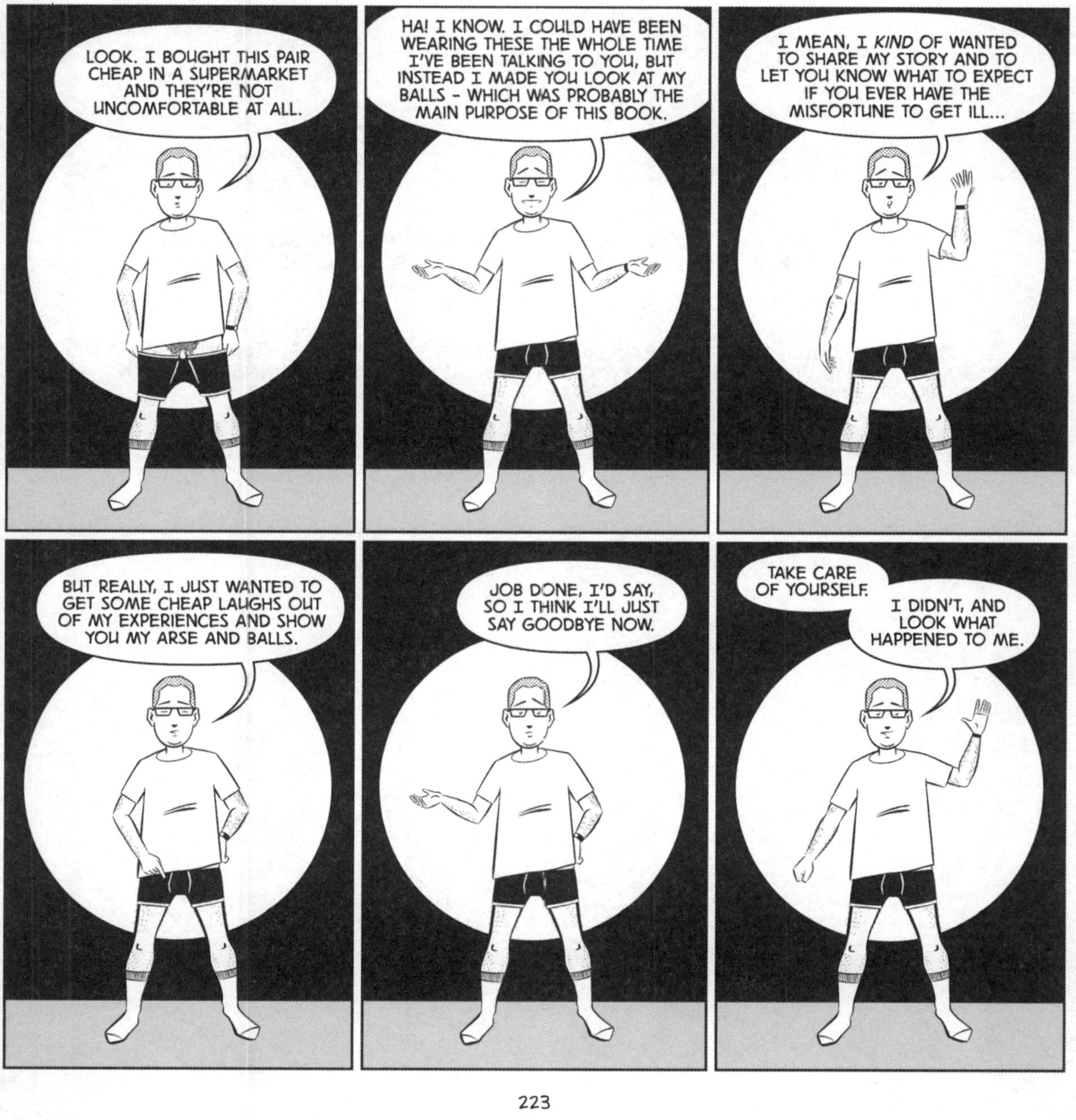
LOOK. I BOUGHT THIS PAIR CHEAP IN A SUPERMARKET AND THEY'RE NOT UNCOMFORTABLE AT ALL.
HA! I KNOW. I COULD HAVE BEEN WEARING THESE THE WHOLE TIME I'VE BEEN TALKING TO YOU, BUT INSTEAD I MADE YOU LOOK AT MY BALLS - WHICH WAS PROBABLY THE MAIN PURPOSE OF THIS BOOK.
I MEAN, I *KIND* OF WANTED TO SHARE MY STORY AND TO LET YOU KNOW WHAT TO EXPECT IF YOU EVER HAVE THE MISFORTUNE TO GET ILL...
BUT REALLY, I JUST WANTED TO GET SOME CHEAP LAUGHS OUT OF MY EXPERIENCES AND SHOW YOU MY ARSE AND BALLS.
JOB DONE, I'D SAY, SO I THINK I'LL JUST SAY GOODBYE NOW.
TAKE CARE OF YOURSELF.
I DIDN'T, AND LOOK WHAT HAPPENED TO ME.

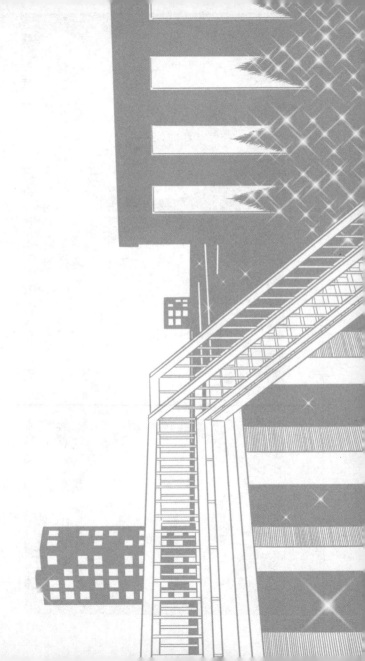

DEDICATED TO MY WIFE, **DR LESLEY MASON**, FOR HER LOVE, SUPPORT AND
PATIENCE DURING THE MAKING OF THIS BOOK AND FOR THE LAST 23 YEARS.

THANKS ALSO TO: ILYA, PAUL RAINEY (WHO SUGGESTED THE TITLE), MARTIN EDEN,
MARK MITCHELL, ROL HIRST, ANDREW CHEVERTON, ANDY OLIVER, CORINNE PEARLMAN,
WOODROW PHOENIX, MEG ROSOFF, NICOLA STREETEN AND ANDREW McALEER.